P9-BIN-481

Motor Learning and Control

Motor Learning and Control
A Neuropsychological Approach

George H. Sage
University of Northern Colorado

ꢀꢀꢀ
Wm. C. Brown Publishers
Dubuque, Iowa

Book Team

Edward G. Jaffe
Senior Editor

Lynne M. Meyers
Associate Developmental Editor

Edgar J. Laube
Production Editor

Geri Wolfe
Designer

Mavis M. Oeth
Permissions Editor

Faye M. Schilling
Visual Research Editor

Aileene Lockhart
Consulting Editor

wcb group

Wm. C. Brown
Chairman of the Board

Mark C. Falb
President and Chief Executive Officer

wcb

Wm. C. Brown Publishers, College Division

Lawrence E. Cremer
President

James L. Romig
Vice-President, Product Development

David Wm. Smith
Vice-President, Marketing

David A. Corona
Vice-President, Production and Design

E. F. Jogerst
Vice-President, Cost Analyst

Marcia H. Stout
Marketing Manager

Linda M. Galarowicz
Director of Marketing Research

William A. Moss
Production Editorial Manager

Marilyn A. Phelps
Manager of Design

Mary M. Heller
Visual Research Manager

Dedicated to
My wife, Liz
My daughters-in-law, Kathy and Trina

Contents

Preface

*W*ithin the past fifteen years there has been a growing interest in motor skill acquisition and control. This interest has been manifested in basic research designed to promote better understanding of motor behavior, as well as in the rapid growth of professions that deal with the development of effective and efficient motor behavior.

This book is designed to serve as a textbook for courses concerned with motor learning and control. The purpose of the book is to describe the basic knowledge that has accumulated in this field of study and to relate this information to possible applications in education, industry, and other professions that deal with problems of motor learning and control.

Special emphasis is given to the important role that the nervous system plays in movement behaviors. This role has received relatively little attention in previous texts on this subject. The physiological psychology approach of this text attempts to integrate neurophysiological and behavioral information, since a knowledge of the functioning of the nervous system is necessary if a beginning is to be made toward understanding the intricacies of skilled motor behavior. This is not to imply that the neural correlates to all motor behavior are known; they are not, and much has still to be learned. But the future holds much promise, and when advances are made toward better understanding about skilled human behavior, chances are very strong that they will be made by scholars who possess a thorough knowledge of the neurological basis of reflex and voluntary mechanisms that control human movement.

Only the essentials of neuroanatomy, neurophysiology, and neurochemistry have been selected for use in this book. The emphasis in this book is only on the study of the neural systems mediating skilled motor behavior; thus no attempt has been made to present a comprehensive treatment of neurology and neurophysiology.

It is anticipated that this book will most likely be used as a text in physical education, physical therapy, and industrial psychology classes. It is difficult to bridge the gap between basic research findings and applications to teaching, coaching, rehabilitation, and other situations where motor behavior occurs. I have been conscious of this, so I have tried not to overstate the applications of research to applied motor activities in a strained attempt to pretend that we know just how to apply all existing knowledge. I will admit, however, that I have occasionally taken some liberties with basic research in making generalizations or describing implications for motor skill acquisition and performance.

This book is appropriate for both advanced undergraduate classes and graduate classes. Indeed, earlier photocopied versions of the manuscript have been used successfully at both levels.

A book like this represents not the work of one but a community of scholars. There are numerous researchers in several disciplines who have made profound and enduring contributions to our understanding of motor behavior. It is impossible for me to acknowledge individual indebtedness to all the writers of articles, monographs, and books that I have consulted, much as I should like to mention every author by name. I have attempted to indicate the sources of original information and ideas that I have used. Such a task is large, however, and the possibility of error is great. The references at the end of the book are a means by which I have attempted to give credit to those whose works I consulted. I wish to extend a special word of thanks to the following scholars whose critiques of earlier drafts of this volume generated improvements that I trust they will recognize:

Robert W. Christina, *Penn State University;*
Patricia Del Rey, *University of Georgia;*
William S. Husak, *California State University,* Long Beach;
H. N. Zelaznik, *Purdue University;*
Muriel R. Sloan, *University of Maryland,* College Park;
Peggy A. Richardson, *North Texas State University.*

The actual preparation of the book involved considerable work, and I am particularly grateful to Connie Beard for her painstaking deciphering of my handwritten drafts and her efficient typing in preparing the manuscript for publication.

This book was completed while I was a visiting professor at the U.S. Military Academy. I am grateful to Colonel James Anderson, Chairman of the Department of Physical Education, for giving me the opportunity to spend a year at West Point.

The dedication of this book signifies my indebtedness to my wife for her unfailing support and understanding. It also signifies my affection for my daughters-in-law.

Motor Learning and Control

Introductory Concepts

1

Introduction to the Study of Motor Behavior

The study of **motor behavior** specifically concerns motor skill acquisition, **motor control,** and **motor performance.** Most texts devoted to learning, control, and performance emphasize verbal skills. Since verbal behavior is of great importance in human affairs, this emphasis is well founded. In this text, however, our primary concern is with motor skills, or motor behavior. Of course, language itself depends on muscular movement—the very act of talking is a complex motor task—but we shall not examine this type of behavior here; instead, motor behavior such as that found in the execution of sports, dance, industrial, and military skills will be our focus.

The field of motor behavior consists of a body of knowledge, compiled by the use of the scientific method, about the psychological aspects of human motor behavior. As such, it may be viewed as a subfield of psychology.

In order to provide the reader with an overview of the subject matter of this text, a brief explanation of the development of general psychology follows. Then, since the particular approach of this text is that of physiological psychology, a description of the focus and development of this field of study is given. The chapter concludes with an overview of what the study of motor behavior is all about and a description of the development of this field of study.

The Study of Psychology

Psychology, as a scientific field of study, is the study of human behavior. It is an attempt to learn about and understand behavior. The word *behavior* is used broadly to encompass a variety of human activities such as sensing, perceiving, attending, learning, and motor acts. Applied, or professional, psychology is the application of the knowledge of basic psychology in specific situations or to certain problems. The use of psychological facts and theories in teaching movement activities such as games, sports, and dance skills is one application of psychology.

For centuries people have speculated about the causes of human behavior and have tried to make sense of their experiences of themselves and of others. But psychology, as a separate academic discipline, is a rather young science, emerging in the latter years of the last century. The initial impetus for separate university departments of psychology came from Europe. Wilhelm Wundt is considered the founder of modern psychology because in 1879 he opened the first formal psychological laboratory in Leipzig, Germany and began publishing the first journal of experimental psychology in 1881.

American universities were quick to develop psychology departments. At Johns Hopkins University, G. Stanley Hall founded the first formal psychology laboratory in 1883 and was instrumental in establishing the first American psychological journal in 1887, the *American Journal of Psychology*. In most cases, the early psychologists were actually academically trained philosophers and were members of university philosophy departments. In the transition to separate departments of psychology, many universities listed a department of "philosophy-psychology" for several years.

In the first decades of this century, psychology witnessed an exciting onrush of new theories and research. Sigmund Freud developed and published his work on psychoanalysis, which has been one of the most powerful forces in psychology in the twentieth century. Growing out of the work of the Russian physiologist, Ivan Pavlov, and the American psychologist, Edward Thorndike, a large group of American psychologists led by John B. Watson adopted behavior as the subject matter of this discipline during the 1920s. This approach emphasized observable phenomena instead of hypothesized or nonobservable phenomena. The behaviorists rejected the notion that the introspective[1] study of conscious experience was the province of psychology. A third major force in psychology emerged at about the same time that Watson and his followers were advancing the cause of behaviorism. This approach, called Gestalt psychology, emphasized that the understanding of behavior should be the study of experience in all its complexity, rather than the molecular study of sensations and actions then common in psychological laboratories. Gestalt psychology is considered to be the forerunner of contemporary cognitive psychology. These three systematic approaches to the study of human behavior have been the foundation and focus in American psychology for the past seventy years. Of course, other theoretical perspectives have vied for recognition and respect during this period; at the present time numerous theoretical positions have their own followers and advocates.

As the discipline of psychology has developed, it has come to act as a unique bridge between the biological sciences and the social sciences. On the one hand, it is allied closely to the biological sciences, such as physiology, neurology, anatomy, and biochemistry, and many of its findings and theories derive from these sciences. But psychology is also closely related to such social sciences as sociology, anthropology, and history. This division results in two major approaches to psychological study. The first is aligned with the biological sciences, the second with the social sciences. Psychology is a distinct science, even though it uses information from other fields of study. In fact few, if any, disciplines do not borrow basic content from other disciplines.

---

[1] Introspection is a word used to refer to the description of one's own conscious processes.

The Physiological Psychology Approach of This Text

We possess several approaches to studying human behavior. Each has its unique techniques and procedures and each has a rich heritage of research findings and theories. The basic orientation of this text is called physiological psychology, and it is aligned with the biological science branch of studying human behavior. Physiological psychology is at the intersection of the neurosciences (neuroanatomy, neurophysiology, neurochemistry) and psychology. In describing the physiological psychology approach, we shall contrast this perspective with two other popular approaches in psychology: behaviorism and cognitivism.

The accumulation of knowledge in the field of psychology is similar to that followed in other disciplines, and research is conducted employing the variables of unique interest. In psychological research, just as with research in other disciplines, two major categories of variables are employed, independent and dependent variables. Before proceeding with the discussion of approaches to studying behavior, an explanation of these two categories of variables is essential; research in which these two types of variables are employed is the foundation on which knowledge in every field of study is accumulated and advanced.

Variables and Their Uses

A variable is any condition that can change in quantity or quality. Examples of important variables to motor behavior are sex, age, intelligence, anxiety, level of aspiration, and amount of feedback. **Independent variables** are controlled and manipulated by the investigator in an experiment. **Dependent variables** and their changes are consequent upon changes in the independent variables. An independent variable is the presumed cause of the dependent variable, the presumed effect.

In psychology, behavior, or a response of some kind, is typically the dependent variable. In a typical experiment, the investigator manipulates independent variables and observes the effects on dependent variables. For example, when motor behavior investigators study the effect of different feedback techniques on learning, they may manipulate feedback (the independent variable) by using different feedback methods and observe the variation in learning rate (the dependent variable) as a presumed result of variation in the independent variable. If one wished to ascertain the effects of a certain drug on motor performance of some kind, the drug would be the independent variable, and the performance would be the dependent variable. The most commonly used dependent variable in motor behavior research is performance.

Behavioral Psychology

In one approach to the study of human behavior, psychologists have focused on the relation between environmental stimuli and human behavior, omitting from their work cognitive psychological processes and complex structures and systems of the nervous system. With this approach, psychologists manipulate environmental stimuli (independent variables) and study the behavioral responses (dependent variables). This approach commonly goes under the rubric of behaviorism, which was the heir to the stimulus-response connectionist approach pioneered by Pavlov and Thorndike. **Behaviorism** focuses on the objective and observable components of behavior—the stimulus and response events. Investigators using this approach are content to assume the existence of some neurological mechanisms related to the organizing and information-processing events that are believed to occur in the organism. But they do not give much attention to these neural activities, and they rarely consider the neurophysiological processes associated with motor activity.

John B. Watson gave behaviorism its name, but B. F. Skinner, the famous Harvard psychologist, perhaps best represents the behaviorist tradition. Skinner believes that since we cannot observe what goes on inside the brain during learning, we should not worry about how information is transmitted and stored and concentrate, instead, on creating the behavior that indicates that one possesses the information. According to him, behavior should be broken down into small pieces, reinforced systematically, and in due course shaped in a way that adds up to learning (Skinner 1968).

Cognitive Psychology

In another approach, psychologists also manipulate the environment (independent variables) and study the behavioral response (dependent variables) with little concern for the underlying neural mechanisms, but they are concerned with explaining those higher mental processes not easily explained using the behaviorist paradigm (research strategy). This approach is called **cognitive psychology,** a descendant of Gestalt psychology, pioneered in the 1920s. It is characterized by a relative lack of concern with stimulus-response relationships or neural activities. The primary focus is on such topics as perception, problem solving through insight, decision making, and "understanding." In all of these processes, cognition[2] is of central importance. Thus, like behaviorism, cognitive psychology arose as a reaction against the introspection of much nineteenth-century psychology; but unlike behaviorism, it does not abandon the study of the mind and consciousness. Wolfgang Kohler was the first of the cognitive psychologists, while Jerome Bruner of Harvard is perhaps the best known of the current cognitivists.

---

[2] Cognition is a general concept embracing all forms of knowing. It includes perceiving, thinking, imagining, reasoning, and judging; it means putting things together and relating events.

Physiological Psychology

A third approach to the study of human behavior, and the approach that will be used in this text, is a physiological psychology approach. Physiological psychology goes by several names: biopsychology, neuropsychology, and psychobiology.

Human **physiological psychology** is the study of the physiological mechanisms underlying behavior. Physiological psychologists are concerned primarily with the neurophysiological events that correlate with psychological processes such as perceiving, thinking, learning, and motivation. Since it is the nervous system—primarily, the brain—that regulates and controls behavior, physiological psychologists direct much of their research effort to understanding the structure and functions of the nervous system and how they relate to behavior. Although physiological psychologists generally focus on neural structures and functions in an effort to understand behavior, they are still concerned with behaviors that involve the whole organism, just like other psychologists.

Two major research strategies are employed by physiological psychologists in order to advance our understanding of behavior (see figure 1.1). In the first, the independent variables are physiological manipulations, while the dependent variables are behavior such as learning or performance. The typical physiological manipulations are ablation, lesioning, electrical stimulation, and chemical applications. Ablation refers to the surgical removal of a particular part of an organism's nervous system. Lesioning involves destroying a part of the nervous system. In both cases, after employing the technique study is made of the resulting impairment or alteration in behavior. These techniques have yielded important information about what parts of the nervous system are responsible for particular kinds of behavior. Normally such techniques are not possible with humans, but illnesses or injuries to

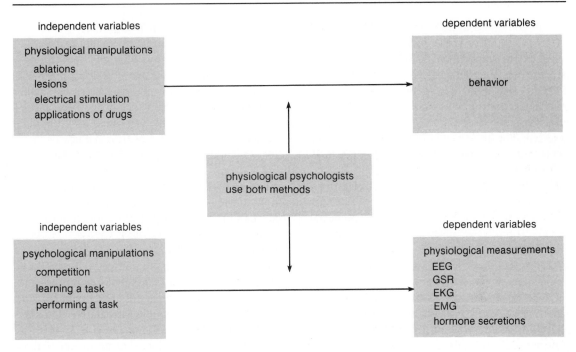

Figure 1.1 *Independent and dependent variables*

humans frequently destroy or require the removal of certain structures in the nervous system. In these cases investigators can study the postoperative effects on a patient's behavior. Study of the loss of ability and changes in behavior helps physiological psychologists determine the role of the surgically removed structures.

Since the nervous system is essentially an electrical system, it is possible to stimulate nerve cells by an outside electrical source, and this is done in electrical stimulation research. Typically, a small electrode is inserted into a particular site in the nervous system, and a weak electric current is sent through the electrode. The investigator then observes the results. Work of this kind has provided psychologists with enormously valuable information about nervous system function.

As with all body tissue, numerous biochemical events are continually taking place in the nervous system. Therefore, chemicals play an important role in behavior. Physiological psychologists frequently explore the effects of various chemical substances on behavior. They can administer chemicals orally, intravenously, or via implanted electrodes and observe the behavioral effects.

In the second major strategy used by physiological psychologists, the independent variables are behavioral manipulations such as learning a task or performing a task under certain conditions, and the dependent variables are the physiological effects.[3] Here, the investigator creates situations calling for behavior of some kind under

---

[3] A field of study that uses this strategy exclusively is called psychophysiology.

certain conditions and then observes the effects on neural activity. These effects are often measured by the responses of heart, blood pressure, perspiration, muscle tension, and hormonal secretions since all of these structures or activities are under control of the nervous system. The electrical activity of the brain itself is also often assessed. The brain is continuously active in the living organism and is therefore spontaneously emitting electric signals. This electrical activity may be monitored by placing surface electrodes on the skull and recording the signals with a special instrument called an electroencephalograph (EEG). It has been found that humans emit several very distinct electrical patterns depending upon whether they are relaxed, excited, thinking, or sleeping.

Physiological Psychology and Other Approaches to the Study of Behavior

Before concluding this discussion on the physiological psychology approach, two important points need to be made. First, concepts such as behaviorism, cognitivism, and physiological psychology exist only as convenient labels for classifying the focus and interest of various investigators and their work. No one approach is completely satisfactory for answering all the questions about human behavior. And psychologists using one of these approaches occasionally employ the theories, research strategies, and techniques of the other approaches in their quest to discover new information about human behavior. Second, there are very few studies of motor behavior—in sports, games, dance, industry, physical therapy, or other leisure or occupational situations in which human motor behavior occurs—where a physiological psychological perspective has been employed. Inferences from research done in the laboratory must be made when attempting to employ a physiological psychology approach to motor behavior in real-life, dynamic situations.

The position taken in this text is that, regardless of the paucity of motor behavior research from a physiological psychology perspective, the study of motor behavior must first focus on a study of the neurophysiological mechanisms underlying motor behavior. These mechanisms are, in the end, responsible for all human behavior. More specifically, it is the nervous system that guides and directs behavior. Any thorough interpretation of behavior is dependent upon a basic understanding of the structures and functions of the nervous system. Without it we would not be able to see, think, move, or perform any of the complex activities that we associate with human endeavor. Thus, our approach seeks to ascertain how the nervous system regulates and controls behavior and psychological processes, recognizing that much is still unknown about how the nervous system functions to control motor behavior. But the underlying premise of this approach is that it will enable us to understand better the relations and interactions between neurophysiological responses and motor behavior. Recently, many physical educators, coaches, and physical therapists have taken an interest in findings in physiological psychology. This is a promising trend. Professionals in these fields can no longer afford to ignore the findings of such research.

Historical Roots of Physiological Psychology

Although the field of physiological psychology is relatively young as an interdisciplinary science, interest in the brain and its relation to behavior goes back many centuries. The great Greek philosopher Aristotle was curious about the site of human intellectual faculties and concluded that the heart must be the seat of our sensory experience and behavior. By the seventeenth century it was well established that the brain and nervous system played an influential role in behavior, but details of how this system worked were still speculative. René Descartes, one of the most profound thinkers of the century, proposed a creative theory of the integrative activity of the nervous system. According to Descartes, animal spirits (fluids)—the most active particles of the blood that are filtered out in the brain and collected in the ventricles—are set in motion in the ventricles of the brain by extended stimuli. These spirits can be directed through tubes to the appropriate muscles to produce movement. Although a far cry from what we know today about how the brain causes movement, Descartes's ideas were influential in emphasizing the control of behavior by the brain.

It was in the laboratories of several German physiologists and physicists during the nineteenth century that physiological psychology acquired its scientific roots. Müller's pioneering work on the physiological basis of sensory experience, Helmholtz's theories on the physiological basis of color vision and of auditory pitch discrimination, and the work of Fechner on methods for measuring psychological responses to physical stimuli laid the conceptual basis for modern physiological psychology.

Other nineteenth-century researchers advanced the understanding of brain-behavior relationships. The functions of the various parts of the brain were ascertained by surgical removal of part of the brain. Pierre Flourens was a pioneer in this work. Electrical stimulation of the brain to determine function began in this period with the publications of Fritsch and Hitzig. The late nineteenth century also witnessed the discovery of the brain wave for which Caton is given credit.

The present century has seen unparalleled advances in physiological psychology. These advances have largely come from the work of a brilliant and dedicated group of researchers, combined with spectacular technological developments. The result has been a continuing series of significant contributions to our understanding of the brain-behavior relationships. We shall be discussing many of the theories and discoveries of these researchers throughout the text. They will not be treated here because their relevance will be more evident if discussed in conjunction with the topic to which they apply.

The Study of Motor Behavior

The study of motor behavior can be viewed as a subfield within the discipline of psychology. As a field of study, it is an attempt to learn more about the psychological factors involved in motor learning, control, and performance. The primary concern of scientists working in this subject area is with understanding and advancing knowledge about human movement. They may or may not also be interested in the solution of practical problems. Scientists of any discipline consider the pursuit to knowledge a worthy endeavor, regardless of its practicality.

A fundamental difference exists between the scientist who discovers knowledge and the professional who applies it. In the case of physics, the physicist (the scientist) discovers the laws of mass and volume, while the engineer (the professional) applies the laws to practical problems, such as those of building a bridge. In another case, the bacteriologist who discovered penicillin was a scientist seeking an understanding of the world of microscopic organisms; the physician who prescribes penicillin is acting as a professional, applying knowledge discovered by the scientist. No value judgment is intended as to whether one role, that of the scientist or the professional, is the more worthy. Indeed, in any field of study both roles are essential for the systematic advancement of the field.

Scientists studying motor behavior have a threefold purpose. First, they seek to understand the behavioral dimensions of human movement. Explanation is the second purpose. As a result of understanding the subject matter, they want to be able to explain behavior. Their third purpose is prediction. As a result of understanding and the ability to explain behavior, they want to be able to predict behavior. Indeed, the aims of every science are understanding, explanation, and prediction.

Just as with many scientific subject areas, there are many applications for motor behavior knowledge and many people are working to advance the applied aspects of this subject. Applications of the basic subject matter of motor behavior are employed in several occupational fields. Industries frequently obtain the services of industrial psychologists to study the human factors involved in performing work. This often results in the redesign of equipment or job tasks to make the movements more effective and efficient for workers. The military has employed motor behavior specialists for the same purposes. In recent years the space program has made extensive use of movement specialists in preparing astronauts and their equipment for space flights. Robotics is a rapidly growing field that is playing an increasingly important role in industry, aerospace, and the military. Robotic devices, or robots, are machines with manipulators that can be programmed to do a variety of manual tasks automatically, and motor behavior specialists are working at the forefront of this area.

Other professionals who apply motor behavior subject matter are physical educators, coaches, athletic trainers and physical therapists. For several reasons the study of motor behavior plays an essential role in the training of people working in these professions. In the case of physical educators and coaches, a thorough understanding of perception, learning, motivation, and other psychological factors is essential in order to predict and control the behavior of students in the gymnasium, on the playing field, in the swimming pool, and in other areas. Psychological variables constitute the most obvious and modifiable types of conditions in the educational process. The effective physical educator and coach must be a skilled practitioner in the educational application of motor behavior subject matter. For the athletic trainer physical therapist, attempting to retrain a patient in the use of body segments rendered dysfunctional due to accident or disease, knowledge of motor control and learning subject matter is crucial.

In this book, illustrations for the application of this subject matter are directed toward the physical educator and coach since many readers of this text will enter these professions. Most studies, examples, and implications that are presented are related to human movement in games, sports, and dance situations.

Development of the Field of Motor Behavior

Scientific investigation into motor control and learning has been largely conducted by experimental psychologists, but during the past two decades physical educators have become some of the most active researchers in this subject. Indeed, at present several of the most distinguished scholars in motor behavior are physical educators. Four periods of distinct character can be identified in the growth of the field. The period from 1890 to 1927 was a time of definition and exploration of the dimensions of this subject. During this era Woodworth (1899) identified some of the fundamental principles of rapid limb movement. His work was one of the first systematic approaches to understanding motor skills. Two other noted researchers of this period, Bryan and Harter (1897; 1899), studied Morse code skill acquisition and proposed principles of motor learning, some of which are still relevant today.

The second period, 1927 to 1945, was an era of considerable increase in the sophistication of experimental work and of the emergence of several theoretical formulations. Much of the research on motor skills during this period used time and motion studies in industrial settings with a view toward making the movements of workers more efficient and effective. Within physical education, the development of motor ability tests and the attempt to relate scores on these tests to motor learning reached faddish proportions (Brace 1927; Cozens 1929; McCloy 1937).

The third period of motor skills research extended from 1945 to the mid-1960s and was characterized by an explosion of research and publication. This period received its initial impetus from World War II in work associated with the armed services. Research increased because of the great need to select and train efficiently airplane pilots and operators of other special machinery, and the need to design display panels and other instruments that could be used with ease. After World War II motor behavior researchers were generously supported by financial grants from various branches of the armed forces and by other governmental agencies to continue the work started during the war.

The most recent trend in motor behavior research began in the mid-1960s and can be viewed as a shift in emphasis from a task orientation to a process orientation (Pew 1974). Early motor behavior work focused on the effects of certain independent variables such as practice schedules, feedback modes, fatigue, or motivational techniques on learning and performance outcome, with little concern for the underlying processes involved. The newer approach, the process orientation, concentrates on the underlying neural mechanisms and cognitive processes that contribute to learning and control. One of the consequences of this trend has been to bind research more closely together. The approach of this text can be understood as being congruent with the current trend in motor behavior.

Summary

The study of motor behavior focuses on motor skill acquisition, control, and performance. This field of study is a subfield of psychology, which is the study of human behavior.

We employ several approaches to the study of motor behavior, but the approach of this text is that of physiological psychology. Physiological psychology is concerned with the neural mechanisms underlying behavior. As such it is at the intersection of the neurosciences and psychology. The orientation of this book, then, is toward the neural events that correlate with motor learning, control, and performance.

Motor behavior scientists have three major purposes in studying motor behavior: understanding, explanation, and prediction. There are a number of leisure and occupational applications in the field of motor behavior.

Scientific study into motor control, learning, and performance has been largely conducted by psychologists, but during the past two decades physical educators have become some of the most active researchers in this subject. The initial major impetus to motor behavior research came during World War II, and interest has continued until the present. The most recent trend in motor behavior has been a shift in research emphasis from a task orientation to a process orientation.

2

Concepts and Methodology in Motor Behavior

*E*very field of study has its particular vocabulary and unique methods for compiling information. Familiarity with them facilitates reading and makes understanding the literature of a field more meaningful. In this chapter, concepts that are frequently employed in motor behavior research are defined and discussed because they will be used throughout this book. Also, several topics related to data collection and analysis in physiological psychology and motor behavior are described.

Terminology Used in Motor Behavior

Motor Learning

Learning can be viewed as a neural change that occurs as a result of experiences with stimuli in the environment. That is, it is the internal process assumed to occur when a change in performance takes place. The entire set of events that underlie learning cannot be viewed directly, so learning must be inferred from changes in behavior; it is, therefore, typically defined in behavioral terms. In this context, **motor learning** is defined as a relatively permanent change in behavior that is a result of practice or experience, and not a result of maturational, motivational, or training factors. Many changes in motor behavior occur naturally as the individual grows and develops, and certainly motor behavior can be radically modified by motivation, but these types of behavioral change are not considered motor learning. Moreover, training, which involves systematic and progressive alterations in physiological systems that increase or modify behavioral capacities (such as strength and endurance) produces changes in behavior, but these changes are not considered motor learning.

Learning anything new must involve changes among the billions of neurons in the brain. It is a fundamental fact that the changes in behavior called learning are in the last analysis a result of changes in the nervous system. It is unwise to study motor learning without studying the nervous system because all of the remarkable functions of learning are mediated by this system. However, it must be pointed out that at present scientists have not yet formulated a comprehensive theory of motor learning in terms of either behavior or neurophysiology, although significant advances have been made in the past decade.

The literature on motor learning contains several terms that are used interchangeably with motor learning, or instead of motor learning, in discussions of motor skill acquisition. The three most commonly used are psychomotor learning, perceptual-motor learning, and sensorimotor learning. In general, these terms do not define different domains of behavior. In some cases, it is merely by personal preference that an author uses a given term. On the other hand, some writers use a certain term to emphasize a particular aspect of skill learning. For example, when the perceptual or integrative processes of motor tasks are studied, the term *perceptual-motor* is frequently used. When sensory cues influencing learning are to be emphasized, some writers use the term *sensorimotor*. But basically all movement behavior, other than simple reflexes and movements, involves the sensory and integrative as well as the motor systems of the body. Although terms such as *perceptual-motor learning* may aid researchers in identifying specific areas of emphasis in skill acquisition, it is not necessary to use the word *perceptual* in a general discussion of motor learning and performance. Indeed, if motor learning is defined as changes in behavior resulting from practice or experience, the word *perceptual* may be redundant.

Motor Performance

Motor performance, as distinct from motor learning, is the observable behavior exhibited when one performs a motor task. A measure of motor performance is the score that one achieves on a given trial or practice period (or a game in sports). For example, the time of ten seconds is the performance of a sprinter during a given race. Fifteen out of twenty field goals attempted by a basketball player during a game can be viewed as performance. Performance is a temporary occurrence that fluctuates due to many variables, among them motivation and fatigue.

Motor Control

During the past decade there has been a trend toward an emphasis on understanding the reflex and voluntary mechanisms that control human movement—that is, the processes underlying movement. This focus on the controlling mechanisms in skilled behavior is referred to as **motor control.** A motor control emphasis in the study of motor behavior and the physiological approach of this text have much in common.

Motor Behavior

Motor behavior is a generic term used when no distinct importance between motor learning, performance, or control is necessary.

Skill

Skill has several connotations and has been used in various ways in the motor behavior literature. One common usage of the word is as an act or task, and another is as an indicator of proficiency.

Skill as an Act or Task

When skill is used with reference to a motor act or task, it consists of a number of perceptual and motor responses that have been acquired by learning. The jump shot can be referred to as a motor skill: It is a task made up of a series of perceptual and motor responses designed to bring about a specific goal—the ball going through the basket. Swimming, hitting a golf ball, and serving a volleyball are other examples of skills in the motor domain and are frequently called motor skills.

Skill as an Indicator of Proficiency

The acquisition of a motor skill is a process in which the learner develops a set of motor responses into an integrated and organized movement pattern. Each motor skill demands a new set of spatially and temporally organized muscular actions. By spatial organization we mean

that the appropriate muscles must be selected; temporal organization refers to the fact that muscle contractions or relaxations must occur at the appropriate time. Skill as an indicator of proficiency implies that a person exhibits competence in carrying out a task that can be defined in terms of its desired goal. Such a person is called skilled or skillful. Paul Fitts (1964), a prominent motor skills investigator before his untimely death, said:

> By a skilled response I shall mean one in which receptor-effector-feedback processes are highly organized, both spatially and temporally. . . . Spatial-temporal patterning, the interplay of receptor-effector-feedback processes, and such characteristics as timing, anticipation, and the graded response are thus seen as identifying characteristics of skill.

Operationally, definitions of skilled are usually given in terms of overt responses to controlled stimulation. The responses are scored on the basis of errors, correct responses, rates, and amplitudes.

The word *skilled* can also be used to describe a relative level of proficiency. For each motor task one is judged to be highly skilled, poorly skilled, or having average skill, depending upon the performance criteria standards for the task. Level of skill does not fluctuate much from one performance to the next. Of course, over many performances the skill level may change. In learning a task an individual can go from a poorly skilled to a highly skilled level by regular practice.

Characteristics of Skillful Motor Performance

A skilled performer is characterized as one who can produce an output of high quality (such as fast or accurate) with a good deal of consistency. The novice typically executes the movements of a task slowly, while the proficient performer moves much faster. The skillful person's performance tends to be of high quality in achieving the goal, while the novice makes many errors. The beginning typist types only about twenty words per minute and makes many errors, while the skillful typist may type over a hundred words per minute with very few errors. And the proficient performer typically exhibits a consistency of performance, while novices tend to be erratic.

Skilled performance is also characterized by an appearance of ease, a smoothness of movement, an anticipation of variations in the stimulus situation before they arrive, and an ability to cope with these and other disturbances without disrupting the performance. Indeed, increasing skill involves a widening of the range of possible disturbances that can be coped with without disturbing the performance. Novice tennis players stroke the ball in jerky movements while seeming to be involved in a frantic game in which they cannot quite keep up. They are caught unprepared by slightly unusual shots by their opponents. Skillful players, in contrast, seem to move with ease. They are in proper position sooner than the beginner and they anticipate and react to situations with unhesitating movements. There are no surprises, in the sense that surprise involves a lack of readiness for a situation. These characteristics are undoubtedly a function of the improved selective attention and perceptual skills acquired by the skilled performer.

Skilled motor performers are moving to accomplish a purpose, although their ultimate movement goal may not be discernible because many movements are performed to obscure the ultimate objective. For example, football running backs who charge into the line after receiving a fake handoff from the quarterback keep their hands folded close to their stomachs to conceal the fact that they do not have the ball.

Motor Ability

Motor ability and skill are not synonymous concepts. Motor ability is a trait or capacity of an individual that is related to performance on a variety of skills and that is rather enduring and permanent after childhood. Biological forces are presumed to be primarily responsible for an individual's basic motor abilities. Abilities, then, serve as the basis for the development of skills, which are specific responses for the accomplishment of a task. A skill is learned through practice and depends on the presence of underlying abilities. Balance, speed of reaction, and flexibility are examples of abilities that are important for the execution of a variety of skills, such as the tennis serve, forward roll, and football block. The topic of motor ability will be covered in detail in chapter 16.

Classifying Motor Tasks

Several systems of classification have emerged in an effort to impose some order on the many different types of motor skills. We shall consider only four of these categories, since they are the most relevant to the topics covered in this book. The first is based on the extent to which the entire body is used; the second is based on the distinctiveness of beginning and ending of movements; the third is based on the stability of the environment during movement; and the fourth is based on whether the pace of movement execution is under the control of the performer.

Gross and Fine Motor Skills

In the literature on motor behavior one frequently finds words used to denote the parts and the extent of the body involved in a movement pattern. Motor tasks are frequently described as fine or gross skills, but there is no standardized criterion on which to identify a skill in these terms. Cratty (1973) suggests that motor skills might be placed on a continuum, from the fine to the gross, with a classification made "with reference to size of the muscle involved, the amount of force applied, or to the magnitude of space in which the movement is carried out."

Generally, actions that involve total body movement and multilimb movement, such as walking, jumping, swimming, shooting a jump shot, or making a tennis serve are considered **gross motor skills. Fine motor skills** are performed by small muscles, especially of the fingers, hand, and forearm, and frequently involve eye-hand coordination. They involve the manipulation of tools and small objects or the control of machines. Tasks such as typing, sewing, handwriting, piloting an aircraft, or operating a rotary-pursuit apparatus in a psychological laboratory are considered fine motor skills. These latter tasks are also called manual or manipulative skills by some writers.

Discrete, Serial, and Continuous Skills

Some skills are considered to be **discrete,** others are **serial,** and others are **continuous.** Discrete tasks are characterized by a recognizable beginning and ending. They involve only a single exertion, such as shooting an arrow or throwing a baseball. A task is serial in nature when the beginning and ending of components can be identified, but events follow each other in sequence, such as a gymnastics routine on the high bar or uneven parallel bars. Continuous skills are repetitious movements, such as running and freestyle swimming.

Open and Closed Skills

Several years ago the British psychologist E. C. Poulton (1957) suggested that human skills might be classified as either open or closed, depending on the extent to which a performer must conform to a prescribed standard sequence of movement during execution and the extent to which effective performance depends on environmental

Table 2.1 Examples of sports in which open or closed skills dominate

Sports in which closed skills dominate	Sports in which open skills dominate
1. Golf	1. Soccer
2. Diving	2. Basketball
3. Shot putting	3. Baseball
4. Gymnastics	4. Hockey

events. The idea of a continuum, from motor skills that are predominantly habitual to those that are predominantly perceptual, was advanced by a British physical educator, Barbara Knapp (1961). **Closed skills** require a consistency of movement pattern and are performed under an unchanging environment. Where environmental conditions are stable or stationary, the learner is attempting to become consistent in producing the most effective movement. A gymnastic stunt, a platform dive, a shot put or discus throw are all examples of closed tasks. **Open skills,** on the other hand, are externally paced in the sense that they must be done under varying environmental conditions each time they are executed; they require a flexibility of movement response. A shortstop's throw to the first baseman is always different because the shortstop always fields the ball from a different location on the field. The handball player is never able to use exactly the same movement pattern for two shots. Proficiency in open skills requires a diversification and versatility of movement to meet the demands of the particular task (table 2.1).

Gentile and her colleagues (1975) have developed an elaborated model of the open and closed skill continuum. In this model, type of movement and the nature of the environmental control are the primary focus. Types of movement are categorized according to body movement or stability and manipulative or nonmanipulative demands, while environmental

Table 2.2   *Taxonomy based upon environmental and movement requirements*

Nature of environmental control	Nature of movement required by task			
	Total body stability		Total body transport	
	No LT/M	LT/M	No LT/M	LT/M*
Closed (spatial control: stationary environment)	Sitting Standing	Typing Writing	Walking Running	Carrying or handling objects during locomotion Javelin throw
Open (temporal/ spatial control: moving environment)	Standing on a moving train Log rolling Riding an escalator	Reading a newspaper on a moving train Skeet shooting Batting in baseball	Dodging a moving object Walking in a moving train Dancing with a partner	Run and catch a moving object Throwing on the run Dribbling in basketball

Source: Gentile, A. M. et al. "Structure of motor tasks."
Mouvement, Actes du 7e symposium en apprentissage psycho-moteur et psychologie du sport. October 1975, pp. 11–28.

*LT/M = Independent limb transport and manipulation, usually involving maintaining or changing the position of objects in space.

controls place varying degrees of spatial and temporal regulation on performance, with skills classified as primarily open or closed. (table 2.2).

Self-Paced and Externally Paced Skills

In the execution of some motor tasks, the pace is under the control of the performer, so these tasks are called **self-paced.** Bowling, golfing, and swimming are examples of self-paced tasks. Other tasks require that the performer respond to external objects, so these tasks are said to be **externally paced.** The fielder in baseball or softball must respond to the flight of the ball while catching a fly ball, the tennis player hitting a backhand stroke is responding to the trajectory of the ball, and the defensive player in basketball is responding to the maneuvers of the offense.

Interdependence of Categories

It is obvious that any given motor task will overlap several of these categories. For example, a motor skill could be classified as a fine, discrete, closed, externally paced skill. Merely classifying skills is not a very useful exercise, but a knowledge and understanding of the classifications can be helpful in reading the literature in motor behavior.

Research Methods in Physiological Psychology

As noted in the first chapter, the goal of physiological psychology is to understand how the nervous system regulates and controls behavior. Researchers in this field have devised unique research methods to achieve their goal. Several of these techniques will be described to provide the reader with an overview of them. (A detailed description of these techniques is beyond the scope of this book.) But first an important point needs to be made. Lower animals are frequently used in the experiments for several obvious reasons: Parts of the brain are sometimes surgically removed or destroyed, and many times the animals have to be sacrificed so that a study of their brains can be made. These procedures certainly could not be carried out with human subjects. Physiological psychologists do not believe that the brains of lower animals are the *same* as those of humans, but there are similarities; knowledge acquired about brain-behavior relationships from other species provides *clues* to this relationship for humans. Moreover, neuroscientists attempt to corroborate their findings on other species through clinical research with humans.

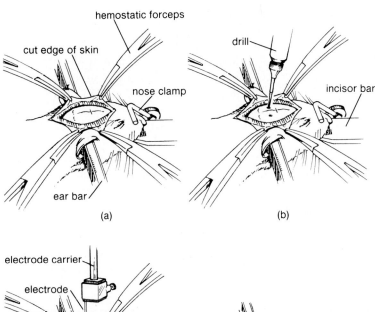

hemostatic forceps

cut edge of skin

nose clamp

ear bar

(a)

drill

incisor bar

(b)

Figure 2.1 *Making a bilateral lesion: (a) skull exposed; (b) bilateral holes drilled in calculated position; (c) electrode inserted to calculated depth; (d) suturing skin.*

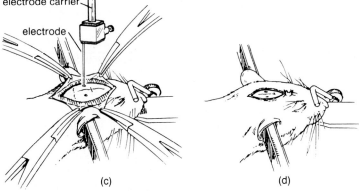

electrode carrier

electrode

(c)

(d)

Ablations and Lesions

Two techniques that physiological psychologists use extensively are **ablations** and **lesions.** The former refers to the removal of part of the brain, and the latter refers to destroying or functionally disrupting part of the brain. In both cases the effects of the procedure on behavior are assessed after the treatment.

In making the ablation, surgical procedures are employed to remove tissue from a specific site in the brain. For making lesions in the brain, researchers drill a hole in an appropriate place in the skull and lower a wire electrode, insulated except at the tip, into the desired position. An electrical current strong enough to destroy tissue is passed through the wire, producing a localized lesion (figure 2.1).

Electrical Stimulation

Instead of removing or destroying part of the brain and observing the behavioral consequences, neuroscientists also electrically stimulate specific brain structures—thus activating the brain cells nearby—to gain an understanding of their function. In this technique, an electrode insulated at the tip is lowered through a hole drilled in the skull and into the brain. An electrical current weak enough not to damage cells but strong enough to activate them is then passed through the electrode. This procedure can take an acute or chronic form. In the acute form, the animal is stimulated during the surgery. In chronic preparations, the electrode is permanently anchored

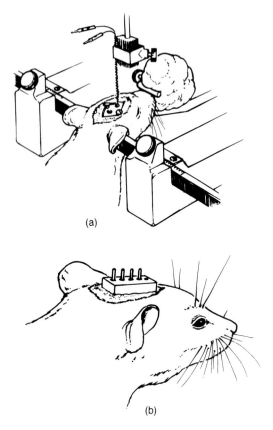

(a)

(b)

Figure 2.2   *(a) Implanting an electrode in an animal's brain; (b) animal with electrode cable connector base.*

in place, and stimulation is accomplished through wires connecting the electrode with an electrode holder permanently attached to the skull (figure 2.2).

Chemical Stimulation

Brain cells can be stimulated by chemicals as well as by electric current. Chemical stimulation is a modification of the electrical stimulation procedure. A thin tube, called a **cannula,** is inserted into the animal's brain instead of an electrode. Chemicals are delivered to a specific site in the brain through the cannula. This technique is valuable in ascertaining the effects of various chemicals on brain cells.

Recording Electrical Activity in the Brain

The brain continuously emits very low voltage electrical fluctuations, or brain waves, that vary in amplitude from a few microvolts up to 200 microvolts and in frequency from near 0 to 50 hertz (Hz).[1] Equipment that amplifies and records the electrical activity of the brain is called an **electroencephalograph** (EEG). It allows investigators to make determinations of brain activity from electrodes pasted on the scalp. Electrodes of this type record large populations of cell firing, but a modification of this procedure uses electrodes implanted in the interior of the brain to record the firing pattern of single brain cells. (Brain waves displayed graphically as fluctuations of voltage over time are called electroencephalograms.)

Four types of brain waves have been identified, each related to a particular form of consciousness (figure 2.3). The brain waves are called alpha, beta, theta, and delta. Alpha waves are synchronous, high amplitude brain waves with frequencies of 8 to 13 Hz. They are associated with an awake but relaxed, resting state. Beta waves are desynchronized, low amplitude waves, with frequencies from 13 to over 40 Hz. They are correlated with behavioral arousal and mental concentration on a task. Theta waves are desynchronized, erratic amplitude waves in the range of 4 to 8 Hz. They are associated with deep concentration, memory retrieval, and creative thinking. Delta waves are synchronous, high amplitude waves in the range of 0.5 to 4 Hz. They are associated with deep sleep.

Recording Electrical Activity in the Muscle

Muscle action during movement is sometimes a focus of interest in physiological psychology, especially when studying motor control and learning processes. The most frequently used technique

---

[1] Hertz refers to cycles per second. One Hz = 1 cycle per second.

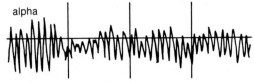

Alpha waves, 8 to 13 cycles per second, are often symmetrical, with large amplitude.

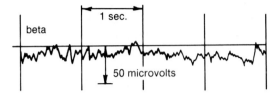

1 sec.

50 microvolts

Beta waves are fast—from 13 to 40 cycles per second and higher—and have small amplitude.

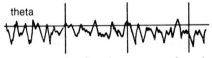

Theta waves, 4 to 8 cycles per second, are less regular, with lower amplitude than alpha waves.

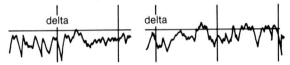

Delta waves, 0.5 to 4 cycles per second, are irregular. The first strip shows theta followed by a large delta wave, with several delta waves in the second tracing.

Figure 2.3   *Typical EEG patterns.*

for recording the electrical activity associated with muscle activity during a response is electromygraphic (EMG) measurements. With the EMG, measurements are made either at the surface of the body near a muscle of interest through electrodes placed over the muscle, or directly from the muscle by penetrating the skin with needle electrodes. Most EMG measurements are used to obtain an indication of the amount of activity of a given muscle, or group of muscles, instead of an individual muscle fiber. Hence the EMG pattern is typically a summation of the muscle fiber firing of the muscle group being measured.

Research Methods in Motor Behavior

Many questions about motor behavior are of interest to researchers as well as to physical educators and coaches. The effects of certain types of practice schedules, mental practice, and incentives on learning rate or the effects of fatigue, certain drugs, or rewards on performance are some of the types of questions that interest both the scholar and the professional. But how can objective answers be obtained? If one wishes to ascertain how certain factors affect motor learning and performance, one is immediately confronted with the problem of objective investigation.

A number of strategies can be used. One might ask the performers, but they are a poor source of objective information. One might ask the teachers or coaches, but they, too, are unreliable sources. The investigator can form opinions based on observation, but this, too, has many weaknesses. One might select two individuals or groups and study how a certain variable is manifested as the individual or groups performed, but many factors might account for possible differences—even if the observations are precisely quantified. For example: The two groups might have differed in initial skill; practice trials and practice time might have differed; environmental conditions or instructions might have differed (assuming instructions were not the variable being studied). In all of these situations, one or more extraneous factors in the study can obscure the independent variable in which the investigator is interested or give a distorted view of reality.

In order to make valid and reliable inferences from observations, the investigator must seek a strategy better than any of the above. At the heart of science is the experiment, and the major aspect of experimentation is controlled observation. Experiments in many disciplines are typically carried out in a laboratory because the laboratory allows for good experimental control of subjects, of observations, and of important variables under study.

Systematic control, observation, and isolation of factors are the chief reasons why a great deal of motor learning and performance research is done in the laboratory. Ideally, motor behavior research findings from the laboratory should be verified in "real-world" settings—the gymnasium, athletic field, or natatorium. Until this is done, however, principles that explain learning and performance in the laboratory can be extended to serve as guides to the teacher-coach of motor activities. Of course, it should be understood that motor behavior research should not always be expected to result in immediately applicable, practical, and specific implications for the teacher. The study of motor behavior is not just another name for methods of teaching, although it often does and should play a supportive role.

In conducting controlled laboratory research on motor behavior, it is usually necessary to start the study with subjects who are at a novice level. Consequently it is desirable to use unpracticed and unfamiliar tasks. Most typical sports activities are therefore inappropriate since they do not satisfy the criteria of unpracticed and unfamiliar tasks. Virtually all adolescents and adults have had prior experience with these activities; typical sports movements have already been learned to some extent. So it is customary in the motor learning laboratory to employ so-called novel tasks—tasks that differ from those in the learner's usual repertoire of skills.

Motor skill learning and performance research with human subjects has largely been limited to a few laboratory tasks. Some of the earliest and least sophisticated laboratory tasks used in motor behavior work were ball tossing and juggling tasks. Over the past fifty years other tasks have been employed. We shall describe a few of the most used tasks.

Motor Skills Research Tasks

Countless motor tasks have been employed in research on motor learning and performance. In general, the tasks can be classified into four categories: tasks for measuring time and speed, tasks for measuring accuracy, tasks for measuring extent of performance, and secondary tasks.

Tasks for Measuring Time and Speed

Two of the most important variables of motor behavior are speed of reaction and speed of movement. The most frequently employed measures of these components of motor behavior are reaction time, movement time, and response time, and each has been used a great deal in motor behavior research.

Reaction Time **Reaction time** (RT) is the time that transpires between the presentation of a stimulus and the initiation of a response. For example, if a subject is seated before a display panel with a finger on a response key and is asked to release the key as soon as a light on the panel goes on, the time lapse between the time the light goes on and the key is released is the RT. During RT neural impulses are transmitted to the brain, processed there, impulses transmitted to muscles, and movement started.

RT can be fractionated into component parts based on neurophysiological function. In research one goal is to ascertain which part of RT is related to the receptor, to afferent pathways, to central processing, to efferent pathways, and finally to muscle action. One technique employed to achieve this goal is to fractionate RT. Some investigators have divided RT into premotor and motor parts. Premotor RT is the interval from the onset of the stimulus until the first change from baseline to increased electrical activity at the motor-point region of the muscle, as measured by electromyographic (EMG) recordings; motor RT

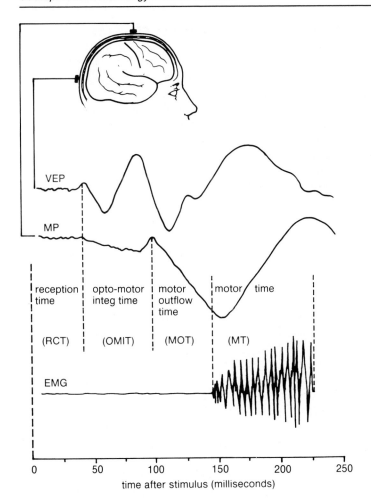

Figure 2.4 *Schematization of visual reaction-time model (VEP=visual evoked potential, MP=motor potential).*

VEP

MP

reception
time

(RCT)

opto-motor
integ time

(OMIT)

motor
outflow
time

(MOT)

motor   time

(MT)

EMG

0   50   100   150   200   250

time after stimulus (milliseconds)

is the interval from the increased electrical activity at the motor-point region of the muscle until movement is actually initiated (Botwinick and Thompson 1966).

Other fractionations of RT have involved measuring the interval from the application of the stimulus until the first change in cortical activity in the brain, measured by electroencephalograph recordings (figure 2.4). It has long been known that RT to auditory stimuli is faster than RT to visual stimuli by about fifty milliseconds (msec). Recently it has been discovered that auditory stimulus activity reaches the cerebral cortex eight to nine msec after stimulation, while a visual stimulus takes twenty to forty msec to reach the cortex. Since both sensory pathways are about the same length, presumably the difference is a function of differences in transduction speed.

The basic equipment needed for measuring RT is:

1. A timer, usually a chronoscope, that records time in hundredths or thousandths of a second and that is activated by a stimulus (typically a buzzer or a light).
2. A reaction or response key that, when released or depressed, stops the time (figure 2.5).

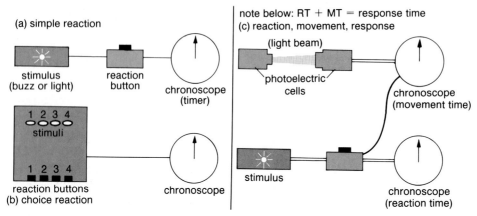

Figure 2.5   *Instruments for measuring speed of response characteristics.*

Figure 2.6   *Instruments for measuring reaction time and movement time.*

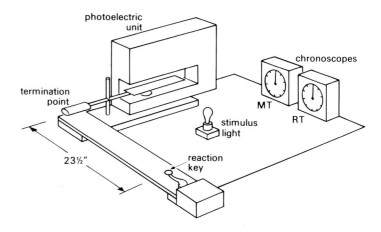

Wherever speed of execution is important, knowledge about RT is useful. Of course, there are innumerable places in the world of work and of recreation where speed of execution affects performance. The study of RT is of interest for the information it generates about individual differences and the factors that affect speed. RT experiments are important also because of the information they generate about the functioning of the nervous system, such as theories about attention, perceptual processing capacity, processing speed, and response programming.

Movement Time and Response Time **Movement time** (MT) is the time taken to complete a task after it has been initiated (not when the stimulus is applied), and ends when the movement of the body terminates the task. **Response time** is a term used to indicate the combined time of both RT and MT. It is the total time from presentation of the stimulus to the completion of the task (figure 2.7).

Since movement time and response time are also frequently measured while doing RT research, instruments used to measure MT and response time also include response keys and

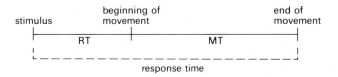

Figure 2.7   *Reaction time (RT), movement time (MT), and response time.*

chronoscopes, but they may include a photoelectric cell or microswitch and one or more additional timers as well (figures 2.5c and 2.6).

In a typical experiment in which RT, MT, and response time are all measured, a stimulus activates chronoscopes A and B. Chronoscope A is stopped when the subject initiates movement (measuring RT). Chronoscope B terminates when a light beam of the photoelectric cell is broken by an arm, hand, or leg of the subject (indicating response time). To calculate MT, RT is subtracted from response time. Of course, chronoscope B can be wired to start when movement is initiated, and stopped when movement ends. In this case, the time on chronoscope B will indicate MT. In this situation, the sum of the time recorded on the two chronoscopes provides the response time. A third chronoscope could be used to start with the stimulus and terminate with movement through the photoelectric cell. This would record the response time on one chronoscope.

The various components for time and speed are clearly evident in many sports skills. In track races, from the firing of the starter's pistol until the runners make their first movements from the blocks is the RT; the time from the first movement until runners break the tape is their MT; and the time from the firing of the starter's gun to the breaking of the tape (the time measured in track and most other timed sports events) is the response time. In sports where a ball is used, the performers must make various reactions to the ball. Many sports require fast reactions to opponents' maneuvers, and in team sports the actions of teammates also require a response. In sports such as basketball, soccer, field hockey, and volleyball, a performer may have to react to twenty or thirty stimulus situations in less than a minute.

In baseball the distance from the pitcher's rubber to home plate is 60'6'', and if a ball travels the distance in 0.6 seconds (not unusual with a fastball pitcher), it is traveling about 10 feet every 0.1 second. Batters with an RT of 0.2 seconds will be able to view the ball 10 feet longer than batters with a 0.3 second RT before they have to start their swings. This will, of course, give them a decided advantage over batters with a slower RT. One's efficiency in interacting with the environment in each of these cases is limited by the amount of time it takes to initiate movement.

Tasks for Measuring Accuracy

Accuracy is another variable important to motor behavior because many motor skills require that the performer do something with a minimum of error. In motor skills such as bowling, archery, and pistol shooting, accuracy is the sole criterion by which performance is evaluated, and becoming skillful in these tasks means becoming more accurate. There are many dimensions of accuracy. For example, performance may be judged by accuracy in hitting a stationary or moving target, such as in pistol shooting and trap shooting. Accuracy in moving with a specified speed or producing a specified force are other examples.

Several laboratory tasks have been used to assess performance accuracy. One of the most used laboratory instruments in which accuracy is

Figure 2.8 *A rotary-pursuit apparatus. The subject attempts to keep the metal stylus on the target on the turntable while it is revolving. Time on target is measured by a timer, while the number of times the subject is on target is recorded with a counter.*

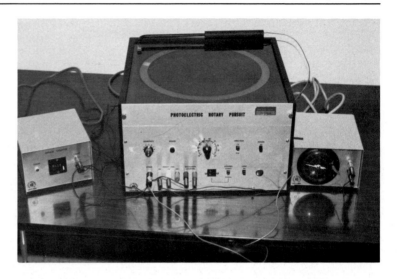

assessed is the rotary-pursuit apparatus, a tracking task in which the subject attempts to maintain contact with a moving target (figure 2.8). The rotary-pursuit apparatus consists of a turntable with a light as the target. The subject attempts to keep a photosensitive stylus in contact with the light target as the turntable rotates. An electric clock measures the amount of time that the stylus is in contact with the target during a given time trial. Performance is usually measured by time-on-target (TOT); for a given trial of thirty or forty seconds, the time that the subject maintains contact with the target constitutes TOT, the accuracy score. As subjects learn to make the correct movements to maintain stylus contact with the light, their TOT increases. More elaborate models of this task allow for automatic timing of the on- and off-target time, variable speed, and direction control of the turntable, and more complex orbital patterns of the target can be used.

Another task in which accuracy (in this case balance accuracy) is assessed is the stabilometer. This device looks like a very short teeter-totter. The subject takes a standing position on the platform and attempts to keep the unstable platform in a level position. Performance scores are kept in terms of either the time-on-target (the target being balance) or the number of times the edge of the platform touches the stabilometer foundation (each touch is considered an error) during

a trial. A practice trial can be set for any specific time (usually twenty to thirty seconds) (figure 2.9).

Over the past ten years, one of the most-used instruments in motor behavior research for studying the processes of motor control and learning has been linear positioning tasks. A typical linear positioning task is shown in figure 2.10. The apparatus consists of four steel rods mounted in wooden blocks at either end. The blocks are fastened to a wooden base. Two steel rods are positioned parallel to one another while two other rods are positioned below in a similar fashion. A ball bearing sleeve runs on each of the upper rods and supports a small slide so that it can move freely along the length of the rods. This provides essentially frictionless movement of the slide in a horizontal direction. A similar slide is located on the bottom pair of rods. Placement of this slide along the rods prevents the upper slide from moving beyond the lower slide. This arrangement allows target positions to be set anywhere along the trackway. A pointer extends downward from each slide. The pointer ends just above a scale marked in millimeters mounted on the base of the apparatus. Subjects are usually blindfolded, provided with a criterion distance or location along the rod to move, and then evaluated by their accuracy in achieving this distance or location.

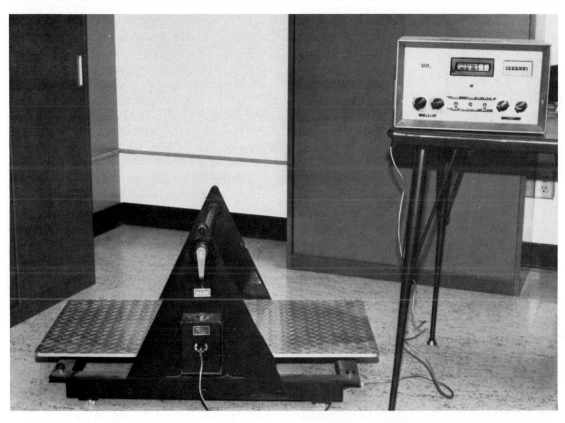

Figure 2.9   A stabilometer. This instrument consists of a horizontally pivoted board upon which a subject stands with feet straddling the supporting axle. The subject attempts to keep the platform balanced as long as possible during each trial. Time on balance and number of times off balance during each trial (usually 20 to 30 seconds) is recorded by a timer.

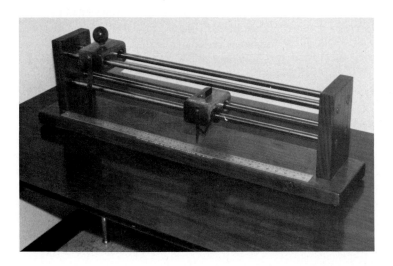

Figure 2.10   A linear positioning task. The lower block is used by the experimentor to set the criterion position. The upper block is used by the subject to move to the criterion position. Typically, the subject is blindfolded while being tested.

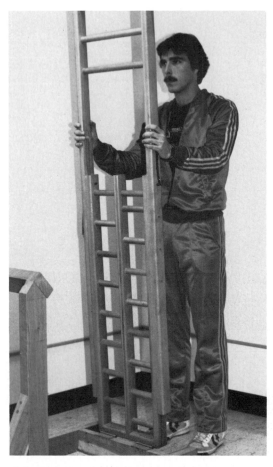

Figure 2.11 *The Bachman ladder. This is a free-standing ladder. The subject climbs as high as possible on each trial until toppling over, then begins climbing again. Trials may be timed, for example, 30 seconds, or each attempt to climb may be counted as a trial. The score is the number of rungs climbed in a trial.*

Tasks for Measuring Extent of Performance

Skills are often measured by the extent of performance, such as the distance an object is thrown, the force exerted over a given period of time, or the number of subtasks completed in a given time. Here, the work performed is scored and a performance measure obtained.

The laboratory task that has been most popular over the past twenty years for assessing extent of performance is the Bachman ladder climb (figure 2.11). The Bachman ladder is a free-standing ladder that a subject attempts to climb. The object is to climb as many rungs as possible before toppling over. A score is kept of the cumulative rungs that subjects climb, for example, in a thirty-second trial. Each time subjects topple off the ladder during a trial, they return to the starting position and begin climbing again. A second method of scoring this task is by the number of rungs climbed in a single trial. In this case, when balance is lost the first time a trial ends and the number of rungs climbed is counted.

Other tasks in which extent of performance is measured are those in which objects are thrown for distance, such as a ball throw for distance, or tasks in which the performer is given a specific time to perform a task and a score is kept of the performance. A one-minute basketball lay-up task is an example. The number of baskets made in the specified time would constitute the score. This is actually a combination of speed and extent tasks.

Trends in Motor Behavior Research Tasks

An increasing trend in motor learning research is the use of computerized experimentation. The selective mathometer, originally designed by Clyde E. Noble in 1952, is now fully automatic. This apparatus is used in human selective learning experiments. All events are automatically recorded by counters and by a continuous printout recorder (figure 2.12).

Many researchers have designed their own tasks to meet their specific research needs. A review of the tasks that have been employed in recent motor behavior research will reveal an incredible variety of tasks developed to respond to the unique questions of a particular study.

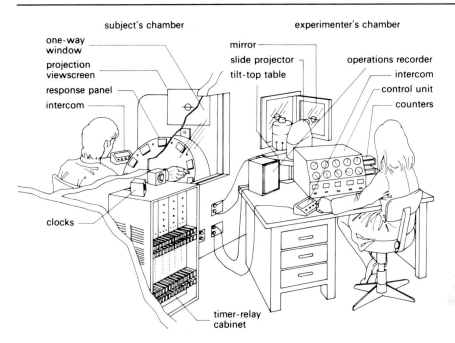

Figure 2.12   *The selective mathometer, an instrument for research in human selective learning.*

The highest forms of motor skill involve tasks in which one movement pattern is superimposed upon another, such as shooting a basketball while moving or throwing a football to a sprinting end. Performances of this kind are extraordinarily complex. Although it would be highly beneficial to study the learning factors of such behavior, only limited work of this kind has been done because of the bewildering technical difficulties involved in controlling and analyzing the stimulus and response variables involved in these situations. Relatively few motor learning studies have been conducted in dynamic situations such as in the gymnasium, playing field, or swimming pool. Rather, research has been more concerned with studying variables that cut across many motor tasks and identifying general principles that apply to many specific tasks. Variables such as practice, feedback, motivation, and transfer are examples.

Secondary Tasks

Occasionally, researchers employ tasks in which the performers are highly skilled, so differences between performers or groups of performers are subtle and difficult to measure. In such cases, investigators have used secondary tasks that are performed simultaneously with the primary task. Performance measurements are then made on the secondary task. The underlying theory behind this approach is that as performers become more proficient at a task (the primary task), the less attention they have to devote to its execution. This being the case, the more highly skilled performers are on a task, the less disruptive this is to their performance of a secondary task. Thus, when the primary task does not provide sensitive measures of differences among performers' scores, secondary task scores can become the performance measurement focus (Brown 1962; Kerr 1975).

Table 2.3   *Performance measures*

Type of Performance	Examples of Performance Tasks	Measurements
Speed	Amount of time to: —react to a stimulus —run 100 meters	Reaction time in msec. Movement and/or Response time in seconds, minutes, hours
Accuracy	Number of baskets made or missed out of 20 shots, e.g., 15 out of 20	
	Time-on-target on a rotary pursuit task or time-on-balance on the stabilometer	Time in seconds on target or balance
	Degrees or millimeters (or inches) deviation on a positioning task	Amount of error
Extent	How high and/or far was an object thrown or hit	Inches, feet, yards
	How much force was generated	Weight, pounds
	Frequency of response execution	Number of responses
	Number of rungs climbed on the Bachman ladder	Number of responses

Measuring Performance

Motor performance, as distinct from motor learning, is the achievement, or score, on a motor task; it is simply a measure of one's behavior. A performance score on the 100-meter dash might be 10.5 seconds and fifteen free throws out of twenty attempts is a performance score. Regardless of the type of motor task, then, performance scores are the measures that are used in assessing a performance. These scores are related to the types of tasks being performed (table 2.3).

When a task requires speed of reaction and movement, performance scores are recorded in milliseconds, seconds, minutes, or hours to complete the task. Tasks requiring accuracy are scored by the time a performer is performing accurately, or the amount of deviation, or error, from the target. Movement extent scores are typically in terms of inches, feet, or yards an object was projected or the amount of weight or force that was exerted. This is not an exhaustive list of performance measures, but rather an illustration of the most common measures.

The Peculiar Case of Measuring Error Scores

In motor skills that are measured by some index of accuracy, deviations from the target are considered as errors. For example, a performer who attempts to throw a basketball at a target and misses the target by five inches is recorded as having committed a five-inch error; a performer who is asked to move the slide of a linear positioning task fifty centimeters, but who moves fifty-five centimers, is said to have made a five-centimeter error. But the amount of error in a response is only one form of error score. It actually may not be the most relevant for a particular situation because both the amount and the nature of errors may be of interest to the researcher. Thus, several error scores are commonly used in motor behavior research. The three most frequently used error scores are **absolute error** (AE), **constant error** (CE), and **variable error** (VE). Each is calculated differently and each yields different information. The issue of error scores, and which error score is most appropriate, is extremely controversial, and it is beyond the scope of this text to enter into a discussion of this issue. Readers interested in the calculation of various error scores and the uses of each might consult the following sources: Schutz and Roy (1973), Henry (1974; 1975), Newell (1976), Schutz (1977), Safrit, Spray, and Diewert (1980).

Measuring Motor Learning

As noted previously, motor learning is a relatively permanent change in behavior that is the result of practice or experience, and is *not* the result of maturational, motivational, or training factors. It is assumed that the change in observable behavior is the result of some change in the nervous system—some biochemical or structural change—that now enables the individual to perform in a certain way.

Learning cannot be observed directly, but only inferred by observing behavior or performance. Although motor learning must be inferred from performance scores, merely using performance scores as indicative of learning is inappropriate since performance obviously can fluctuate due to such factors as motivation, fatigue, boredom, noise, and temperature. Thus, there is a dilemma in assessing learning, which is a *relatively permanent* change in performance, because it must be inferred from performance scores, which are transitory. While no satisfactory solution exists, there are several ways in which performance scores can be used to demonstrate a relatively permanent change in behavior. Each method has certain strengths and weaknesses, and we now have an active controversy about the best method of measuring motor learning. Without going into details on this controversy or trying to suggest an ideal method, the commonly used methods are described below. All have been used in motor learning research.

Performance Curves as Measures of Learning

Motor performance on a task can be measured and a score obtained of the performance. In motor behavior research, numerous performance scores are typically obtained on each subject. These scores can then be plotted on a graph to illustrate the pattern of performance for individual subjects or for the average performance of a group as a whole. These records of performances, when published in the motor behavior literature, are usually called learning curves, but a more correct terminology is **performance curves** because performance variations do not necessarily reflect learned capabilities. However, the performance curve does allow one to make subjective assessments of learning.

On performance curve graphs, customarily the horizontal axis shows the units of practice, such as number of trials or the amount of time spent in practice. The vertical axis depicts the performance as measured by some index. These performance indexes can be classified into roughly three types, depending upon what aspect of performance is measured. One type is an error index. Here performance is recorded by errors, and a decrease in the number of errors is plotted. A second type is a time index. The decreasing amount of time necessary to perform the task or the increasing time that correct performance occurs is plotted. A third type is an accuracy index wherein some measure of accuracy, such as hitting a target, is plotted. The scores can be recorded in actual scores or in percentage of success, according to a standard of some kind.

Shapes of Performance Curves Performance curves that appear in journals or books usually represent scores of a large group of subjects whose performance on each trial has been averaged for the group. The curve formed by this method tends to be rather smooth. This gives the impression that

Figure 2.13   *Typical performance curve for two groups involving performance on a rotary-pursuit apparatus.*

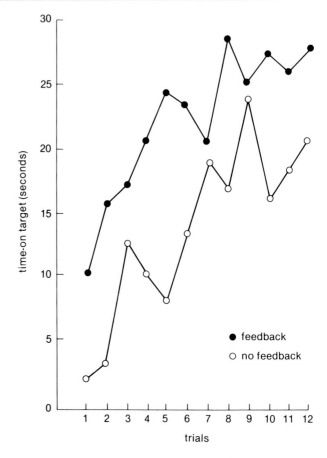

skill improvement progresses at a regular pace in a highly predictable manner, whereas, in fact, an individual's performance on a motor skill is erratic. Figure 2.13 shows rather typical performance curves as two groups practice a motor skill.

When a large number of performances are averaged, the result is usually a smooth, regular curve. Performance curves assume various shapes depending on such things as the complexity of the task, practice schedules, feedback, motivation, and other conditions present during the performance (figure 2.14). There is no single performance curve. A curve that shows rapid initial improvement, followed by decreasing gains from practice, is called a curve of decreasing returns, or a negatively accelerated curve. This kind of curve usually results when the task is relatively easy and mastery of the movements occurs rapidly. When a curve indicates little improvement

initially, then a period of rapid improvement, it is called a curve of increasing returns, or a positively accelerated curve. This kind of curve is typical of a task requiring unique movements that take some time to learn, but once they are learned performance improves quickly. An S-shaped curve shows little initial improvement followed by a period of rapid improvement and then a decreasing return curve. This S-shaped curve is most likely the continuation of a positively accelerated curve, that is, practice continues until performance approaches its maximum potential. A linear curve is essentially a straight line. The curves described above refer to curves on which correct responses or accuracy are plotted, for they all indicate increasingly adept performances as proficiency improves. A curve on which errors are plotted shows a declining characteristic.

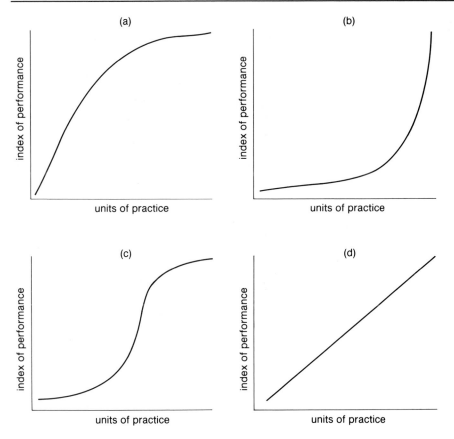

Figure 2.14   *Learning curves. (a) negatively accelerated curve; (b) positively accelerated curve; (c) s-shaped curve; (d) linear curve.*

When using a performance curve to derive inferences about learning, one should be sensitive to two of the most salient trends in performance: improvement in proficiency and increases in consistency. In the former, the performance scores should show a steady increase. For example, accuracy scores should show an increase in achieving the target; speed scores should show a decrease in time to complete the task. In the latter, the performance scores should show a decrease in variability; practice trial to practice trial scores should be more consistent, less erratic.

Performance Plateaus A curious feature of performance curves that has been the subject of much discussion and debate is the so-called **plateau.** A plateau is a period during which relatively little improvement in performance takes place. Sometimes a learner reaches a certain level of performance and remains there for some time without much improvement, then again shows improvement. The notion that plateaus are an essential characteristic during skill acquisition was first proposed by Bryan and Harter (1899) in one of the pioneer studies on skill. In their experimental findings on learning to send and receive

Morse code as a function of practice, they discovered that as practice continued the performance seemed to show a plateau, or level of performance where little or no improvement showed up on the performance curve over many trials. They explained plateaus in this way:

A plateau in the curve means that the lower-order habits are approaching their maximum development, but are not yet sufficiently automatic to leave the attention free to attack the higher-order habits.

The belief in the necessity of plateaus, as proposed by Bryan and Harter, was widely accepted for many years. Even today one hears physical educators and coaches refer to the performance of their students as being "at a plateau." However, subsequent experimentation on the plateau has led some scholars to refer to this phenomenon as the "phantom plateau." In other words, they have not found plateaus to be an essential feature of learning (Keller 1958). Other investigators have found that plateaus often do occur during skill learning under certain conditions such as fatigue, methodological changes adopted by the learner, or discrete changes in the environment. While learning complex skills, plateaus frequently occur as individuals attempt to construct complex movements from simple patterns.

Plateaus are still a puzzling issue. Although they are definitely not essential features of skill learning, they may, and in fact do, occur under certain conditions. A variety of factors result in periods during which there is little or no measurable improvement in performance.

Learning Formulas for Measuring Motor Learning

A performance curve allows one to make a subjective assessment about learning, but other methods are more precise and permit statistical treatment within and between individuals and groups. Several formulas have been used in the motor behavior literature. In the *total learning score method,* all performance scores on all trials are added, including the initial and final scores.

In the *difference in raw score method,* the difference in raw score is obtained by subtracting the initial score (typically scores on the first two or three trials) from the final score (typically scores on the last two or three trials). The formula is: (Sum of last N trials) minus (Sum of first N trials). N is an arbitrary number of trials, usually two or three. In the *percent gain of possible gain method,* the learning score is computed by dividing the actual gain from the initial score to the final score by the possible gain from the initial to the highest possible score. The formula is: (Sum of last N trials) minus (Sum of first N trials) divided by (Highest possible score on N trials) minus (Sum of first N trials).

Transfer Designs for Measuring Motor Learning

In research studies involving an estimate of the relatively permanent effects (learning effects) of an independent variable, as distinct from the performance effects, a **transfer design** is often used to assess learning. Transfer designs are typically used in experiments in which the learning effects of some independent variable (such as a particular form of feedback or a particular motivational technique) is employed with one group of learners (experimental group) and not the other (control group). After an initial series of practice trials, called the practice phase, both groups are given a rest. This is done to allow the temporary effects of the independent variable to be dissipated. Then both groups are transferred to a common level of the independent variable; that is, in the transfer phase both groups practice the task with the same value of the independent variable (Adams and Reynolds 1954). Any difference in performance scores between the groups that remains after the rest and the transfer to a common level of the independent variable represents the relatively permanent effects of the independent variable and serves as the basis for determining the effects of that variable on motor learning. The transfer design provides a useful technique for assessing the effects of independent variables on the learning of motor tasks.

Dunham (1971; 1976) has suggested an elaboration of the basic transfer design called a double transfer design, since two experimental and two control groups are used. At the transfer phase, one of the experimental groups shifts to a control group condition and the other continues practice under the experimental condition. One of the control groups shifts to an experimental group condition and the other continues practice under the control condition. This design has much to offer, but has not been used very often, probably because it requires twice the number of subjects as does the basic transfer design.

Measuring Retention

Remembering that explicit in the definition of learning is the term *relatively permanent,* proficiency that has been retained can be said to be learned; indeed, retention refers to the persistence of proficiency on a task after a period of no practice. You may be wondering, then, why this section on measuring retention is not a part of the section on measuring learning. The answer is that most measures of learning are made on performances that are not widely separated in time. For example, when trends on a performance curve are used as subjective estimates of motor learning, typically the practice trials have occurred in a single session. Or, if they have occurred in more than one practice session, the practices were held on consecutive days. Even when a transfer design is employed to eliminate temporary conditions that may be affecting performance, and to obtain a truer learning score, the lapse of time between the practice trials and the transfer trials is usually a few minutes, hours, or at the most a day or two. On the other hand, measurement of retention of motor skills is typically done after considerable lapses of time between the practice or skill acquisition phase and the retention test. Retention intervals typically vary from a day or so to several years.

The reason that learning is not typically measured by a retention test administered after a prolonged interval of no practice is that a long lapse of time introduces a new and very important variable into the situation: forgetting. Forgetting is viewed as the opposite of learning, since learning refers to the acquisition of some skill, while forgetting refers to the loss of that proficiency. Thus, while *relatively permanent* is an essential component of the definition of learning, persistence or permanence of learning that may have occurred with practice or experience is not typically assessed by learning measures.

Having said this, we shall describe one type of retention test that has been used as a rough estimate of learning. If a test is administered to a learner before any practice trials are taken, then after the practice trials have been completed, and again after an extended interval of no practice, one can compare the original test score and the score obtained at the end of the practice phase with the original score and the retention test score. The first scores indicate performance effects, while the latter two scores indicate any relatively permanent effect of the practice. Exactly how much learning has occurred cannot be resolved by this method.

The more common usage of retention tests is to ascertain information about the persistence, or lack of persistence, of an acquired proficiency— meaning that basically such tests are about memory or forgetting. Since the processes of memory and forgetting will be discussed in chapter 15, we shall be concerned with only the measurement issue in this section.

Retention, like learning, must be inferred from performance scores, and several methods of measuring retention have been used. Three of these methods are the absolute retention method, percent-of-gain method, and savings method.

Absolute Retention

The simplest retention test is **absolute retention,** which is the level of performance on the first trial(s) of the retention test after the retention interval. It is simply performance after the retention interval. No formula is used to analyze this score. Usually a performance curve is plotted of the performance scores throughout the practice trials and then a bar is drawn on the curve to represent the retention interval. The scores of the first trial or two after the retention interval are then plotted on the performance curve to illustrate graphically the results.

Percent-of-Gain

Here retention is assessed after a period of no practice and is recorded as a percentage of the proficiency level just before the retention interval. The proficiency level before the retention level is considered to be 100 percent, and the proficiency after the no-practice period is a percentage of original learning. If performers are able to hit a target ten times out of ten tries before the retention interval and eight times out of ten tries after it, their retention is 80 percent.

Savings

This technique involves tabulating the number of trials the learner requires to reach a certain level of proficiency, the criterion level; then after the retention interval the number of trials required for the learner again to reach the criterion level of proficiency is counted. The difference between the original level and the retention trials is considered the retention **savings.** Using this technique, if a learner requires 100 trials to attain the criterion of ten target hits out of ten tries, and then requires forty trials after the retention interval, the savings is sixty trials, or 60 percent.

As with learning scores, there is an active controversy among motor behavior researchers about the most appropriate measurements of retention. Each retention testing technique is flawed by a variety of factors that are not easily resolved (Schmidt 1972).

Summary

Every field of study has its particular vocabulary of concepts and unique methods for conducting research. Familiarity with them makes reading and understanding the literature of that field more meaningful. This chapter describes these concepts and methods.

The terms *motor learning, motor performance, motor behavior,* and *motor control* are used frequently throughout this text. While there may be a tendency to think of them as having the same meaning, they are not synonymous. Motor learning is a relatively permanent modification in behavior that is inferred from improvement in performance as a result of practice or experience. It is assumed that some biochemical or structural change in the nervous system underlies modifications in behavior. Motor performance is the observable behavior that is exhibited when one performs a task. Motor control refers to the reflex and voluntary mechanisms involved in skilled behavior. Motor behavior is a generic term for any kind of movement activity.

The word *skill* has two common usages: The first is as an act or task, and in this context it consists of a number of perceptual and motor responses that have been acquired by learning. The second is as an indicator of proficiency, and in this context is the implication that a person exhibits competence in carrying out a task— such a person is said to be skilled.

Motor ability is a general trait or capacity of an individual that is related to performance on a variety of skills and that is rather permanent. Abilities serve as the foundation for learning specific skills.

We use several classifications of motor skills: gross-fine, discrete-serial-continuous, open-closed, and self-paced–externally paced. Any given motor skill will overlap several of these categories.

In physiological psychology, the most frequently employed research techniques are ablation, lesioning, electrical stimulation, chemical stimulation, and recording electrical activity of the brain.

Motor skill learning and performance research has largely been limited to a few laboratory tasks. For measures of reaction and movement speed, reaction time and movement time instruments have been used. Accuracy is an important variable in motor behavior because many skills require that the performer do something with a minimum of error. The rotary-pursuit, stabilometer, and linear positioning tasks are frequently used for studying movement accuracy. Skills are often measured by the extent of performance. The laboratory task that has been most popular for assessing extent of performance has been the Bachman ladder. Many researchers design their own equipment to meet their specific research needs.

We have a dilemma in assessing learning because learning is a relatively permanent change in performance and because it must be inferred from performance scores, which are transitory. A variety of procedures have been used to infer motor learning from performance scores, none of which is completely satisfactory.

Retention is typically measured by one of three methods: absolute retention, percent-of-gain, or savings.

3

A Physiological Psychology Model of Motor Behavior

*I*n attempting to understand the complexities of motor behavior, it is helpful to have reference to a conceptual framework. In this chapter, you will find a framework that identifies the basic functional and neurological components of motor behavior. The framework is in the form of a model. A **model** is a unifying structure that facilitates the conceptualization of some phenomenon, and it functions to provide a pattern or guide to how a system works. The basic notion behind model development is that first it identifies the components of a functional system and then affords an overview of how that system functions. Once one is familiar with the components of a system and how they work, one can begin to understand how to control the system, modify it, and predict how the system will respond if certain variables or forces are applied to it.

This chapter serves as a prelude to the next twelve chapters. Concepts and ideas about motor behavior introduced in this chapter are covered in more detail in the succeeding chapters.

Basic Components of a Movement Model

Any approach to model building abstracts the common characteristics from a multitude of activities and categorizes them into components of function that are more easily understood. Reference to the model is then made to determine the relative functioning of each component with respect to the entire system. The model proposed here is based on a review and synthesis of other models for motor behavior (Gentile 1972; Marteniuk 1976; Welford 1976; Gallistel 1980; Kinsbourne 1981). However, most of these other models do not give any attention to the neural mechanisms underlying the phenomena of motor behavior.

The general assumption incorporated in our model is that complex motor behavior can be viewed as an **information-processing** activity guided by feedback control mechanisms that enable adaptive processes to occur. In this perspective of human motor behavior, the individual is viewed as an active, problem-solving, decision-making, processor of information. This view has come to have increasing influence in the human sciences.

An information-processing system has two important characteristics. First, the processing can be broken down into a series of stages; second, processing at each stage is limited. In viewing motor behavior from this perspective, information in the form of physical energy (from light or sound, mechanical or chemical) impinges on the individual and serves as a stimulus to the sense organs. Thus the word *processed* means that information in the form of **stimuli** is coded into electrical energy at the sensory receptors, where it takes the form of electrical impulses that are sent over sensory nerve cells to the central nervous system (CNS). In the brain and spinal cord, present information is integrated with stored information (memories). This processing results in information (electrical impulses) being sent to the muscles and glands to produce a response. The

response produces feedback information (nerve impulses) to control and direct the immediate response, or it may produce adaptive behavior for future responses to a similar stimulus situation.

Information from the environment is picked up by structures of the nervous system, transmitted over nerve fibers, integrated and interpreted by nerve cells. Muscles and glands are activated by the mediation of nerve cells. Hence it is obvious that recognition of the critical role of the nervous system must be an integral feature of any model of motor behavior. Indeed, a meaningful model of motor control, learning, and performance is unlikely to emerge without consideration of the functions of neural mechanisms. Therefore the composite of the model to be described in this chapter is called a physiological psychology model.

Functional Components

Before presenting the complete physiological psychology model, it may be well to review two simple models that illustrate the basic functional and neurological components of motor behavior. The first model relates to the functional components and is shown in figure 3.1.

Input is made up of all the stimuli impinging on a person at any given time. The total amount of input is sometimes referred to as the display. There are relevant and irrelevant stimuli in a display; relevant stimuli are those that are important for the present moment, and irrelevant stimuli are those not needed or used for the immediate situation. **Decision making** refers to the process of integrating and interpreting input and determining the appropriate response that should be made to relate the stimuli to the response. **Output** is the response (or behavior) in the form of muscular action or glandular activity. **Feedback** refers to the information that is received during or after a movement. Feedback may be intrinsic to the task wherein the movement execution itself produces feedback information. Or the feedback may be augmented, as it is when an instructor gives information about the consequences of a movement.

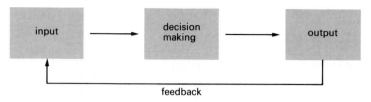

Figure 3.1   *The basic functional components of motor behavior.*

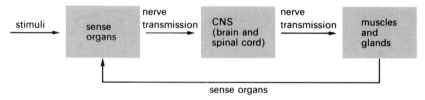

Figure 3.2   *The basic neurological mechanisms for motor behavior.*

Neurological Components

From the simple functional model, we can consider the neurological mechanisms that are related to the components above. A simple model of this kind is shown in figure 3.2.

In relating this model to the first one, we see that input is received via the sense organs. The brain and spinal cord serve the decision-making function, and output is mediated by the muscular and glandular system. Feedback is mediated by the various sensory organs. The information moves from one part of the model to the other parts via neural transmission.

Since an understanding of neural processes requires a knowledge of the structures and functional activity of the nervous system, the next two chapters contain condensed and simplified introductions to neuroanatomy and neurophysiology. These chapters are intended to provide an overview of the structures and functions of the nervous system and an appreciation of some of the physiochemical events that occur in it.

A Physiological Psychology Model

We are now ready to examine an elaboration of these simple models. This detailed model, shown in figure 3.3, more precisely illustrates the functions and neural mechanisms for motor behavior.

The components of this more elaborate model are described below, but first it may be well to begin by stating what this model *does not* represent. It does not specify *all* of the various components that make up the human perceptual-motor system—it is greatly oversimplified. The human neuromotor system is too incredibly complex to identify all of the mechanisms and their interrelationships. Moreover, much is still unknown about how the system *really* works. While more elaborate and complex models of motor behavior have been developed, when placed in a schematic diagram, such as figure 3.3, they tend to look like the wiring diagram for the Boeing 767 and are virtually uninterpretable for the general student of motor behavior.[1]

---

[1] Readers wishing to review descriptions and illustrations of more sophisticated models are referred to Marteniuk (1976), Welford (1976), and Gallistel (1980).

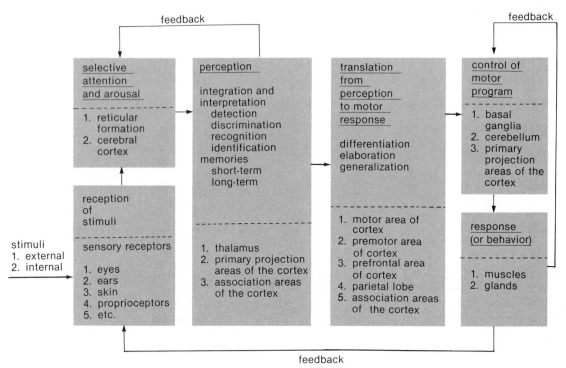

Figure 3.3 A model of the functional and neural mechanisms for motor behaviors.

Stimuli

Motor behavior involves the integration of several kinds of information: (1) about the present environment; (2) about what is to be achieved; (3) about previous experiences with a task; (4) from the movement task itself; and (5) about the results of the performance itself. This information serves as stimuli to the individual.

Successful motor behavior depends on an individual's ability to pick up stimuli within the environment and to transmit this information to various parts of the body for a response. Various stimuli impose upon the motor performer in sports: visual stimuli in the form of teammates, coaches, and opponents; auditory stimuli such as the sounds of balls being hit, voices of teammates, coaches, opponents, and starting signals; and mechanical stimuli imposed by the pressures

of opponents in boxing and wrestling and the pressure of water in swimming. Of course, many other stimuli could be mentioned.

Stimuli that impinge upon the individual are of two basic varieties, external and internal. External stimuli are in the form of light energy, sound energy, mechanical energy, thermal energy, and so on, originating outside the organism. One form of internal stimuli arises from mechanical or chemical energy operating from within the individual. For example, pressures on internal organs by movement stimulate receptors in the muscles and joints of the body, and hormones serve as chemical stimulators for certain target cells of the nervous system. Another form of internal stimuli arises from the cognition, or thinking, mechanisms in the brain. One extraordinary feature of the human nervous system is this self-generation of information—what we call thinking and imagination. Stimuli (external and internal) are transmitted as electrical impulses throughout the nervous system over nerve fibers via an electrochemical process.

Motor behavior normally relies heavily upon the functioning of various sensory systems, especially the visual, auditory, and proprioceptive[2] systems. During the initial stages of motor learning, the individual relies heavily upon visual information, but as performance becomes habitual it is likely that proprioceptive feedback, or "feel," becomes more important. The role of vision in motor behavior is discussed in detail in chapter 9, while the role of proprioceptors is taken up in chapter 10.

Neural Mechanisms for the Reception of Stimuli

The neural mechanisms for reception of external and one form of internal stimuli are the sensory receptors throughout the body. It is through the sensory systems that we are in contact with our environment. They are sensitive to a wide variety of stimuli that impinge upon the organism. (Stimuli that are formed in the cognitive mechanisms will be discussed later in this chapter in relation to motor program formation and control.)

For external stimuli, the first task of the sensory receptors is to **transduce** (change from one form of energy to another) the stimulus energy into electrical energy. This process is accomplished in different ways by the various sensory systems. The next task is to transmit the electrical current produced by the stimulus into the CNS. The process of transforming external stimuli into nerve impulses is described in chapters 5 and 6, and the structure and functioning of the visual and proprioceptive sensory systems are discussed in chapters 8, 9, and 10.

---

[2] The proprioceptive system is composed of sensory receptors located in the muscles, tendons, joints, and inner ear. This system is described in chapter 10.

Selective Attention

The individual cannot and does not consciously process all stimuli in the immediate environment. One of the most critical factors in motor behavior is the ability to select and attend to only the relevant stimuli in the environment and to ignore the irrelevant stimuli. It is possible for one to direct one's attention to any stimulus in the display by choice, but normally the multitude of stimuli from the various senses are largely ignored. Only a very limited range of stimuli is selected for attention out of the many bombarding the sensory systems.

This division of stimuli into relevant and irrelevant information occurs very rapidly, so that the processing of certain stimuli is enhanced or inhibited. Evidence of various kinds strongly indicates that the sensory systems and the CNS have limited capacity for handling data, and many of the sensory data are irrelevant to appropriate behavior. Hence only a part of the incoming information is selected for conscious processing, and attention is focused on only a part of the stimulus display. The topic of **selective attention** is examined in detail in chapter 7.

Neural Mechanisms for Selective Attention

There is considerable controversy in the neurophysiological literature as to what are the neural mechanisms of attention. In particular, does attention involve a peripheral "filtering" or central "gating" of sensory inputs, or is the cerebral cortex[3] the primary center for selective attention? The possible neural mechanisms and the issue of their contribution to selective attention is taken up in chapter 7.

Arousal

Arousal refers to the state of wakefulness or alertness of the individual. A certain amount of arousal is necessary for optimal motor learning and performance. Arousal facilitates the cerebral cortex and enhances transmission throughout the brain, making it more effective in

---

[3] The cerebral cortex is the outer layer of cells in the brain.

processing incoming sensory information. Arousal also activates various mechanisms throughout the body to prepare the body for action.

Arousal can be viewed as having two dimensions: a background level and a stimulus-specific level. First, the background level of arousal refers to the general state of the individual that varies with the time of day, spontaneous neural activity, and many other factors. The stimulus-specific arousal response is triggered by novel and changing stimuli as well as by cortical activity such as thinking about a certain thing.

The stimulus-specific arousal response brings about an alert, even emotional state of the individual. There is growing evidence that some aspects of stimulus-specific arousal are important for optimal performance, memory storage, and enhanced rates of learning. This is described in more detail in chapter 7.

Neural Mechanisms of Arousal

It was Moruzzi and Magoun (1949) who first identified the neuroanatomical basis for arousal. Their ideas have been extended in recent years by many other scholars. The primary location of arousal structures is in the brainstem and midbrain. These neural mechanisms are discussed in chapter 7.

Perception

The process by which sensory information is organized, integrated, and interpreted to produce meaning of the incoming data and the formulation of a movement response involves **perception.** Perception is essentially an organizing process, and past experiences play a leading role in this process. The process of perception involves detection, discrimination, recognition, and identification of incoming information for an interpretation. Then the oncoming information takes on meaning. Perception is an important component in motor behavior because all complex motor learning and performance require perceptual function. Perception is examined in detail in chapter 7.

The idea that incoming information has to be combined with previously encountered information implies that previous experiences are somehow retained in the nervous system. Memory refers to the retention and subsequent retrieval of information and as such comprises a major element of perception. Memory is a very significant aspect of perception, but also cuts across other components of this motor behavior model and consists of several stages itself. Therefore, chapter 15 is devoted to memory.

Neural Mechanisms of Perception

The various stimuli that impinge upon the individual are processed by a complex system at various levels of the nervous system, from the sense organs to the highest centers in the brain. All the sensory systems are important in perception because they provide the raw material out of which perception arises. Other mechanisms responsible for perceptual activities are located in various subcortical structures of the brain, and in various regions of the cerebral cortex. These all play decisive roles in the analysis, coding, and storing of information. They will be identified and discussed in chapter 7.

Translation from Perception to Motor Response

A response to perception in the form of motor behavior can be understood as a translation process, a translation from perception to a series of detailed muscular units. Perceptual information must be converted to muscle commands to produce a movement pattern. One of the central questions in motor behavior study is how a movement response is actually selected and prepared for execution.

The translation of current information into an appropriate **motor response** obviously involves memory—not only for ascertaining the meaning of current information, but memory of previous responses that have been made to similar data in similar situations and the consequences of those responses.

There is an active controversy about how the translation from perception to motor response occurs. The issues and controversies of this topic are discussed in chapters 12, 13, and 14.

Neural Mechanisms for Translation to Motor Response

The neural mechanisms for the formation of voluntary movements are quite complicated and are certainly not formed in narrow areas of the cerebral cortex, as once believed. Subcortical mechanisms participate in the creation of a voluntary movement, with each mechanism performing a highly specific role in the whole functional system. Traditionally, the focus in motor formulation has been on the role of the cerebral cortex. However, recent research has shown quite convincingly that several structures in the brain contribute to formulating motor behavior. Details of these structures and functions are described in chapters 12, 13, and 14.

Control of Motor Responses

Once a specific response has been selected, the individual must produce the appropriate movement pattern. Historically, there have been two major explanations for the control of movements. The first emphasizes the role of sensory feedback during a movement, and the second proposes that movements are structured and executed by "motor programs." These two proposals will be described in chapter 14.

Neural Mechanisms for Motor Response Control

Various neural mechanisms are undoubtedly responsible for the movement control function. It is clear that three interconnected parts of the brain—the motor areas of the cortex, the cerebellum, and the basal ganglia—act together to control movement. During the past decade neuroscientists have focused on lower neural centers in the control of movement. Evidence is rapidly accumulating that demonstrates important motor control functions in the spinal cord and even the muscles themselves. The neural mechanisms for motor control are the subject of chapters 13 and 14.

Output

The activity of muscles and glands constitutes the behavior (or response) that has been brought about by all the preceding processing activity. In the case of muscles, movement activity occurs; in the case of glands, hormones or other secretions occur.

Neural Mechanisms for Output

The nervous system is in intimate contact with muscles and glands and is the primary mechanism for the control of these two systems. Output in the form of nerve impulses stimulates muscle fibers, causing them to contract and thus produce movement, and stimulates glandular cells, causing them to secrete hormones or other products that tend to serve supporting roles for movements. The details of the interrelationships among the nervous system and muscles and glands is described in chapters 5 and 12.

Feedback

All motor behavior involves strong feedback effects, whether one is considering spinal reflexes or complex movements such as a basketball jump shot. The model presented here posits feedback as essential to some extent in various components of motor behavior.

Response-produced feedback is used not only to make certain that a movement is carried out as intended, but, more important, to correct errors if the movement is unsuccessful. Thus, stimuli produced by the learner's own behavior appear to play a critical role in the acquisition of skilled motor behavior. The movement-produced feedback enables the learner to correct systematically errors from practice trial to practice trial in order to develop a motor pattern that coincides with the learner's intentions. Feedback, then, is not only a feature of the ongoing movement, but various types of feedback that occur at the completion of movements are important in enhancing motor learning.

Neural Mechanisms for Feedback

A fundamental characteristic of the central nervous system is the feedback loop. At all levels of the central nervous system and within each level, numerous feedback loops exist to integrate and coordinate ongoing activities.

Feedback for human movement is mediated by all of the sensory systems. Movement stimulates sensory receptors in the muscles, tendons, joints, and inner ear, and the nerve impulses that are set off by movement are powerful sources of feedback. Seeing and hearing the consequences of movements also constitute important sources of feedback.

Problems of Human Movement Models

One of the problems in presenting models of human behavior is that they convey the notion of a static system. Nothing could be further from the truth. The human neuromuscular systems are constantly active. All of the components in the model are in a continuous state of activity and change. Another problem with models of human behavior is that they are much too simplified for what actually is occurring. The human nervous system is fantastically complex, and our understanding of its intricate functions is still quite incomplete. Nevertheless, a model like the one described here can help us gain a clearer understanding of the components of motor behavior.

Summary

A model is a unifying structure that facilitates the conceptualization of some phenomenon and provides a guide for how a system works. The model of motor behavior described in this chapter views motor behavior as an information-processing activity. The functional components of the model are input, decision making, output, and feedback. Neurological components that correspond to the functional components are sense organs, the central nervous system, and muscles and glands. When analyzed in more detail, stimuli are transduced into nerve impulses by the sensory receptors. This information in the form of nerve impulses is further processed by being subjected to the selective attention, arousal, and perceptual mechanisms extending throughout the central nervous system. It is then translated into a motor response. Most of the brain plays a role in this process. Once a specific response has been selected, an individual produces the appropriate movement pattern, with the activity of muscles and glands constituting the behavior. Finally, all motor behavior involves strong feedback effects, which once again involve the sensory systems.

Basic Functioning of the Nervous System

4

Anatomy of the Nervous System

*T*his book is concerned with the ways in which the nervous system mediates the analysis of information from the external and internal environments and the organization of motor behavior. As a prelude to this approach, it is necessary to present an outline of the gross structure, microstructure, and general principles of operation of the nervous system as a foundation for understanding later concepts. This chapter describes the basic anatomy of the nervous system, the next is concerned with neural transmission, followed by a description of the integration mechanisms of the nervous system. Only the most elementary facts about how the nervous system functions in motor behavior are introduced in these chapters. More detail about the functions of the specific parts of the nervous system will be provided as the need arises.

Since special terminology is employed in **neuroanatomy** when describing the location of structures, the first section of this chapter presents the most common terms and their meanings. There follows a description of the structural and functional unit of the nervous system, the neuron, and then the major structures of the nervous system are identified and briefly described.

Terminology Used in Neuroanatomy

Before we begin our examination of the nervous system, it is necessary to have an understanding of some of the terminology used when describing the *location* of certain structures in the body. It is customary to discuss the location of parts of the body in relation to three imaginary planes (figure 4.1). The sagittal plane divides the body into right and left parts. A sagittal plane that divides the body into right and left halves is called a median plane. The coronal plane is at right angles to the sagittal plane and divides the body into front and back. The horizontal plane divides the body into upper and lower parts, so it is at right angles to the other two planes. Other commonly used terms and their definitions are listed in table 4.1.

The Neuron

Like every other system in the human body, the nervous system is made up of individual cells. These cells are specialized to carry out a unique task, the transmission of nerve impulses from one cell to another. The structural and functional unit of the nervous system is the **neuron,** or nerve cell. It is the individual component of which the whole nervous system is built. Like all of the body's cells, neurons are designed in ways that are appropriate to their functions, which are primarily receiving, conducting, and transmitting information. A membrane surrounds the gelatinous protoplasm within the neuron, much like a skin surrounds a sausage. Protoplasm is a fluid substance containing a number of chemicals, granules, and other substances. The three main parts of a neuron are the cell body, dendrites, and the axon (figure 4.2).

Cell Body

The cell body, also called the soma, is the metabolic center of the cell. It contains the nucleus, which is responsible for regulating the various processes of the entire cell. Extending out from the cell body are one or more fibers, some of which are microscopically short while others are over a meter in length. Neuron cell bodies are located mostly within the brain and spinal cord, which together make up the central nervous system (CNS). Some are found in ganglia (singular, ganglion), which are clusters of cell bodies outside the CNS. Clusters of cell bodies within the CNS are called nuclei.

Dendrites

A dendrite is one type of nerve fiber extending from the cell body. A neuron can have anywhere from one to thousands of dendrites projecting outward from the cell body. These fibers typically divide like the branches of a tree into a number of small fibers before terminating. **Dendrites** are the major receptive surface of the neuron. All incoming information from other neurons arrives on the dendrites and cell body. Dendrites have more surface area than the cell body because they branch extensively, so the majority of incoming information is received at the dendrites. This information is subsequently conducted to the cell body.

Axon

The second type of neuron fiber is called an **axon,** and it is attached to the cell body at a point called the initial segment. (This location on an axon is also called the axon hillock. We shall use both terms throughout the book.) There is only one axon for each neuron, but an axon typically gives off many side branches, called collateral fibers.

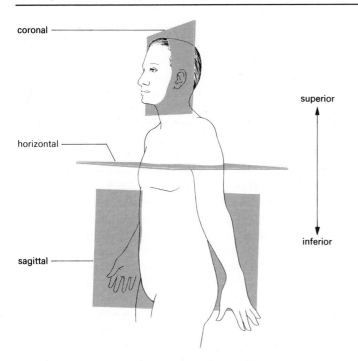

coronal

horizontal

sagittal

superior

inferior

Figure 4.1   *Anatomical planes in the anatomical position.*

Term	Definition
Superior, cranial	Toward the head
Inferior, caudal	Toward the feet
Anterior, ventral	Toward the front of the body
Posterior, dorsal	Toward the back of the body
Medial	Toward the middle of the body
Lateral	Toward the side of the body
Peripheral	Away from the center of the body
Ipsilateral	On the same side of the body
Contralateral	On the opposite side of the body

Table 4.1   *Neuroanatomical terminology*

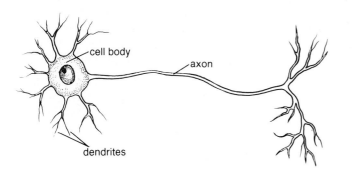

cell body

axon

dendrites

Figure 4.2   *A neuron, the structural and functional unit of the nervous system.*

The end portions of an axon are called presynaptic terminals (other terms are telodendria, boutons, and knobs), and each axon may have numerous presynaptic terminals because it may have given off many collateral branches. The axon presynaptic terminals typically end on dendrites and cell bodies of other neurons, or on muscles and glands throughout the body.

The functional connection between the presynaptic terminals of an axon and another neuron is called a **synapse.** We shall have more to say about synapses in the next chapter.

Neuron Function

One of the major purposes of the neuron is to pass messages, or impulses, from one part of the body to another. It does this by an electrochemical process whereby an impulse, much like an electric current in a wire, is propagated from neuron to neuron. The impulse is transmitted from one part of the body to another by a sequence of dendrite or cell body to axon to dendrite or cell body of another neuron, linked together through many neurons. This forms the conduction pathway of the nervous system. The nervous system functions exclusively by these neuron chains.

Classification of Neurons

We have two methods for classifying neurons. One is based on location and function, the other on structure. In the first method, neurons are classified as afferent, efferent, or interneuron. **Afferent** neurons carry nerve impulses from the sensory receptors into the spinal cord or brain. These afferent neurons are also called **sensory neurons.** On the other hand, **efferent** neurons transmit impulses from the CNS out to the effector organs—the muscles and glands. Effector neurons passing

to muscles are commonly called **motoneurons.** The **interneurons** originate and terminate wholly within the CNS, and over 95 percent of all neurons of the nervous system are of this type.

Neurons are also classified by structure, specifically the number of fibers extending from the cell body. Some neurons have only one fiber process and are called unipolar. In unipolar neurons, only the axon is connected to the cell body, without dendrites. Unipolar neurons are located in the spinal and cranial nerves and carry afferent signals from the sensory receptors. The single fiber process, the axon, divides into central and peripheral branches very close to the cell body in a T-shaped manner.

A second type of neuron has only two fiber processes and is thus called bipolar. Bipolar neurons are rather rare, being found in only two or three sites in the nervous system. The most common type of neuron in the human nervous system is the multipolar neuron, in which numerous dendrites and an axon extend from the cell body. Multipolar cells are found throughout the nervous system (figure 4.3).

Neuroglia

Within the CNS is a special type of nonneural cell that performs primarily nutritive and supportive functions for neurons. These cells, called neuroglia (or just glia), outnumber neurons ten to one and are in close proximity to the neurons. They literally glue the CNS together. Since these cells are not involved in the information transmission functions of the nervous system, they will be of no further concern to us.

The Peripheral Nervous System

The nervous system is customarily divided into two general parts, based on spatial location. One part is called the **peripheral nervous system** (PNS). The PNS lies outside the bony projection

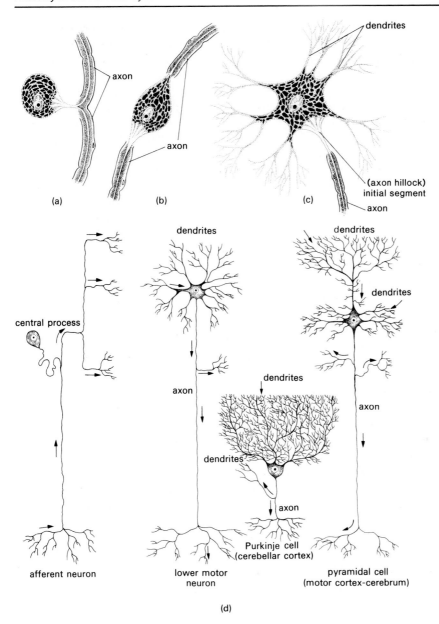

dendrites

axon

axon

axon

dendrites

(axon hillock)
initial segment

axon

(a)   (b)   (c)

dendrites

dendrites

central process

dendrites

dendrites

axon

dendrites

axon

dendrites

axon

Purkinje cell
(cerebellar cortex)

afferent neuron

lower motor
neuron

pyramidal cell
(motor cortex-cerebrum)

(d)

Figure 4.3   Three main types of neurons. (a) a unipolar
neuron; (b) a bipolar neuron; (c) a multipolar neuron;
(d) schematic illustration of some principal forms of
neurons which are found in particular parts of the nervous
system.

of the skull and vertebral column and consists of all those nerve fibers that enter or leave the brainstem and spinal cord and innervate (supply) the sensory receptors, muscles, and glands. These fibers are enclosed in cablelike structures called **nerves.** The second part of the nervous system is called the central nervous system (CNS) and it is composed of those neural structures lying entirely within the vertebral column and skull. The major structures of the CNS are the brain and spinal cord. Essentially, the PNS represents lines of communication, whereas the CNS is the center of coordination and the place of determination of the most appropriate response to incoming impulses.

The PNS is further divided into somatic and autonomic systems. The somatic peripheral system controls all the skeletal muscles—the muscles we contract when we make voluntary movements or when involuntary adjustments in posture and other reflexes are made. The autonomic nervous system, in contrast, controls the heart, smooth muscles (blood vessels, digestive and reproductive organs, and so on), and glands. Each system also contains sensory components. Sensory input to the somatic system is from skin, joint, and muscle receptors and includes touch, pressure, temperature, joint angulation, and muscle tension. Sensory input from the autonomic system is from smooth muscles, heart, and glands and is generally less precise than the somatic sensory input.

Nerves

The PNS originates in thirty-one pairs of spinal nerves, which emerge between the spinal vertebrae, and twelve pairs of cranial nerves, which leave the brainstem. A nerve is a bundle of nerve fibers, not including the cell bodies, bound together by well organized connective tissue sheaths

and lying outside the CNS. Thousands of nerve fibers are necessary to form a nerve. Nearly all nerves contain both afferent and efferent nerve fibers, so they are called mixed nerves. Thus, within a nerve some fibers will carry impulses toward the CNS while others will carry impulses away from the CNS.

Of the thirty-one pairs of spinal nerves, eight are cervical, twelve thoracic, five lumbar, five sacral, and one coccygeal. The number and names of the spinal nerves correspond closely to those of the vertebral column. This column consists of thirty-three vertebrae, named according to the regions of the body they occupy. Spinal nerves pass through lateral openings between the vertebrae called intervertebral foramina (singular, foramen) (figure 4.4).

Upon emerging from the intervertebral foramina, spinal nerves divide into a complex network of branches that then supply segments of the skin and muscles with nerve fibers. Many of the nerves form plexuses (networks or tangles of nerves) or junctions, from which peripheral nerves arise to actually supply the various skin areas and muscles.

Each spinal nerve supplies fibers to a specific segment of the body. Such segments are called dermatomes. Since we have thirty-one pairs of spinal nerves, there should be thirty-one pairs of dermatomes. But since the first cervical nerve has no dorsal root, it does not innervate a dermatome. Therefore the body actually has thirty pairs of dermatomes.

On a dermatome chart, each dermatome is labeled by the spinal nerve that innervates it. For example, dermatome L_2 means that part of the body innervated by the second lumbar spinal nerve. There is, of course, some overlapping between contiguous dermatomes. Thus, if one spinal

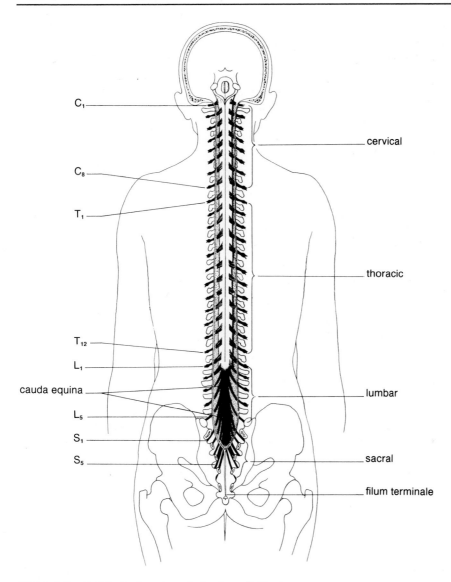

Figure 4.4 *Vertebral column in posterior view with the surface of the spinal cord exposed.*

Figure 4.5 *A dermatome. Each numbered area represents an area of the skin supplied by the spinal nerve of the corresponding number. The letters C, T, L, and S refer to cervical, thoracic, lumbar, and sacral.*

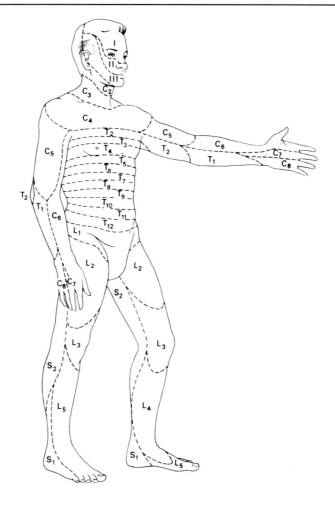

nerve becomes nonfunctional, the region of the body that it once innervated does not become inoperative (figure 4.5).

Twelve pairs of cranial nerves arise from the lower centers of the brain, especially the brainstem. They carry sensory information to the brain from the eyes, ears, nose, mouth, and from the same general sensory receptors found in the spinal nerves. These nerves also project motor fibers to control movements of the eyes, mouth, face, tongue, and throat, and they supply the major outflow for the control of smooth muscles and glands in the visceral regions of the body. Their structure and function are not of major interest for our purposes.

The Central Nervous System

The brain and spinal cord make up the **central nervous system.** CNS structures are protected by the skull, the spinal column (vertebrae) and its ligamentous connections, and the cerebrospinal fluid. The foramen magnum ("large opening") is an opening at the base of the skull. It is through this opening that the brain connects with the spinal cord (figure 4.6).

The structures of the CNS basically function to carry out two tasks: (1) to transmit information about the environment and the body to the

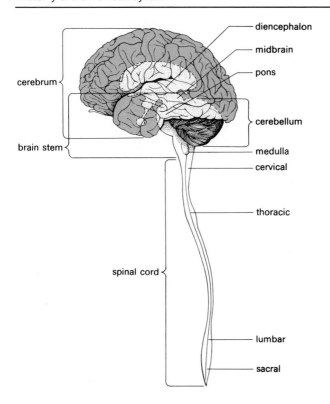

diencephalon

midbrain

pons

cerebrum

cerebellum

brain stem

medulla

cervical

thoracic

spinal cord

lumbar

sacral

Figure 4.6   *The central nervous system (CNS) and its major parts.*

brain where it is recorded, stored, and compared with other information; (2) to carry information from the brain to muscles and glands, thus producing movement or bodily adaptations to environmental demands.

The Spinal Cord

The nervous system works as a mechanism for information input, coordination and processing, and output. The **spinal cord** has an essential role in in both the input and output phases. It carries to the brain all sensory information from the body and all motor commands sent down from the brain to muscles and glands. It is, therefore, primarily a transmission pathway. But it also has important reflex functions as well. The cord makes possible smooth sequences of extension and flexion of the limbs and it coordinates the movements of all four limbs when they are employed in standing, walking, and running.

The spinal cord, which is about as thick as an adult's little finger, joins the brain at the brainstem through the foramen magnum. It occupies the vertebral canal, formed by the vertebrae, which gives it protection and support. The cord extends from the foramen magnum to the level of the first or second lumbar vertebra. Below this level, separate nerve trunks and roots of nerves continue to run through the vertebral column. This mass of nerves in the vertebral canal below the spinal cord resembles the tail of a horse, hence its anatomical name, cauda equina (see figure 4.4).

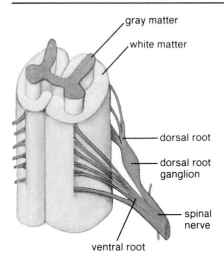

gray matter

white matter

dorsal root

dorsal root ganglion

spinal nerve

ventral root

Figure 4.7 *The spinal cord, showing ventral and dorsal roots and the emergence of a spinal nerve.*

In cross section, the spinal cord consists of a center portion and an outer part. The former is in the shape of a butterfly (or H) and is gray in color. The anterior horns of the gray matter are customarily known as the vertebral horns, while the posterior horns are called the dorsal horns of the spinal cord. This gray color is a result of tight packing of neuron cell bodies. The outer part of the cord surrounds the gray matter and is white in color because it is made up of nerve fibers rather than cell bodies (figure 4.7).

Each spinal nerve of the pair that arises from each spinal cord segment begins as a series of nerve fibers from the dorsal and ventral horns of the spinal cord. The ventral horns of the gray matter contain cell bodies, the axons of which project outward through spinal nerve to connect with muscles and glands. The dorsal horns contain interneuron cells that receive incoming signals from sensory neurons, transmitting them to the brain and other levels of the spinal cord. These latter, or intracord signals, are carried over relatively short distances and support a variety of spinal cord reflexes.

The fibers from dorsal and ventral horns at each spinal cord segment leave the cord and pass through the intervertebral foramina. Just before the fibers of the two horns unite to form a spinal nerve, we find an enlargement on the dorsal root called the dorsal root ganglion. This ganglion contains the cell bodies of sensory neurons. As noted above, cell bodies of the ventral root fibers are located in the ventral horn of the spinal cord (figure 4.8).

Inside the CNS a bundle of nerve fibers is called a tract. The spinal cord has numerous tracts for carrying impulses from the sensory receptors to the brain and from the brain to the muscles and glands. The outer portion of the cord, the white matter, consists of these upward- and downward-coursing tracts that subserve sensory and motor functions.

The Brain

John C. Eccles (1977), a Nobel laureate in neurophysiology, said that the human **brain** "is without any qualification the most highly organized and most complexly organized matter in the universe." It is the master control, the guiding force behind all human actions. This organ regulates heart and respiratory rates, controls body temperature, and performs numerous other duties without our really being aware of them. The brain is responsible for the range, diversity, and complexity of human behavior. Without it, we would not be able to see, think, move, or perform any of the complex activities we associate with human endeavor.

The brain was described by one writer as "two fistfuls of pinkish-gray tissue, wrinkled like a walnut and something of the consistency of oatmeal." It weighs about 3.5 pounds, but although

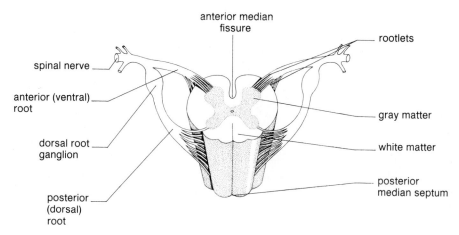

Figure 4.8   *A spinal cord segment.*

it makes up only about 2.5 percent of the total body weight, it receives 15 percent of the total blood supply and uses about 25 percent of all the oxygen consumed by the body. Indeed, it requires a steady supply of oxygen. If the flow of blood to the brain is interrupted for as little as fifteen seconds, loss of consciousness can result; interruption of blood flow for more than four minutes causes irreversible damage to brain cells and can cause death.

Since the early 1900s, textbooks have compared the brain to a telephone switchboard. More recent books use the analogy of a computer. Both analogies are functionally useful for illustrative purposes—the brain functions as a switchboard and computer—but they are technically inaccurate. No switchboard or computer can accomplish anything like the miracles of scrutinizing, sorting, coding, and remembering performed by the brain.

The brain can be conveniently subdivided into three parts: the brainstem, cerebrum, and cerebellum. It also contains several small cavities, called ventricles.

The Brainstem

Inside the base of the skull the central areas of the spinal cord expand into a very complicated region of tracts and nuclei called the **brainstem.** This region of the brain is responsible for many involuntary and metabolic functions. Some of the brainstem nuclei subserve important, highly complex reflexes, such as the orienting reflex, a stereotypic response to novel stimuli that involves head turning, eye movements, arousal, postural adjustments, and autonomic effects including heart rate and respiration changes.

The major structures of the brainstem are the medulla, pons, midbrain, and diencephalon. There is also a complex mixture of cell bodies, fibers, and nuclei spread throughout the brainstem that is collectively called the brainstem reticular formation.

Medulla   The **medulla** is the superior extension of the spinal cord and contains a number of sensory tracts for information ascending to the brain

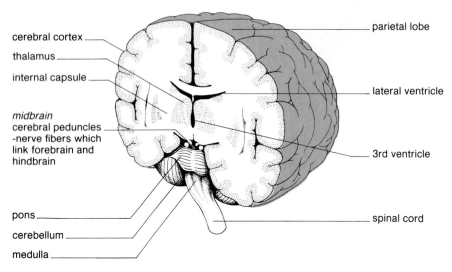

cerebral cortex

thalamus

internal capsule

midbrain
cerebral peduncles
-nerve fibers which
link forebrain and
hindbrain

pons

cerebellum

medulla

parietal lobe

lateral ventricle

3rd ventricle

spinal cord

Figure 4.9   *Coronal section through brain.*

and motor tracks for information descending toward muscles and glands (figure 4.9). The medulla also contains a collection of neurons and nerve tracts that serves an important function of providing regulation of vital internal processes, such as respiration, blood pressure, and heart rate. Finally, the medulla possesses nuclei from which cranial nerves emerge. The cranial nerves carry sensory signals from sensory systems in the head and upper body and motor signals for the control of these same areas.

The Pons   The **pons** is a highly convoluted structure. It is an integration center for sensory information from muscles and joints. The word pons, meaning bridge, is derived from the thick band of transverse fibers (fibers crossing from one side of the midline to the other) that make up its ventral portion and serve in part as a bridge between the hemispheres of the cerebellum (see figure 4.9). Functionally, this ventral portion of the pons interconnects the cerebellum with motor areas of the cerebrum.

The dorsal part of the pons contains the terminations of the cochlear nerve (nerve from the ear). Also, the nuclei of the vestibular nerve are found here. These later nuclei play an important role in reflex control of the head, neck, and eyes.

Together, the ventral and dorsal parts of the pons contain several nerve tracts and collections of nuclei that allow for coordination and involuntary influences on automatic movement and posture.

Midbrain   Above the pons lies an area of the brain known as the **midbrain.** This area constitutes the top of the brain stalk and comprises several structures. The largest portion of its area contains the cerebral peduncles (a stemlike part), which are comprised of fibers connecting the cerebral cortex to the pons or the spinal cord. The medial parts of the midbrain contain all the various pathways that ascend to the thalamus. The roof of the midbrain includes two pairs of small hemispheres called the superior and inferior colliculi. The first is involved in reflex movements caused by visual stimulation, the latter in reflex

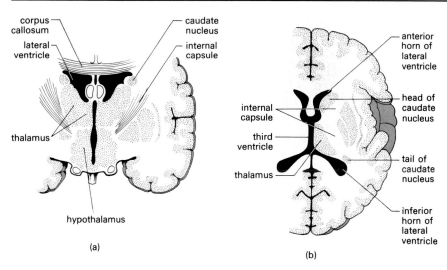

Figure 4.10 (a) Coronal section through cerebrum; (b) horizontal section through cerebrum.

movements caused by auditory stimulation. This area also contains other small nuclei that have connections with the cerebellum, cerebral cortex, and several of the cranial nerves (see figure 4.9).

Diencephalon From an evolutionary standpoint, the oldest areas of the brain lie in its center and extend up into the cerebrum like a clenched fist, with the cerebrum enclosing them. At the core of the brain is the area known as the **diencephalon** (di-en-sef-ah-lon), which connects the cerebral hemispheres with the midbrain. This area consists of a variety of structures that lie on either side of a narrow internal cavity, the third ventricle (a small cavity). We need mention only two of those structures, the thalamus and the hypothalamus (figure 4.10)

The thalamus consists of a large grouping of nuclei that is located on either side of the third ventricle. This structure is shaped somewhat like two small footballs. One part of the thalamus is concerned with relaying information from the sensory systems for vision, hearing, touch, joint and muscle receptors, and perhaps pain, to the cerebral cortex. Another part of this structure does not seem to be involved in relaying specific sensory impulses, but does appear to play an important role in the arousal of the individual for activity. Some of the nerve fibers from the cerebral cortex and the cerebellum also terminate in the thalamus.

The hypothalamus is made up of a group of small nuclei located close to the base of the brain and to the "master gland," the pituitary. In spite of its small size, the hypothalamus contains the highest integrative centers for the control of the autonomic nervous system. It is involved in such functional activities as the regulation of body temperature, endocrine gland activities, and emotional behavior in general. The hypothalamus is by far the most important center in the brain in the elicitation and coordination of motivated behavior.

Figure 4.11 *The reticular formation and structures which are associated with it.*

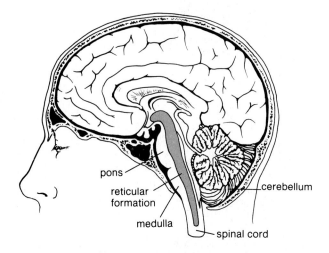

pons

reticular
formation

cerebellum

medulla

spinal cord

Reticular Formation Extending throughout the brainstem is a set of neurons and nuclei called the reticular formation (see figure 4.11). This network of cells receives input from several sources: All of the sensory systems, which give off collateral fibers, synapse on reticular formation neurons. Nerve fibers from higher brain centers also make synaptic connections here. The neurons of this structure are also sensitive to stimulation from drugs and certain endocrine products.

The two major output fiber networks of the reticular formation are directed to spinal and cranial neurons and to higher brain centers, especially the cerebral cortex. Stimulation by descending reticular fibers can cause either a decrease or an increase in the firing of neurons controlling the skeletal muscles. The ascending reticular fibers seem to be critically involved in the control of sleeping and waking, and appear to play an important role in attention and activation of the individual for cognitive and motor activity.

The Cerebrum

The **cerebrum** is the large umbrellalike dome of the brain that is divided into two cerebral hemispheres by the longitudinal fissure (a groove or furrow). The two hemispheres are symmetrical, one on the right and one on the left, with the fissure between them, running from front to rear.

The cerebrum is further divided by the central fissure (also called the fissure of Rolando) that extends laterally across the midportion of each hemisphere. Another fissure, the lateral fissure (also called the fissure of Sylvius), is deep and runs laterally directly below the central fissure. The lateral and central fissures help to mark off the four major regions of each cerebral hemisphere. These regions are called lobes (figure 4.12).

The frontal lobe is anterior to the central fissure. This area increases in size most dramatically with the ascent of the phylogenetic scale. In the cat or dog, the area forward of the central fissure is very small, but in humans the frontal lobe amounts to half the lateral area of the cerebrum. The parietal (pa-ri-e-tal) lobe is behind the central fissure and extends back to the parieto-occipital fissure. The occipital lobe makes up the posterior aspect of each cerebral hemisphere. The division between the parietal and occipital lobes is not clear-cut because the fissure separating the two is not as large and deep as those separating the other lobes. Below the lateral fissure is the temporal lobe, which makes up the remaining portion of the lateral surface of the hemispheres.

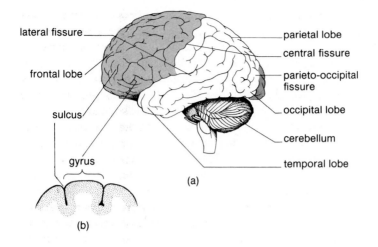

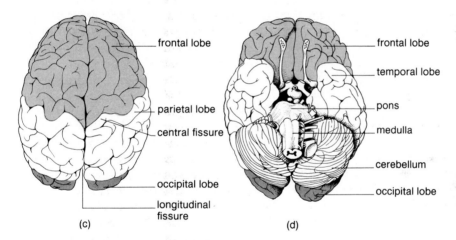

Figure 4.12   *(a) The cerebrum and its lobes; (b) cross section of the cortex; (c) the cerebrum from above; (d) the cerebrum from below.*

The Cerebral Cortex

The outermost layer of the cerebrum is called the **cerebral cortex** and is composed mostly of tightly packed cell bodies of neurons. The cortex is only about one-fourth inch thick, but of the approximately 14 billion neurons in the human nervous system, 9 billion are found in the cortex.

As animals ascend the phylogenetic scale, the surface of the cortex increases in area and be-comes folded. Humans have a very large cortex, so large in fact that it virtually covers and encloses the other structures of the brain. In order to fit into the skull, the cortex has numerous folds, or convolutions. The convolutions are called gyri (singular, gyrus), while depressions, or grooves, between the gyri are called sulci (singular, sulcus), or fissures if they are quite deep.

All sensory systems project their signals to the cortex, each to a specific region. A great deal of motor control of muscles and glands arises from other regions of the cortex. Basically, the cortex mediates three important aspects of behavior: (1) the reception and interpretation of sensory information; (2) the organization of complex motor behaviors; (3) the storage and utilization of learned experiences.

The cerebral cortex and other functional components of the nervous system are linked together by an elaborate circuitry of pathways and interconnections forming a network of communication. The nerve fibers that make up these pathways extend into and out of the cortex, or interconnect various parts of the cortex, and generally can be divided into three categories: projection-motor fibers, association fibers, and commissural fibers.

Projection-motor fibers stream into and out of the cortex, passing through a relatively narrow column near the center of the brain called the internal capsule. Ascending fibers transmit impulses from the thalamus to the various sensory projection regions of the cortex. Descending fibers carry impulses from different regions in the cortex to lower-brain centers and to the spinal cord.

Association fibers interconnect different parts of the cortex of each cerebral hemisphere. This extensive fiber network serves to connect each part of each hemisphere with every other part.

The two cerebral hemispheres are united by several commissures (sites of union of corresponding parts) of nerve fibers that cross the midline—similar to the way the two halves of a walnut are connected to the middle. The most prominent is the corpus callosum, which is located at the bottom of the longitudinal fissure and consists of a broad sheet of densely packed fibers (see figure 4.10). The human brain has about 200

million callosal fibers. These fibers connect one point in one hemisphere with a corresponding point at a symmetrically opposite position in the other hemisphere. This arrangement allows the two hemispheres to "keep in touch" with each other. Thus, sensory impulses that reach one hemisphere are almost automatically transmitted to the other; when signals are sent from one hemisphere to muscles or glands, the signals are also sent to the opposite hemisphere to keep it informed of the ongoing activity.

Experiments have demonstrated that one of the functions of the corpus callosum bundle is concerned with the transfer of learning from one hemisphere to the other. In a series of "split-brain" studies over the past twenty years, Sperry and his colleagues (Sperry 1974) have found that learning in one hemisphere is usually inaccessible to the other hemisphere if the connections between hemispheres are severed.

The Basal Ganglia

The term **basal ganglia** is nonspecific. It refers to a group of nuclei (ganglia is really a misnomer) located in the inner layers of the cerebrum, surrounding the lateral aspects of the thalamus. There is no agreement as to what cerebral ganglia constitute the basal ganglia, but the structures most frequently listed are the caudate, globus pallidus, putamen, and amygdala (see figure 4.13; also see figures 12.2 and 12.5).

The basal ganglia neurons project a rich supply of nerve fibers to the spinal cord. They also project up to the cortex areas concerned with organizing movement, and they receive descending signals from cortex nerve cells.

Collectively, the basal ganglia are part of the system for organizing complex motor activity. Damage or disease of these areas results in tremor, abnormal rhythmic movement, and loss of muscle tone.

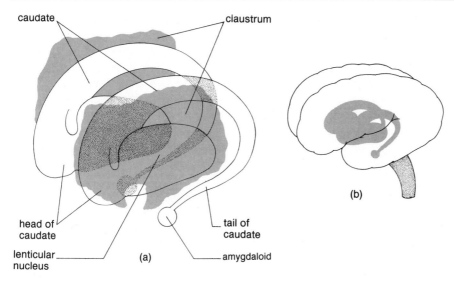

caudate

claustrum

head of
caudate

tail of
caudate

lenticular
nucleus

(a)

amygdaloid

(b)

Figure 4.13   *(a) The positions of the basal ganglia;
(b) location of these structures in the cerebrum.*

The Cerebellum

A view of the brain indicates that the cerebrum is the dominant structure, but lying posterior and inferior to the cerebrum is another structure that looks like a small cerebrum. This structure is the **cerebellum,** meaning "little brain." It lies behind the pons and medulla and is much convoluted in appearance. It comprises two hemispheres, each of which has a cortex and a vast network of internal fiber connnections. Its connections with the rest of the CNS are via three pairs of fiber tracts: inferior, middle, and superior cerebellar peduncles (see figures 4.6 and 4.12).

Although knowledge about the precise functions of the various parts of the cerebellum is incomplete, the cerebellum seems to play an important role in coordinating and monitoring complex patterns of skilled motor activity. This work is carried out through its connections with the cerebral cortex, other brain structures, and the spinal cord. Damage to the cerebellum tends to produce jerky, inaccurate, and uncoordinated movement. We shall discuss the functions of the cerebellum in more detail in chapter 12.

The Ventricles

Within the brain are four hollow openings, called **ventricles,** that are filled with cerebrospinal fluid. (This fluid will be discussed in the next section.) There are two lateral ventricles, a third ventricle, and a fourth ventricle. The lateral ventricles lie on either side of the fissure that divides the cerebrum into two hemispheres. These lateral ventricles connect with the third ventricle located behind each thalamus. At the lower level of the long thin third ventricle, a narrow opening called the cerebral aqueduct connects into the fourth ventricle. At its end, the fourth ventricle narrows and continues as the central canal of the spinal cord (figure 4.14).

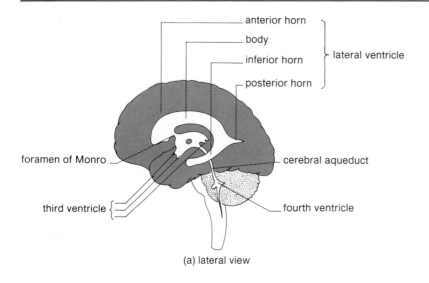

(a) lateral view

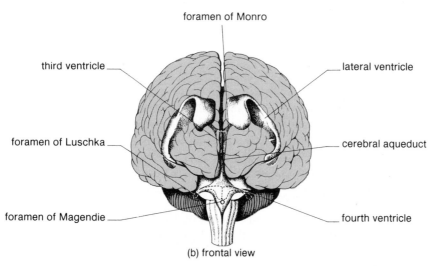

(b) frontal view

Figure 4.14   *Ventricles of the brain.*

Meninges and Cerebrospinal Fluid

The brain and spinal cord are protected by layers of nonnervous tissue called **meninges.** There is an outer layer, called the dura mater, a middle layer composed of the arachnoid membrane, and an inner layer, the pia mater, which is closest to the brain. The dura mater is a tough, fibrous membrane that lines the inner surface of the skull and vertebrae. It is basically a bone lining. The in-

nermost of the meninges is the pia mater, a soft, tender membrane that lines the brain and spinal cord. Between the dura mater and pia mater is the arachnoid membrane (figures 4.15 and 4.16).

Cerebrospinal fluid (CSF) fills the space between the arachnoid membrane and the pia mater around the entire brain and central canal of the spinal cord. The brain and spinal cord virtually float in this solution (figure 4.17).

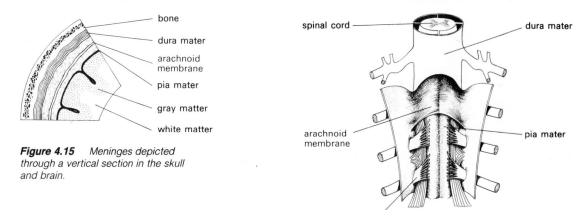

Figure 4.15 *Meninges depicted through a vertical section in the skull and brain.*

Figure 4.16 *The meninges surrounding the spinal cord.*

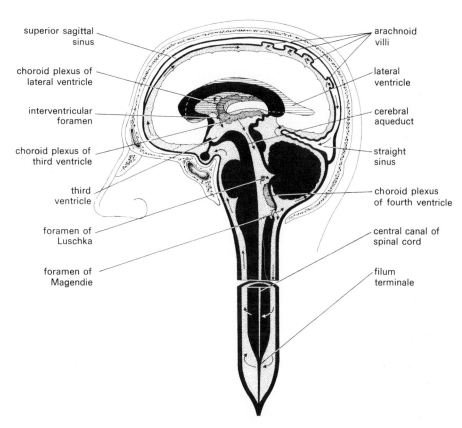

Figure 4.17 *The cerebrospinal fluid and its circulation pathways. CSF circulates within the subarachnoid space and the ventricles.*

CSF has several functions. Surrounding the brain and spinal cord, it provides a protective covering for the delicate nerve cells by acting as a cushion for blows to the head and quick movements of the head. It also helps to keep the total volume of cranial contents constant. Finally, it appears to play a role in the exchange of metabolic substances between it and nerve cells.

Summary

This chapter describes the anatomy of the nervous system. The nervous system, like all systems of the body, is made up of individual cells. The structural and functional unit of the nervous system is the neuron, which has three main parts: cell body, axon, and dendrites. Neurons are classified as afferent, efferent, or interneuron, based on their location and function. They are also classified by their structure. When grouped this way, the three types of neurons are unipolar, bipolar, and multipolar. One of the main functions of the neuron is to transmit messages in the form of nerve impulses from one part of the body to another.

The peripheral nervous system (PNS) lies outside the skull and vertebral column and is made up of all the nerve fibers that enter or leave the brainstem and spinal cord and supply the sensory receptors, muscles, and glands. This system is further divided into somatic and autonomic systems. Essentially, the PNS represents lines of communication from the PNS to the CNS.

A nerve is a collection of nerve fibers bound together by connective tissue. Nerves lie outside the CNS. There are thirty-one pairs of spinal nerves and twelve pairs of cranial nerves. Each spinal nerve supplies fibers to a specific segment of the body. A segment of the body that is supplied by a spinal nerve is called a dermatome.

The CNS is made up of the brain and spinal cord. It has two basic tasks. First, it transmits information about the environment and body to the brain. Second, it carries information from the brain to muscles and glands. The spinal cord joins the brain at the brainstem. It occupies the vertebral canal formed by the vertebrae and it extends from the brainstem to the level of the first or second vertebra. In cross section, the cord has a center portion in the shape of a butterfly and an outer portion surrounding the center section.

The brain is encased within the skull and weighs about 3.5 pounds. It can be subdivided into three parts: brainstem, cerebrum, and cerebellum. The major structures of the brainstem are the medulla, pons, midbrain, and diencephalon, with the reticular formation extending through all of these structures.

The umbrellalike dome of the brain that is divided into two hemispheres is called the cerebrum; it is further divided into regions called lobes. The cerebral cortex is the outermost layer of the cerebrum and is composed mostly of tightly packed cell bodies of neurons. A group of nuclei located in the inner layers of the cerebrum is called the basal ganglia. Basal ganglia are part of the system for organizing complex motor activity.

Lying posterior and inferior to the cerebrum is the cerebellum, or "little brain." It has two hemispheres, each of which has a cortex. The cerebellum seems to play an important role in coordinating and monitoring patterns of skilled movements.

Layers of nonnervous tissue, called meninges, cover and protect the brain and spinal cord. Cerebrospinal fluid (CSF) circulates throughout the entire brain and central canal of the spinal cord within the ventricles. CSF provides a protective covering for the CNS structures and it probably plays a role in the exchange of metabolic substances between it and nerve cells.

5

Neural Transmission

*A*ll human behavior depends upon the biochemical and physiological processes of the nervous system. This system is made up of neurons whose purpose is to receive and send messages, in the form of nerve impulses, from one part of the body to another. The overall function of the nervous system is to integrate and control all the body's activities. In order to do this, neurons receive and respond to stimulation; they also transmit signals from one neuron to another.

In chapter 4 the basic features of a neuron were described. In this chapter we consider how a neuron conducts a nerve impulse along its own axon and how a nerve impulse is propagated from one neuron to another. We also consider how nerve impulses are transmitted to muscle fibers, bringing about muscle contraction.

Conduction of Nerve Impulses

One of the unique features of a neuron is that it is designed to conduct an electric current. In order to understand how the neuron accomplishes this task, one must understand several features of electricity and nerve cells.

The functioning of a nerve cell depends upon the electric events that take place across the membrane of the cell, which in turn depend upon the presence of charged particles called **ions.** There are two types of electric charges. It is customary to refer to them as positive and negative charges. Characteristic of these charges is that positive charges repel positive charges and negative repel negative, but positive and negative charges attract each other. Thus, when positive and negative charges are separated, an electric force draws the opposite charges together. Why this is so is unknown; it is a fundamental property of matter.

Now, if oppositely charged particles are allowed to come together, work will be done—a force will be exerted over distance because Work = Force × Distance (W = FD). Therefore, when oppositely charged particles are separated, they have the potential of doing work if they are allowed to come together. The movement of electric charge is called electric current, and voltage is defined as the amount of work done by an electric charge when moving from one point in a system to another.

Resting Membrane Potential

So it is that the first requirement in producing an electric current is that positive and negative charges must be separated. This is accomplished in a neuron because the membrane is semipermeable and acts as a selective barrier to ionic movement, and it has an active transport mechanism that helps to maintain ionic imbalance. The result is that the inside of the membrane becomes electrically negative with respect to the outside. A potential is established.

To be more specific, the surface of the membrane of a neuron separates two aqueous solutions that have very different ionic concentrations. In the resting state of a neuron there is a greater concentration of sodium ions (Na^+) on the outside of the membrane than on the inside because they are actively transported outward through the membrane by a mechanism called the "sodium pump." Further, these ions are too large to pass inward through the membrane in its resting state. Inside the cell membrane is a concentration of various organic ions (A^-), mostly negatively charged proteins or amino acids. They are too large to pass out of the cell membrane. Potassium ions (K^+) are also highly concentrated on the inside of the membrane in its resting state because they are highly permeable to the cell membrane and are pulled to the inside by the negatively charged organic ions found there. Accumulation of potassium ions inside the cell due to the indiffusible organic ions creates a concentration gradient favoring the outward flow of potassium, even against the attraction of the organic ions. But there is a limit to this process, and an equilibrium is reached when the tendency of potassium to diffuse out is balanced by the electric pull of the organic ions. The outward movement of potassium ions does not completely neutralize the state of electronegativity on the inside of the membrane. As a result, the intracellular fluid is negative, about seventy millivolts (mv), with respect to the outside of the cell membrane. This difference is called the **resting membrane potential.** In resting neurons, then, the neuron is literally a battery with its negative terminal on the inside. It now has the potential for performing work—in this case conducting an electric current (figure 5.1).

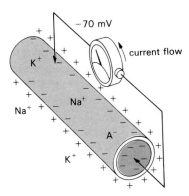

Figure 5.1 *Resting, or membrane potential. Sodium (Na+) ions are in high concentration outside the membrane, while potassium (K+) ions and organic anions (A−) are in high concentration inside the membrane. The potential across the membrane is about—70 millivolts.*

The Action Potential in the Axon

We shall now examine the steps in the propagation of a nerve impulse in the axon. The roles of the dendrites and cell body in the process is quite different and will be discussed later in this chapter.

As described above, membrane polarity is maintained by a differential balance of ions on the inside and outside of the membrane. The membrane voltage of −70 mv produces a strong pressure for inward flow of sodium ions and a strong outward flow of organic ions. However, the resting membrane is impermeable to these classes of ions.

If, however, the membrane of an axon is stimulated, there is a sudden change in membrane permeability, making the membrane highly permeable to sodium. Any stimulus that suddenly increases the permeability of the axon membrane to sodium elicits a sequence of rapid changes in the membrane. If the stimulus lowers the resting potential to a critical level (called the threshold potential, usually around −55 to −60 mv) in the axon (that is, if the internal voltage of

the axon changes from, say, −70 to −55 mv), an explosive action occurs. The increased permeability causes sodium ions to flood in through the membrane at a rapid rate. The potential difference in the membrane is not only neutralized, but is relatively reversed in less than a millisecond. The outside briefly becomes negatively charged 30 to 40 mv in relation to the inside of the membrane. This entire sequence of changes that the axon membrane goes through when it has been stimulated strongly enough to alter the membrane to a threshold potential is called an **action potential** (figure 5.2). The action potential occurs in two separate stages: **depolarization** and **repolarization.** The conduction of the action potential along an axon is actually the nerve impulse.

The nerve impulse, as seen by a spike on an oscilloscope, changes the permeability of the membrane immediately ahead of it and establishes the conditions for sodium to flow into the membrane, repeating the process in an impulse wave until the spike has reached the end of the axon. This process is not unlike the way the fuse in a firecracker burns from where the match is applied on down to the firecracker itself. Thus, when depolarization takes place at one point in an axon, it acts as a stimulus for depolarization elsewhere. Although there are apparently some exceptions, when the action potential travels down the axon, it activates all the axon collateral branches. When the action potential reaches the end of the axon, a reaction is triggered that leads to the release of a transmitter substance. We shall describe this process more fully later in the chapter.

At the peak of the depolarization wave, the membrane becomes impermeable to sodium and simultaneously highly permeable to potassium. This causes a rapid outflow of the potassium ions, thus restoring the original negative charge on the interior of the membrane. A membrane potential develops across the membrane caused entirely by

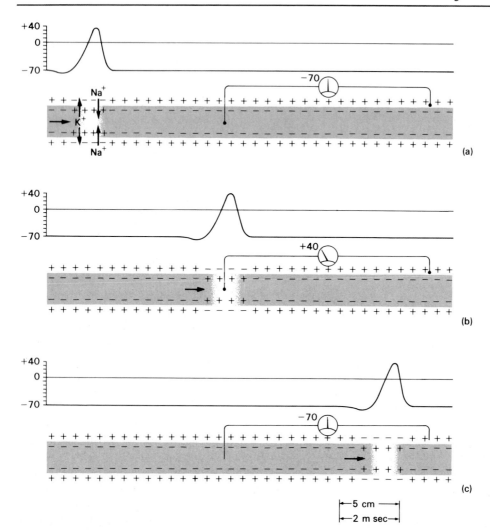

Figure 5.2   *Propagation of an action potential in the axon of an unmyelinated neuron. The arrows show the direction of transmission. In (a) sodium rushes into the axon, causing the membrane potential to be changed locally to positive. At this point, sodium is prevented from passing out of the membrane, but potassium rushes out of the axon and the normal resting potential is now restored (b) and (c). At the point of the action potential (light zone), the potential across the membrane is reversed to about +40 millivolts as measured on a galvanometer.*

the potassium ions. The rapid outflow of potassium is more than capable of returning the membrane potential back to its resting level of −70 mv as the potassium ions move to the outside and establish electronegativity inside the membrane. This is the repolarization phase of the action potential.

In order for the membrane to return to its *original* resting condition, with the large concentration of sodium ions outside the membrane, the sodium ions that diffused to the inside of the cell membrane during the action potential must be returned to the outside and potassium ions returned to the inside. The "sodium-potassium pump" is an active transport mechanism for returning sodium ions to the outside of the membrane and the potassium ions to the inside, thus restoring the original distribution of ions characteristic of the resting membrane potential. Very little is known about the details of how the sodium-potassium pump works.

Action potentials can occur in a neuron as often as several hundred times per second. Over a hundred thousand action potentials may repeatedly be produced in an axon before its ionic supplies are temporarily exhausted.

Refractory Periods

Depolarization and repolarization take place in about a millisecond (one-thousandth of a second, msec). Between the instant of depolarization and complete repolarization, the membrane experiences a period known as the refractory period, which actually consists of two brief periods (figure 5.3).

Immediately after an action potential has occurred at a point along an axon, the axon cannot produce a second action potential regardless of the intensity of the stimulus. This is called the **absolute refractory period.** In firing a rifle, another shot cannot be fired until another bullet is in the chamber and the firing pin drops again. Similarly, there is a short period following one action potential in which another one cannot be set off, no matter how strong the stimulus. In large

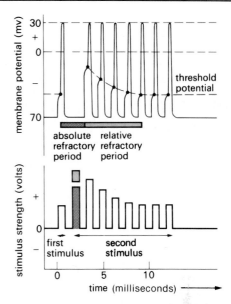

Figure 5.3   *Immediately following an action potential, the axon is absolutely refractory to all stimulus intensities and thus cannot fire another impulse. During the relative refractory period, the intensity of a second stimulus necessary to fire a second action potential must be greater than the resting threshold and decreases as the time between the first and second stimulus.*

axons this period may last 0.5 msec. This continues into a second period, the **relative refractory period,** in which nerve impulses can be generated, but the stimulus must be stronger than threshold level. To illustrate, if the threshold potential for a given axon in its resting state is −55 mv, during the relative refractory period the threshold potential may be −45 mv. Thus, a stimulus to the axon must be more intense to alter the cell's membrane potential to achieve the threshold and cause an action potential than if the axon were in a resting state. The relative refractory period lasts from 4 to 8 msec.

The All-or-None Law

If a stimulus is strong enough to depolarize the membrane at the initial segment of the axon (location where the cell body and axon join) about 15 mv, to −55 mv, the threshold is achieved; an

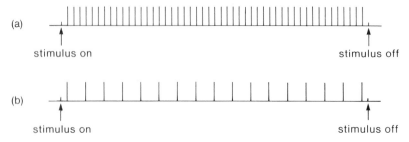

Figure 5.4   *Action potentials in a single nerve fiber in response to the application of two intensities of stimulation. Although the stimulus is suprathreshold, a stronger stimulus (a) produces a higher frequency of impulse firing than a weaker stimulus (b).*

action potential begins and travels the entire length of the axon. This is known as the **all-or-none law,** and the process might be compared to shooting a pistol. As soon as a pull on the trigger is strong enough to drop the firing pin (threshold), the pistol fires. A harder pull on the trigger will not change the velocity of the bullet because the powder charge in the bullet, and not the pull on the trigger, is responsible for the response. The action potential is self-sustaining and maintains a constant amplitude throughout its passage along the axon.

A stimulus that is not strong enough to achieve threshold is said to be subthreshold, while a stimulus stronger than threshold is said to be suprathreshold. It should be noted that the threshold is not the same for all neurons. Some neurons have lower thresholds, and thus respond to weaker stimuli than other neurons. A stimulus that is suprathreshold for some neurons will be subthreshold for others.

The cell body and dendrites differ somewhat in their response to stimulation. The effect of stimulation in these parts of the neuron is graded, resulting in a varying electrical potential being produced as a consequence of varying stimulation. This means that a weak stimulus produces a weak effect and a strong stimulus, a strong effect. This will be described more completely in a later section of this chapter.

Frequency Coding

Because of the all-or-none response in an axon, the amount of response an axon produces is essentially independent of the intensity of the stimulus exciting it. If a stronger stimulus does not produce a stronger action potential response in the axon, what effect does a stronger stimulus have on axon response? The answer is deceptively simple. A stronger stimulus fires the axon more frequently (per unit of time) than a weaker stimulus. Thus, a more intense stimulus produces a greater frequency of impulses in an axon than does a less intense one. This phenomenon occurs primarily because a more intense stimulus can excite the axon while it is still in its initial relative refractory period, while a weaker stimulus cannot. This conversion of stimulus intensity into frequency of impulses is called **frequency coding.** The essence of frequency coding is that a weak stimulus fires the axon at a very slow rate, while an intense stimulus can cause the axon to fire hundreds of times per second (figure 5.4).

Impulse Conduction in Myelinated Axons

Many axons within and outside the CNS are covered with a layer of fatty material known as myelin sheath. **Myelin** is external to the axon cell membrane, extending from just outside the cell body to near the presynaptic terminals. The myelin sheath is formed from a type of satellite cell

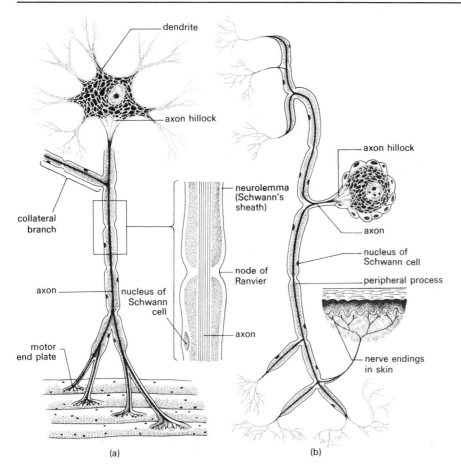

(a)   (b)

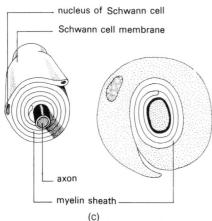

(c)

Figure 5.5 *(a) An efferent (motor) myelinated neuron; (b) an afferent (sensory) myelinated neuron; (c) lateral view of a myelinated axon.*

in the nervous system called a Schwann cell. This cell winds itself around the axon, producing a spiral envelope of many turns and forming a jelly roll-type of structure.

The myelin sheath is interrupted every millimeter or so by gaps called nodes of Ranvier. At the nodes, regular membrane depolarization can occur. But beneath the myelin-sheath membrane, depolarization cannot take place because the myelin sheath is a very effective insulator of the membrane from electrical currents (figure 5.5). At the nodes of Ranvier, nerve fibers show action potentials just like those found in unmyelinated axons. But the myelinated sections do not give action potentials when depolarized. When an action potential occurs at one node, the depolarization wave spreads passively along the internode regions into the next node where, if

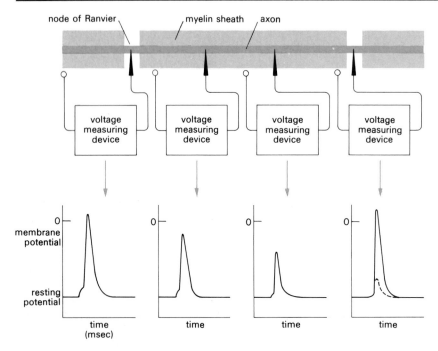

Figure 5.6   *Transmission of an action potential in a myelinated axon. Dashed line in graph on the right shows what voltage would have been at that node if the membrane at that node had not been able to produce an action potential.*

greater than threshold, it acts the same way any other depolarization would and results in a full-sized action potential. Thus, the action potential in myelinated axons moves along the fiber by passive spread in the myelinated regions and by the occurrence of action potentials at the nodes (figure 5.6).

This type of neural transmission is called saltatory conduction and it is valuable for two main reasons: It increases the velocity of conduction along the axon. It also prevents the polarization of large areas of the fiber, thus preventing leakage of large quantities of sodium to the inside of the axon, and thus conserving energy required by the sodium-potassium pump to expel the sodium.

Occasionally, people will suffer a degeneration of myelin. The loss of myelin sheaths, or of the cells that produce them, is implicated in diseases such as multiple sclerosis.

Speed and Frequency of Axon Conduction

The speed of axon conduction is a function of the cross-section diameter and the myelination or nonmyelination of the fiber. Basically, the larger the cross-section diameter, the faster the speed of conduction. Myelinated axons conduct impulses at a faster speed than unmyelinated axons. In unmyelinated fibers from 0.2 to 1.0 microns (a micron is one-thousandth of a millimeter) in diameter, the speed of the conduction is from 0.2 to 2.0 meters per second, depending on the size of the axon. The range in velocities for the normal range of myelinated axons with diameters ranging from 2 to 20 microns is 12 to 120 meters per second (table 5.1).

Axon conduction speed is related to the urgency of the information that it is called upon to transmit. Faster conducting axons are concerned

Table 5.1 *Some examples of the relationship of nerve fiber diameter and speed of conduction.*

Type	Diameter (microns)	Velocity (m/sec)	Function
A (alpha)	12–20	80–130	Motor, proprioception
A (beta)	8–12	40–80	Touch
A (gamma and delta)	1–8	5–40	Pain, temperature
B	3	3–15	Autonomic preganglionic
C	1 or less	0.5–2.0	Autonomic postganglionic

Source: Based on Langley *et al.* 1969.

with the control of movement, especially that involved in mediating rapid reflexes, such as those used for regulating posture. At the other extreme, axons carrying visceral information are small, unmyelinated, and slow conducting. In the evolutionary design of the nervous system, it seems that axon size and myelination have developed in relation to the urgency of the information carried for the survival of the organism.

The number of impulses that can be conducted per unit of time is determined by the refractory periods of the axon, which depends upon the cross-section diameter of the axon. The larger the diameter, the shorter the refractory periods. Thus, at one extreme very large axons can conduct twenty-five hundred impulses per second, and at the other extreme small axons conduct only twenty-five impulses per second.

Response of Dendrites and Cell Bodies to Stimulation

As noted in the preceding section, the distinctive feature of the axon is an active response to above-threshold depolarization—the action potential, or nerve impulse. Dendrites and the cell body *do not* propagate action potentials. Their properties of response are different from those of the axon.

Stimulation of a neuron typically occurs at the dendrites and cell body (this will be described in a later section). But the initial segment of the axon plays a decisive role in the processing of stimulation to the neuron because it is this point on the neuron that determines whether or not the stimulation produces an action potential. Stimulation to the cell must depolarize the initial segment enough to achieve threshold in order for a nerve impulse to be generated.

Stimulation on a dendrite or cell body produces a local depolarization at that point, but the effect diminishes with distance from the stimulus. Thus, if a dendrite or cell body is depolarized ten mv at the site of stimulation, half a millimeter away it might be depolarized by five mv. Response, then, is decremental. A dendrite might be stimulated at some distance from the initial segment of the axon and not affect the resting potential of the axon because the electrochemical disturbance in the dendrite decreases with the distance it travels toward the axon. Only when the total stimulation impinging on the neuron produces enough depolarizing effects at the initial segment of the axon to achieve threshold is an action potential triggered in the axon.

Synaptic Transmission

We have examined the electrical process of the nerve impulse and how it travels along the axon. Now we can consider what happens to the nerve impulse once it reaches the end of the axon.

As an axon approaches another cell, it decreases in size and forms a small terminal called a presynaptic terminal (also called by other names such as telodendria, knobs, and boutons). At the site at which the presynaptic terminal connects with another neuron, there is a submicroscopic gap between the individual cells called the **synapse.** When two neurons make contact with each other, we say that they synapse with each other.

The synapse is a specialized junction between two neurons. It is here that the electrical activity of one neuron influences the activity of the second, producing either excitation and perhaps the firing of an impulse in the second, or inhibition and an inability to fire an impulse in the second. It is at the synapse that the interactions and modifications of nerve impulses that are responsible for determining an organism's behavior take place.

A single axon may have synapses with only a few cells. Or, since axons typically give off many collateral fibers, each of which ends with a presynaptic terminal, it may have synapses with up to several thousand neurons. At the same time, any given neuron may have hundreds or thousands of synaptic contacts on its cell body or dendrites. It has been discovered in recent years that virtually all of the surface of a neuron's cell body and dendrites may have presynaptic terminals from other neurons impinging on it. Notice that presynaptic terminals typically make contact only on the cell body and dendrites of other neurons (there are exceptions) (figure 5.7a).

The number of possible interactions among neurons in a single human brain is greater than the total number of atoms making up the entire universe! Thus, it is in the patterns of interconnections that the integrative processes—such as perception, memory, motivation, and consciousness—occur.

The submicroscopic space that completely separates the presynaptic terminal and the postsynaptic neuron is called the synaptic cleft. The distance between the cell membranes at this point is about 200 angstroms. (An angstrom is one hundred-millionth of a centimeter, or five hundred

times narrower than a human hair). When a nerve impulse arrives at the presynaptic terminal, certain chemicals are released from the terminal. They diffuse across the cleft separating the two neurons and interact with the outer surface of the membrane of the postsynaptic cell. This interaction leads to a change in the permeability of the membrane to certain ions. The resulting reaction in the postsynaptic neuron may then cause it to fire a nerve impulse. This series of events at the synapse occurs within a millisecond or so. The more frequently a presynaptic terminal fires, the more **transmitter substance** that is released into the synaptic cleft and the more likely the postsynaptic neuron will be triggered into firing (figure 5.7b).

Presynaptic terminals contain a number of circular structures, or tiny sacs, called vesicles. The vesicles contain a substance that serves as a chemical transmitter of the nerve impulse. Apparently, when a nerve impulse arrives at the presynaptic terminal, synaptic vesicles merge with the axon membrane, discharging their contents into the synaptic cleft and thereby delivering a signal that excites or inhibits the postsynaptic cell. The vesicles return to the interior of the presynaptic terminal for refilling.

There are two different types of synapses, classified by their effect on the postsynaptic neuron: excitatory synapses and inhibitory synapses. Some presynaptic terminals secrete an excitatory transmitter substance and when they are active they are said to produce an **excitatory postsynaptic potential** (EPSP). Other presynaptic terminals secrete an inhibitory transmitter substance and therefore produce an **inhibitory postsynaptic potential** (IPSP) when they are firing.

Excitatory transmitter substances increase the permeability of the postsynaptic cell to sodium ions at the point of the synapse. This allows sodium ions to flow rapidly to the inside of the

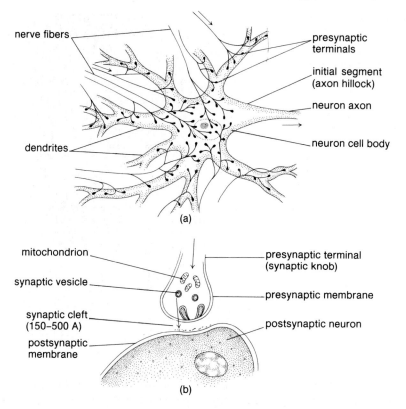

Figure 5.7 *The synapse. (a) presynaptic terminals impinging upon the cell body and dendrites of a neuron. (b) microscope view of a single synapse.*

cell, and the intense ionic movement across the postsynaptic membrane causes some depolarization to occur. As a result, the resting potential of the cell membrane decreases. This does not mean that the second neuron fires off a nerve impulse when it receives excitatory transmitter substances from a presynaptic terminal. It merely means that its resting state has been altered. This will be further explained below. Inhibitory transmitter substances have the opposite effect of excitatory transmitters. Instead of increasing the permeability of the postsynaptic neuron's membrane, inhibitory transmitters hyperpolarize the membrane, which tends to prevent the generation of a nerve impulse in the postsynaptic neuron.

Transmitter Substances

Less than thirty years ago, scientists were aware of only four neurotransmitters. Since then, two dozen or so have been discovered, and some scientists believe that there may be as many as two hundred different neurotransmitters in the nervous system.

One excitatory substance in the brain and at the neuromuscular junction (site where axon presynaptic terminals and muscle fibers connect) is acetylcholine. It is injected into the synaptic cleft to act on the postsynaptic cell membrane. Then, within 1 to 2 milliseconds, it is destroyed by a hydrolizing enzyme, cholinesterase, so that its action is rapidly terminated, and the postsynaptic membrane depolarization occurs as a discrete

event. After acetylcholine is broken down by cholinesterase, the byproducts diffuse back into the
presynaptic terminal where they are reformed
into acetylcholine and packaged in synaptic vesicles, completing the cycle. Other transmitters
undergo a similar process.

The inhibitory transmitter in the spinal cord
is glycine, while at the higher levels of the brain,
gamma amino butyric acid (GABA) is prominent. These transmitters, like the excitatory
transmitters, are packaged in synaptic vesicles
and liberated into the synaptic cleft in a quantal
manner.

Other compounds that are reasonably well
established as being neurotransmitters are sero-
tonin, epinepherine, norepinepherine, and dopa-
mine. They exist in the presynaptic terminals of
neurons located at various sites in the nervous
system.

As a general rule (there are exceptions) all
presynaptic terminals of a single neuron secrete
the same transmitter substance. For example, all
synapses made by a neuron that secrete acetylcholine will secrete the same substance despite
great differences in the location of the cells on
which it synapses. If the effect of a given neuron
is to be excitatory on one neuron and inhibitory
on another, as in reciprocal innervation of antagonistic muscles, an additional (inhibitory) neuron is interpolated between the first neuron and
the one that is to be inhibited.

Excitatory Postsynaptic Potential (EPSP)

As noted above, there are two different types of
synapses. An excitatory synapse increases the
likelihood that the postsynaptic neuron will reach
threshold and fire an impulse. An inhibitory synapse produces changes in the postsynaptic cell
that lessen the likelihood that the cell will fire an
impulse. A neuron is controlled, as it were, by two
opposing operations, excitation and inhibition.

In the dendrites and cell body, where most
synapses occur, the effect of stimulation is to alter
the resting potential maximally at the site of

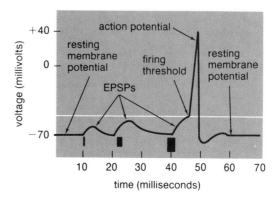

Figure 5.8   *Schematic illustrations of excitatory
postsynaptic potentials (EPSPs). The vertical bar
immediately before each EPSP represents the amount of
synaptic activity producing the EPSP. Note that as the
synaptic input increases, the EPSP increases. When
enough synaptic activity bombards the neuron, the EPSP
reaches firing threshold and an action potential is initiated,
as shown on the extreme right.*

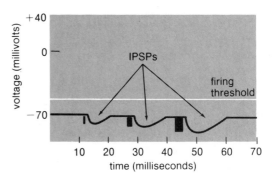

Figure 5.9   *Schematic illustrations of inhibitory
postsynaptic potentials (IPSPs). The vertical bar
immediately before each IPSP represents the amount of
inhibitory synaptic activity producing the IPSP. As the
amount of inhibitory synaptic activity increases, the IPSP
increases (that is becomes more negative). The larger the
IPSP, the less likely it is that the neuron will fire an action
potential.*

stimulation, with the effect diminishing with distance. Excitatory transmitters depolarize the
postsynaptic neuron, driving its membrane potential toward threshold. This state of the neuron
when the membrane is between −70 mv, the
resting potential, and −55 mv, the threshold, is
called the excitatory postsynaptic potential
(EPSP) (figures 5.8 and 5.9).

The size of the postsynaptic potential (EPSP) is proportional to the amount of transmitter released by the presynaptic terminal, or terminals, firing at a given time. Furthermore, since the response of dendrites and cell bodies to a stimulus is proportional to the intensity of the stimulus and response is decremental, the effects of the EPSP diminishes with distance from the synapse. Thus, when a cell body or dendrite receives a transmitter substance at one of its synapses, the EPSP created by that transmitter is reduced as it moves away from synapse. If the EPSP does not reach the threshold at the initial segment of the axon, no nerve impulse is fired.

When excitatory presynaptic terminals secrete their transmitter onto the postsynaptic neuron but fail to cause an action potential in the axon of the postsynaptic cell, the postsynaptic cell is said to be "facilitated." That is, it becomes more capable of being fired with just a little additional stimulation. A neuron in a facilitated condition needs only a little additional excitatory transmitter secreted upon it to raise the EPSP to the threshold. If this occurs, the axon will begin to fire nerve impulses and will continue to do so as long as the stimulus remains above the threshold. If the EPSP rises higher than just threshold, the axon will fire more rapidly.

Excitatory synaptic transmission can be understood as following a specific sequence:

1. Arrival of nerve impulses at the presynaptic terminals;
2. EPSP in the postsynaptic neuron;
3. Summation of separate EPSPs by the postsynaptic neuron;
4. If the summated EPSPs reach the threshold at the initial segment of the axon of the postsynaptic neuron, an action potential is propagated along the axon in an all-or-none fashion.

Inhibitory Postsynaptic Potential (IPSP)

Another important activity that occurs at the synapse is inhibition. Inhibition at the synaptic junctions plays a critical role in the CNS. If it were not for inhibition, excitation would spread throughout the neurons of the CNS, causing a continual state of convulsive activity in the organism.

Some presynaptic terminals secrete an inhibitory transmitter instead of an excitatory transmitter. Inhibitory synapses achieve their effectiveness by generating an inhibitory postsynaptic potential (IPSP) that directly counteracts the depolarizing action of the EPSP. The effect of an inhibitory presynaptic terminal is to hyperpolarize the membrane of the postsynaptic cell with which it has contact, driving the membrane potential away from the threshold, and making the generation of an action potential in the postsynaptic neuron more difficult. The resting membrane potential of -70 mv, under the influence of inhibition, may become -80 mv or more and thus more difficult to fire.

The sequence of events for inhibitory transmission is very similar to the sequence in excitatory transmission. That sequence is as follows:

1. Arrival of action potentials at the presynaptic terminals;
2. The presynaptic terminals release inhibitory transmitter into the synapse;
3. The inhibitory transmitter acts on the postsynaptic neuron to hyperpolarize the membrane.

Since the effects of EPSPs are counterbalanced by IPSPs, the state of a postsynaptic neuron at any moment, that is, how close the cell is to the threshold, is the result of all of the synaptic activity affecting the neuron at that time. Since numerous presynaptic terminals synapse upon one neuron, its firing pattern represents the integrated summation of all the excitatory and inhibitory activity impinging upon it at a given time.

Additional Features of Synaptic Transmission

The conduction of a nerve impulse along an axon is essentially electrical, while across a synapse it is essentially chemical. It is important to note that the nerve impulse that liberated neurotransmitter substance into the synapse and the nerve impulse that is propagated in the postsynaptic neuron are actually two distinct nerve impulses. Thus, there is a slight delay between the time of the arrival of an impulse at a presynaptic terminal and the beginning of a postsynaptic action potential. This is called synaptic delay and is caused mainly by the liberation and diffusion of the transmitter substance to the postsynaptic membrane.

Synaptic transmission has additional unique features. First, there is only one-way conduction at the synapse. Impulses crossing the synapse cannot be transmitted backward through the synapse into the presynaptic terminals of the first neuron. Second, the synapse is more susceptible to fatigue, anesthetics, and stimulants than the neuron itself. Hypnotics, anesthetics, and acidosis all have the effect of depressing the transmission of impulses at the synapse. It is at this point that the so-called nerve gases act by obstructing chemical transmission.

The Neuromuscular Junction

All movement, every action carried out by the body, is a result of impulse transmission from neurons to muscle fibers. Skeletomotor neurons[1] (also called alpha motoneurons) located in the cranial nerves and anterior horns of the spinal cord send out their axons to innervate muscle fibers at a site called the neuromuscular junction,

which is a special type of synapse. The **neuromuscular junction** (also called a motor end plate) is the connection between a presynaptic terminal of a nerve fiber and a skeletal muscle fiber (figure 5.9). This junction functions to transmit nerve impulses from nerve fibers to stimulate muscles for the contraction of muscles.

The events occurring at the neuromuscular junction are similar to those occurring at a synapse between two neurons. Each of the presynaptic terminals of a motoneuron passes beneath the muscle membrane. Between the terminal and the plasma membrane of the muscle there is a synapse somewhat like that found between neurons. When a nerve impulse arrives at the neuromuscular junction, the terminals secrete a transmitter substance into the cleft between the presynaptic terminal and the muscle plasma membrane.

The Motor Unit

Each motoneuron axon branches into several presynaptic terminals, and each terminal innervates a muscle fiber. A skeletomotor neuron (including its collateral branches which end as presynaptic terminals) and all the muscle fibers innervated by it are called a **motor unit** because all the muscle fibers contract as a unit when adequately stimulated by the motoneuron (figure 5.10). Motor units vary greatly in the ratio of muscle fibers to motoneuron, depending upon the precision of movement controlled by the muscle. Small muscles of the eye, which perform very delicate movements, may have a single motoneuron supplying a single muscle fiber, whereas the larger muscles that do not require delicacy in movement may have one motoneuron innervating hundreds of muscle fibers. In the postural muscles the ratio of muscle fibers to motoneurons is about 150:1. Here, each motor unit consists of a motoneuron and some 150 muscle fibers (see figure 5.11).

---

[1] There are two basic types of motoneurons in the skeletal muscles: skeletomotor neurons and gamma motoneurons. Skeletomotor neurons innervate the large skeletomuscle fibers. Gamma motoneurons innervate very small, specialized muscle fibers. This latter type of motoneuron will be described more fully in a later chapter.

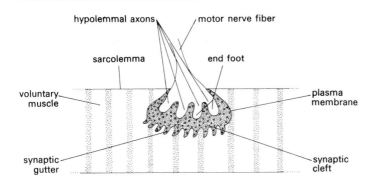

Figure 5.10 *A neuromuscular junction, or motor end plate.*

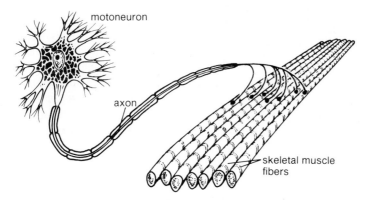

Figure 5.11 *A motor unit consists of one motoneuron and all the muscle fibers with which it communicates.*

The amount of work produced by a single motor unit is quite small and is usually insufficient to produce any observable movement of a joint spanned by the whole muscle of which it is a part. Even in small joints, such as those of the thumb, at least two or three motor units are necessary to make a visible movement.

Normally, small motor units are recruited early when movement is produced and, as the force is automatically or consciously increased, larger motor units are recruited, and at the same time all the motor units also increase their frequency of firing. Contraction of an entire muscle is the result of two factors: the time pattern of contractions (or twitches) arising from the motor units in the muscle and the number of motor units that are activated.

Neuronal Circuits

Nerve transmission normally involves many neurons. In fact, from the time a stimulus is received until behavior is exhibited in response, hundreds or even millions of neurons may be involved. The CNS is organized into many different parts, and it is through the functional synaptic linkups in various parts of the body that neurons from one part of the body, when stimulated, can influence neurons in another part of the body. These linkups of many accumulations of neurons are called neuronal circuits. The neurophysiological knowledge about principles of organization of neuronal circuits is very incomplete. Indeed, there is no complete and detailed understanding of any single neuronal circuit's overall functioning, in terms of properties of the constituent neurons and all of their interconnections.

Summary

The overall function of the nervous system is to integrate and control all the body's activities. It does this through the actions of neurons, which receive and respond to stimulation as well as transmit signals from one to another. The functioning of a nerve cell depends upon the electrical events that take place across the cell membrane. The first requirement for producing the most important electrical event, the action potential, is that ions must be separated to produce a resting membrane potential. This is accomplished in a neuron because the membrane is semipermeable and acts as a selective barrier to ionic movement. Also, it has an active transport mechanism that helps to maintain ionic imbalance.

The fundamental unit of information transmitted from one part of the nervous system to another is a single action potential, or nerve impulse. An action potential is generated when a stimulus of sufficient intensity impinges on a neuron. The information content in the nervous system depends simply on the frequency of impulses carried by a given axon and the connections the axon makes with other cells.

Axons conduct nerve impulses at various speeds. In general, the larger the diameter of the axon, the greater the velocity of impulse conduction. Also, myelinated axons conduct with greater velocity than unmyelinated axons.

Axons fire action potentials on all-or-none basis. Dendrites and the cell body do not propogate action potentials, so they have properties of response different from those of the axon.

The synapse is a specialized junction between two neurons, and it is here that the electrical activity of one neuron influences the activity of the second. It is at the synapse that the interactions and modifications of nerve impulses that are responsible for determining an organism's behavior take place.

The site where motoneurons impinge on muscle fibers is called the neuromuscular junction, which is a special type of synapse. This junction functions to transmit nerve impulses from nerve fibers to muscle fibers to produce the contraction of muscles.

Each motoneuron axon branches into many presynaptic terminals, each of which innervates a muscle fiber. A motoneuron and all the muscle fibers innervated by it are called a motor unit. Contraction of an entire muscle is the result of two factors: the number of motor units that are activated and the frequency of firing of these units.

Sensory and Motor Systems and Their Relationship to Motor Behavior

6

Sensory Integration

*O*ur sensory systems play a crucial role in motor learning and performance. Our simplest movements, the reflexes, are initiated by the senses. Complex movements are often responses to sensory input, and ongoing sensory information is important for control and regulation while movements are underway.

The energy that impinges upon one's sensory receptors provides the raw data out of which "meanings" arise. **Sensation** can be understood as the first stage in a multistage process of bringing order and organization out of the kaleidoscopic environment. For vision, this enables us to see people, trees, and houses; for audition we hear a song being sung, the cry of an infant, the ticking of a clock. This process by which sensory input is organized and interpreted is called perception.

The focus of this chapter is on the ways in which sensory information is received by receptors, transmitted to the brain, and integrated with stored information to form perceptions. This sensory integration process precipitates the responses that the individual then makes.

Sensory Functions

The only means that we have for getting information about our environment is by specialized sensory receptors. That is why our senses are sometimes referred to as our "avenues to the world." They are the source of our knowledge of the world about us, and most behavior is a response to physical stimuli that have activated sense organs. Our sensory systems, then, provide us with the raw information necessary to make effective and efficient movements. Indeed, motor learning and performance are largely dependent upon sensory data.

Although there is some difference among these sensory mechanisms, their basic functional properties are similar. The sensory receptors first respond to a stimulus, which is in the form of energy, such as mechanical, light, or sound. At the receptor, the various forms of energy are transduced (converted from one form of energy to another) into an electrical potential that gives rise to nerve impulses that are then conducted by sensory neuron (also called afferent neuron) axons into the CNS. In the CNS, the impulses are transmitted into various lower-brain centers. Then for most of the senses the impulses are projected into the cerebral cortex.

Throughout the transmission network the neural impulses are recoded because of the complex synaptic connections. Thus, coding[1] and recoding of sensory information occur at all levels of the sensory systems, from the receptors to the cortex. Sensory systems, therefore, should be considered not only as structures activated by various forms of stimuli, but as systems capable of presenting a detailed report of patterns of stimuli received from the environment.

Another important function of sensory input is the maintenance and modification of arousal, alertness, and attention levels. Most of the sensory systems project input into specific areas of the cerebral cortex. However, as these impulses ascend to the cortex, collateral axons send off impulses into a lower brain structure called the reticular formation, which is made up of numerous neurons whose cell bodies lie throughout the brainstem and thalamus. These neurons in turn send a profusion of axons throughout the brain, and when the reticular formation is activated, it enhances arousal by facilitating or even firing neurons in the cortex and other parts of the brain. So varying levels of behavioral arousal, from hyperexcitement to sleep, are partially mediated by the senses.

The sensory systems also have feedback mechanisms, through connections with the motor system, that control responses contributing to the reception of stimuli. For example, visual regions of the brain control eye movements for altering the pattern of light on the visual receptors. Thus, by specific adjustive responses the brain can select its own input. Only a portion of the total stimuli impinging on an individual at one time is perceived and attended to. Without mechanisms for selective attention, we would respond to all stimuli impinging on the body at one time, causing disorganization of behavior.

Normally, more than one sense is used at a time in our interactions with the environment. The senses typically cooperate with and supplement one another. Each sense modality (modality means kind of sensation, such as visual or auditory) contributes its own unique version of an occurrence in the physical world. These versions are

---

[1] A code is a set of nerve impulses for transmission of information, and coding refers to processes resulting in such a set of impulses. Encoding is the act of translation of a stimulus into a code. Recoding refers to coding of information already transformed into impulses into a new or altered set of impulses. Recoding occurs at each synapse.

usually blended into a coherent and unified single impression. When we are introduced to a strange object, we might use our hands to gain information about its size, weight, temperature, and texture. But we also obtain much valuable information about its properties by seeing it. The famous story of the six blind men who touched different parts of an elephant and described what they thought it was illustrates the importance of multisensory information. Sensory data gained simultaneously through the various senses are one means by which we build up an enriched storehouse of perceptions about our environment.

Sensory Limits

In the rise of species from lower to higher evolutionary levels, there is an increasing dominance of sensory organs for vision and hearing over the other sensory receptors. This greatly enriches the quality and quantity of sensory experience. In humans, the sensory systems include a greater number of differentiations than those of any other species. But even with the amazing variety of stimuli to which we can respond, our senses provide us with only an incomplete pattern of information about our environment because our receptors cannot detect certain levels of physical stimuli due to **sensory limits.** We cannot detect, and consequently obtain no information from, sound waves below twenty cycles per second or above twenty thousand cycles per second. In between is the whole spectrum of hearing, both tone and loudness. Light rays in the form of radiant energy travel much faster than sound waves and they supply light for seeing. But there are many wavelengths of radiant energy that human receptors do not detect. For example, radio and radar waves have wavelengths that are too long for us to detect, while X-rays and gamma rays have wavelengths that are too short to stimulate the human eye.

Sensory Receptors and Sensory Neurons

Sensory receptors are the windows of the nervous system. The only way that the nervous system is in contact with the environment is through these receptors. The receptors are in contact with sensory neuron fibers that transform the stimulus energy impinging on the receptor into nerve impulses. The main function of the sensory neuron is to conduct this sensory information, coded as nerve impulses, to the CNS from the periphery of the body.

Sensory neurons tend to be unipolar and bipolar neurons. The initial segment of these neurons is not located near the cell body, but instead is near the terminal of the axon. Action potentials in these neurons typically originate at the terminal and are transmitted toward the cell body and then onward over the other axon and its collaterals of the cell. Sensory neurons that respond to stimulation of the skin have their cell bodies in the dorsal root ganglion near the spinal cord. One axon ending is located in the skin, while the other axon ending of these neurons projects into the spinal cord (figure 5.5b).

The actual structure of sensory receptors varies considerably. Some receptors are the specialized terminations of sensory neurons, while others are separate cells connected to the sensory neuron endings. Moreover, some receptors have accessory structures, such as the lens of the eye or the membranes in the ear, that act to focus, alter, amplify, or localize a particular type of stimulus.

Sensory receptors are generally specialized to respond to a specific type of stimulus, such as light, temperature, mechanical stimulation, or sound. However, most of them can be stimulated by various forms of energy. For example, the visual receptors (rods and cones) normally respond to light energy, but they can be stimulated by intense mechanical stimuli such as pressure on the eyeball. The type of stimulus that a given receptor-type is most sensitive to is referred to as its adequate stimulus. An adequate stimulus, then, is that form of stimulation to which a given receptor has the lowest threshold.

Reception of Stimuli

When a stimulus impinges upon a receptor, it brings about an alteration in the resting membrane potential of that structure that is graded according to certain characteristics of the stimulus, such as intensity, and that is confined to the region of the receptor. This receptor action is analogous to the chemical excitability of dendrites, and the altered membrane potential of a receptor resulting from a stimulus is called a **generator potential.**

A generator potential is a depolarization of the sensory receptor that may, if it attains a certain magnitude, trigger the all-or-none response of the initial segment of a sensory neuron. It always precedes the firing of a nerve impulse from the sensory neuron.

If a subthreshold stimulus is applied to a receptor, a small generator potential develops. If a more intense, but still subthreshold, stimulus is applied, the generator potential will be correspondingly greater. Two subthreshold stimuli applied closely together will summate, and the generator potential they produce will be correspondingly greater. If the combined generator potential is great enough to achieve the threshold potential at the initial segment of a sensory neuron, it fires off. So the initiation of afferent impulses is a two-stage process: The physical stimulus causes a depolarization of the receptor membrane, the generator potential, and, if the stimulus is strong enough, the generator potential initiates an action potential in the sensory neuron that propagates along its axon.

Sensory Adaptation

Many sensory receptors respond strongly to the onset of a stimulus but either completely cease to respond to a steady stimulus after a brief time or respond at a much reduced rate. This phenomenon is called adaptation. **Sensory adaptation** does not result from fatigue at the receptors because if the stimulus is even momentarily stopped and then reapplied, an initial burst of impulse activity recurs and the process is repeated. This would not occur if the receptors were indeed fatigued.

Sensory adaptation is a means by which certain stimuli can be blocked and thus not burden the CNS with irrelevant or redundant information. For example, shortly after putting on one's clothes, the sensation of the clothes against the skin ceases as the touch-pressure receptors adapt to the stimuli. The functioning of the nervous system would become chaotic if all stimuli impinging upon an individual at one time had to be processed by the CNS.

Discrimination of Intensity of Stimuli

Essential to the perception of sensory data is the discrimination of intensity of stimulation. In interpreting sensory information, the nervous system estimates the intensity of sensory data. This interpretation function allows us to tell differences in, for example, degrees of cold or warmth, brightness of light, loudness of sound, and intensity of pain.

Information about stimulus intensity is relayed to the brain in two basic ways. First, an increase in stimulus intensity produces a higher frequency of nerve impulse firing in a sensory neuron. This is called temporal summation. Second, similar receptors of other sensory neurons in the immediate area of the stimulus are also activated as stimulus intensity increases because stronger stimuli typically affect a larger area. This is called spatial summation. To illustrate, touching a surface lightly with a finger brings only a small area of the skin in contact with the surface, and only receptors in that area of the skin are stimulated. But pressing the finger down firmly against the surface increases the area of the skin that is stimulated, thus stimulating additional receptors.

All sensory systems, then, have two methods of coding intensity of stimuli. Increased stimulus strength is signaled by an increased firing rate of nerve impulses in a single sensory neuron and by recruiting of receptors on other sensory neurons in the neighboring area.

Transmission of Impulses to the Brain

Impulses beginning in a sensory neuron pass along nerve transmission pathways that are specific to a certain sensory system. Sensory systems can be divided into those concerned with the distance environment and those concerned with body sensation. The most important of the distance sensory systems is vision because more sensory information reaches the brain over the visual pathways than from all other senses combined. Other distance systems are audition, taste, and olfaction. Body sensations from the skin (touch-pressure, temperature, pain), joints, muscles, and vestibular apparatus (collectively called **proprioceptors**) comprise the **somatosensory** system. Visceral sensations, such as hunger, nausea, and visceral pain, are served by sensory neurons that are part of the autonomic nervous system.

Basically, the transmission network of sensory impulses from the receptor to the brain is similar for all of the sensory systems. Three orders of neurons typically make up the sensory chain: The sensory neuron that transmits the impulse from the receptor into the CNS and on to the first synapse is considered the first-order neuron. The neuron that transmits the impulse up to the thalamus is the second-order neuron. Impulses conveyed from the thalamus to the cerebral cortex travel over the third-order neuron.

The actual transmission networks of sensory systems are more complex than described. However, the details of the various sensory pathways need not concern us here because they will be more fully described in chapters dealing with the sensory and perceptual aspects of specific sensory systems.

Thalamus Sensory Transmission

All sensory impulses (except those of olfaction) pass through the thalamus, synapsing there before ascending to the cerebral cortex. The thalamus could appropriately be called the port of entry to the cortex.

Shaped like two small footballs and lying just above the midbrain in each cerebral hemisphere, the thalamus is actually a series of nuclei (like the seeds of a pomegranate) serving sensory as well as motor functions. Some thalamic nuclei receive direct sensory input, others project motor fibers to lower centers of the brain and spinal cord, and still others have direct cortical connections.

Many of the sensory pathways interact at several levels of the nervous system, and especially at the thalamus. Thus, the thalamus is an important level for sensory integration because many of the nuclei are processing centers of sensory systems that project to the cortex. It is in this structure where the conscious awareness of crude sensation, such as touch, pressure, and pain, are realized. Finer sensory discriminations, which are elevated to the conscious sphere in the cortex, require the input of the information processed in the thalamic nuclei for their final resolution.

One set of neurons in the thalamus does not seem to be involved in relaying specific sensory or motor information, but plays an important role in the control of such processes as sleep, wakefulness, and arousal. This part of the thalamus is called the diffuse thalamic reticular formation and will be discussed in the next chapter.

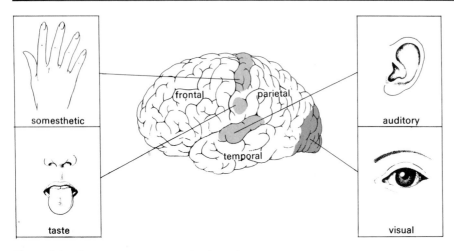

Figure 6.1   *Sensory projection areas for the various sense modalities.*

Sensory Projection Areas

We have seen that stimuli impinging upon sensory receptors are transduced into nerve impulses that are then transmitted into the CNS, where they ascend to the thalamus. This transmission represents the first two orders of the three-order transmission network for sensory impulses. Third-order neurons are located in the thalamus and project their axons into the cerebral cortex. All sensory systems project to the cortex, each to a specific region. The cortex is the last or highest region in the brain where sensory information from the senses is represented.

The regions of the cerebral cortex to which the third-order neurons of a sensory system project are quite circumscribed and are called **sensory projection areas.** The somatosensory projection area is located in the parietal lobe, just behind the central fissure. The visual projection area is found in the occipital lobes, and the auditory projection area is in the temporal lobe (figure 6.1). The fact that the various sensory systems have their own projection areas helps to explain how the brain is capable of differentiating between impulses from the somatosensory system and impulses from the visual system.

The sensory projection areas have certain functions in common. Basically, they analyze the simple aspects of sensations, such as spatial localization of impulses from the sensory neurons and generalized detection of the individual elements of the stimuli. For example, direct electrical stimulation in the somatosensory cortex evokes a generalized tingling in the skin, mild degrees of heat or cold, or numbness in a localized part of the body, such as the hand. Electrical stimulation of the visual projection area evokes flashes of light, colors, or moving lights. These, too, are localized to specific areas of the visual fields in accordance with the part of the visual projection area stimulated.

The localization of sensation in the sensory projection areas is possible because each projection area is mapped out in such a way that stimulation of different regions of the receptor surface leads to stimulation of differing groups of neurons in these projection areas. This produces a coding of locations of objects impinging upon the receptors. Moreover, the aspects of sensory experience that have the greatest functional significance to us, such as the center of gaze for vision and fingertips for touch, have relatively greater cortical representation.

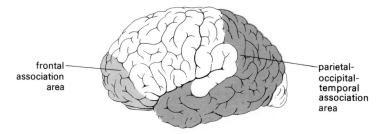

frontal
association
area

parietal-
occipital-
temporal
association
area

Figure 6.2   *Association areas of the cerebral cortex.*

The complete analysis of interpretation of complex patterns of sensory information necessitates that many other areas of the brain work in association with the various projection areas. This does not mean that the projection areas play an insignificant part in sensory interpretation. They have a critical function because when one of these areas is destroyed, the ability to utilize sensory data in that sensory system is diminished drastically. For example, the destruction of the visual projection area in humans causes total blindness. Loss of the auditory projection area results in virtually total deafness.

Interpretation of Sensations

The pathways of neural activity beyond the sensory projection areas are obscure. There are large areas in the frontal, occipital, temporal, and parietal regions of the cortex from which direct sensory information is not received. Indeed, the projection areas of the cerebral cortex occupy less than one-third of the overall cortical area in humans. Input from the projection areas is transmitted to other areas in the cortex and even to subcortical areas for further processing so that "meaning" can be made from the sensory signals.

Association Areas

The areas of the cerebral cortex that do not have direct sensory or motor functioning are collectively called the **association areas** (figure 6.2). These regions of the cortex receive input from the sensory projection areas via the association fibers. Between all of the various areas of the cortex there are billions of neurons and connecting pathways. This profusion of neurons and their fibers connects every part of the cortex with every other part. In addition to the intracortical connections, the interior of the cerebral hemispheres between the cortical layers and the subcortical structures is permeated by a complex network of connecting fiber pathways. This vast network serves as the structural basis for the organization of coherent perceptions and of sequences of nerve impulses that are translated into complex motor patterns.

By *association areas* we are referring to areas adjacent to the sensory projection area, but we are also referring to areas throughout the cerebral cortex. That is, visual information probably activates association areas in the frontal lobes as well as those in the occipital-parietal-temporal lobes. Association areas do not necessarily perform functions associated with a particular sensory system. These areas receive sensory information from many different senses. Furthermore, part of the association areas of the brain are located in subcortical regions, such as the thalamus and basal ganglia, and these regions are intimately associated with cortical association areas.

To summarize, information from the sensory systems is transmitted into the small, circumscribed areas of the cortex, and from each area the signals go to the association areas. Although

Figure 6.3   The phrenologists' view
of the brain.

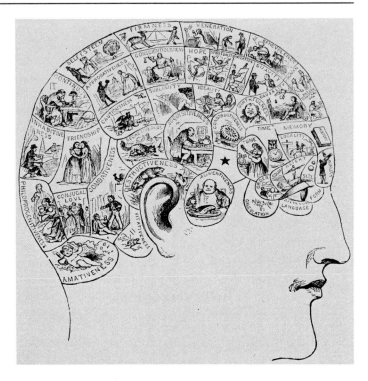

it is not possible to elucidate the specific roles performed by the association areas, it appears that a major function of these areas is to enable the individual to deal effectively with the environment by translating sensory data into information about the environment. A person then combines this information with appropriate stored information (memories), and organizes muscular movements into combinations that will produce specific and effective results.

Integrative Activity in the Brain

The integration of impulses by the various association areas into a meaningful thought or a coordinated movement is still a mystery. But theories about the integrative activity of the brain have existed for centuries. The notion that specific psychological functions can be attributed to specific parts of the brain is known as **cerebral localization,** and it has a long and controversial history. Francis Gall and his followers in the eighteenth and nineteenth centuries advanced the phrenologists' view that the brain was a compartmentalized structure, with separate areas for intelligence, music, affection, and so on. **Phrenology** has been largely discredited by research in the last eighty years (figure 6.3).

Research carried out by Karl S. Lashley, an eminent neurophysiologist, in the 1920s and 30s was instrumental in contributing to a shift in emphasis to more global ideas about brain function. He was a pioneer in the study of the relationship of brain function to memory, learning, and intelligence, especially as they relate to the question of cerebral localization. He trained laboratory animals of various species to perform some task. He then made deep incisions through different regions of the brain (figure 6.4). He reported that these structurally catastrophic conditions caused

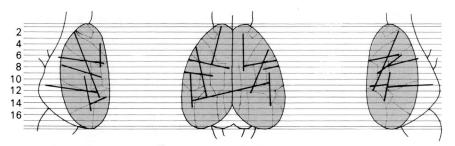

Figure 6.4 *Rats' brains were incised by Karl S. Lashley of Harvard to determine the role of cortical connections in memory. This diagram shows the brain of the rat from the top (center) and both sides. Each heavy line represents an incision made in a single rat. None of the cuts impaired maze-running performance.*

little memory loss to the animals. Lashley's work, in short, offered no support for the notion that specific areas of the brain act as repositories for memory, into which information is stored and from which it is retrieved.

Experiments of this kind on animals and clinical studies of humans led Lashley to formulate his **laws of mass action** and **equipotentiality.** The former suggests that it is the mass of cortical tissue removed, and not the site or specific locus, that determines learning ability. The latter proposes that because the effect of a cortical lesion does not depend upon the specific site, therefore one part of the cortex is equipotential in respect to another (Lashley 1950).

One interpretation about the law of equipotentiality that Lashley never intended is that the cortex is equipotential for every function. Lashley himself admitted that certain intellectual functions, especially those related to specific sensory and motor systems, could be somewhat localized to certain cerebral areas. It is well known that there are specific areas for certain functions such as visual or motor functions. Moreover, neural mechanisms that mediate learning-memory of language in humans apparently possess some anatomical specificity because there is a permanence of certain memory defects in humans, such as agnosia (inability to recognize familiar objects) and apraxia (inability to carry out

purposeful movements in the absence of paralysis), due to temporal lobe impairment. Thus, particular brain regions in humans may play a critical part in the consolidation of memories about certain specific classes of events.

Although evidence exists that certain brain areas may have specialized functions, neuroscientists are moving away from compartmentalizing brain function into highly discrete centers. This is primarily due to the discouraging results of experiments designed to localize behavioral functions (Olds et al. 1972; Thompson 1974).

Our current understanding of the integrative activity of the brain strongly suggests that perceptual-motor activity is in fact the result of the combined functioning of the entire brain. This does not mean, however, that all parts of the brain are equally important in these particular activities, or that we can attribute to any one area a global function, such as intelligence or memory. But it does mean that the specialized contributions of the various areas of the brain are called upon as needed, and the functions of each are employed in the correct order and sequence. Each part of the brain plays its own role in important activities such as the integration of sensations, the development of perceptions, and the organization of voluntary movements.

Hemispheric Dominance in the Brain

It appears that the hemispheres of the brain do not contribute equally to the integration and interpretation of sensory data. The left hemisphere seems to be predominantly involved with analytic thinking, especially language and logic. It appears that this hemisphere processes information sequentially, which is necessary for logical thought since logic depends upon sequence and order. On the other hand, the right hemisphere seems to be primarily responsible for our orientation in space, artistic and musical talents, and body awareness. It appears to process information in a simultaneous, rather than linear, fashion.

People who have had damage to the left hemisphere often suffer loss of language ability (aphasia). Such people talk with difficulty and occasionally they cannot talk at all. Conversely, damage to the right hemisphere often does not interfere with language ability at all, but often causes severe deficits in spatial awareness, musical ability, and in the recognition of other people, especially of their faces.

Neuroscientists have tended to label the left hemisphere the dominant hemisphere because of its primary role in language. Our culture emphasizes verbal and intellectual abilities, thus the bias that the left hemisphere is dominant. In the past decade the concept of **hemispheric dominance** has been replaced by one of functional cerebral asymmetry whereby each hemisphere has a special expertise for a variety of behavioral tasks (Hecaen and Albert 1978).

The left hemisphere has been shown to be the functional hemisphere controlling language and verbal tasks in over nine-tenths of all people, but extreme preponderance of the left hemisphere has nothing, as a rule, to do with handedness. Most left-handed people (70 percent) have speech in the left hemisphere. However, a few (15 percent) have a complete reversal of hemispheric function, and others (15 percent) show a mixed pattern, with both hemispheres having language function (Milner 1974).

The notion that the two hemispheres have specialized functions does not imply that one hemisphere normally functions independently of the other. Since the brain's two hemispheres are connected by commissures, there is a close functional relationship, and the activities of the two hemispheres are not exclusive. Moreover, while hemispheric specialization seems to be an established fact, it is probable that a more conservative estimate of its behavioral importance will ultimately emerge. The present fascination with this topic has produced some ludicrous notions on brain function (Corballis 1980).

Although the two hemispheres normally function in a coordinated but specialized manner, if all of the commissural connections are cut, the separated halves behave as independent brains. Each has its own independent perceptual, learning, memory, and other higher functions, and neither half is aware of what is experienced by the other (Gazzaniga 1970).

Control of Sensory Transmission by the Brain

The brain itself, by means of descending pathways, controls to some extent the incoming sensory data that ultimately reach the cortex. Nerve fibers project down from the higher regions of the brain to brainstem and spinal cord neurons to exert direct control over the progression of sensory impulses. Impulses from these cortical fibers can alter the nature of sensory information that reaches the cortex by exciting or inhibiting neurons in the ascending sensory pathways.

The significance of the descending pathways is not fully known, but since the amount and kind of incoming sensory data can be controlled or "gated" at the lower levels of transmission, the information may be inhibited or facilitated as it proceeds to the cortex. Thus, some sensory data might be prevented from reaching the cortex. It can be seen, then, that some aspects of selective attention, where we attend to one type of sensory input and exclude others, may involve this descending pathway mechanism.

Summary

Sensory systems play an important role in motor behavior. Sensory information must be received, transmitted to the brain, and integrated with stored information to form perceptions. On the basis of our perceptions we respond to our environment.

Our sensory receptors are the only means we have for obtaining information about our environment. Sensory receptors respond to stimuli by transducing the stimulus energy into nerve impulses. The impulses are then conducted into the CNS by sensory neurons. In the CNS, the impulses are transmitted to various brain centers and ultimately to the cerebral cortex.

Although our sensory receptors are capable of responding to a wide variety of stimuli, there are limits to the sensory information that will stimulate them. As a consequence, we are not aware of many stimuli in the environment.

Many receptors respond strongly to the onset of a stimulus, but either completely cease to respond to a steady stimulus after a brief time or respond at a much reduced rate. This is called sensory adaptation and it is the means by which certain stimuli can be blocked and thus not burden the CNS with irrelevant or redundant information.

Information about stimulus intensity is relayed to the brain in two ways: temporal summation and spatial summation. In the first, an increase in stimulus intensity produces a higher frequency of nerve impulse firing in a sensory neuron, while in the second additional sensory neurons are activated as stimulus intensity increases.

All sensory systems transmit nerve impulses over a three-order chain of neurons. The first-order neuron is the sensory receptor and the sensory neuron to which it is attached. Impulses over this order neuron enter the CNS and synapse on the second-order neuron at the first sensory relay. From there, impulses ascend to the thalamus over the second-order neuron. The third-order neuron carries the signal to the cortex.

Each of the sensory systems has a projection area in the cortex into which the third-order signals arrive and where the basic analysis of the sensory information is made. From the projection areas the sensory input is transmitted to other areas in the cortex and even subcortical areas for further processing so that "meaning" can be made of the input. There are large associaton areas in the cortex that are responsible for processing the incoming information and combining it with stored information. Exactly how impulses to the various association areas are integrated into meaningful thoughts or coordinated movement is still unknown.

It appears that the hemispheres of the brain do not contribute equally to the integration and interpretation of sensory data. The left hemisphere is predominantly involved with language and logical analysis, while the right hemisphere seems to be primarily responsible for spatial orientation, artistic talents, and body awareness.

7

Arousal, Attention, and Performance

Key Terms and Concepts
Arousal
Attention
Contingent negative variation
Detection
Discrimination
Evoked potential
Identification
Perception
Perceptual styles
Recognition
Reticular formation
Selective attention
Synesthesia

*T*he previous chapter focused on the reception of stimuli, coding this information in the form of nerve impulses, and transmitting it over defined pathways to the thalamus and on to the sensory projection areas of the cortex. This activity, while it is essential to processing information for eventual perception and behavior, is only part of the story. For effective utilization of sensory input the brain must be in a state of readiness to process the information. A characterization of the brain as aroused or activated is typically used to describe this state. In addition, effective utilization of input requires that only selected aspects of the thousands of stimuli impinging upon us at a moment be attended to, while other stimuli be ignored. This is the process of **selective attention. Perception,** the process of arriving at "meaning" of sensory input, is the culmination of the processes that transmit information over the specific sensory pathways, activate the brain, produce selective attention, and integrate current input with stored memories in the brain. Perception sets the stage for the selection of appropriate motor responses to deal with the situation.

The processes of transmission of sensory information, arousal, attention, and perception are functionally linked. The previous chapter described the first of these processes; the others are discussed in this chapter.

Arousal

Deep within the brain is a kind of inner brain that monitors all incoming sensory data and is richly interconnected with other brain structures, including the cortex. It is capable of controlling the general activation of the cortex as well as the excitability of localized cortical areas. The integrated activity of this system provides the energizing aspects of motivation and general behavior. It is called the arousal system.

Arousal refers to the state of wakefulness or alertness of the individual. A certain amount of arousal is necessary for optimal perceptual-motor behavior. Arousal facilitates the cortex and enhances transmission throughout the brain, making it more effective in processing incoming sensory information. It also activates various mechanisms throughout the body to prepare it for action.

Neural Mechanisms of Arousal

It was Moruzzi and Magoun (1949) who first identified the neuroanatomical basis for arousal. Their ideas have been extended in recent years by many other neuroscientists. The evidence is now rather convincing that it is the reticular formation that is of paramount importance in arousal. This structure has been found to be involved in sleeping, wakefulness, and in fine gradations of attention.

The **reticular formation** consists of a netlike mass of interwoven neurons that extends from the brainstem up to the thalamus (figure 7.1; also see figure 4.11). This network of neurons can be divided into two functional systems: the brainstem reticular formation and the diffuse thalamic reticular system. The cell bodies of the brainstem reticular formation neurons are located at the levels of the medulla, pons, midbrain, and hypothalamus and are surrounded by the pathways and nuclei of the sensory and motor systems. The diffuse thalamic reticular system represents the

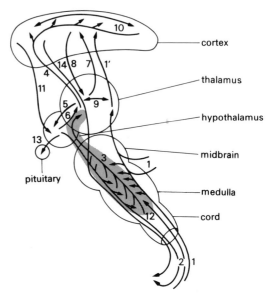

Figure 7.1   *A schematic diagram of the input and output transmission of the reticular formation. The cross-hatched area represents the location of the reticular formation.*

upper continuation of the brainstem reticular formation. The cell bodies of this system spread through various nuclei of the thalamus, and the nerve fibers project to all regions of the cortex.

All sensory systems supply a profusion of collateral axons to both the brainstem and thalamic reticular systems, thus stimulating both components of the reticular formation. It is obvious, then, that almost any kind of sensory signal can stimulate the neurons of the reticular formation. For example, signals from the muscles, skin, eyes, and ear can all cause activation of this mechanism. Furthermore, one important hormone of the body, epinephrine (adrenalin), also has a powerful effect on the reticular formation. All of these input sources have the effect of stimulating reticular neurons.

In addition to sensory systems and hormones, another source of reticular input is found in direct projections from cortical areas of the brain to the reticular formation. There is a vast network of cortical axons to both systems of the reticular formation. Indeed, cortical input to the reticular formation is more widespread than that from any sensory mode. However, the cortical axons to the reticular systems arise only in limited regions of the frontal, parietal, and temporal lobes. These connections serve an important function, though, because they provide a means by which the cortex can indirectly influence cortical cells as well as lower brain and spinal cord neurons. Cortical to reticular formation neurons are both excitatory and inhibitory in influence.

Axons of reticular formation neurons extend throughout the CNS. Reticular formation axons can be classified as either ascending or descending axons. Ascending axons project into certain thalamic nuclei and other subcortical structures, but especially into most of the cerebral cortex. One primary function of these reticular formation axons is to facilitate the higher brain center neurons. When they are transmitting impulses, they are said to have an activating or arousal effect on cortical neurons. For this reason, the ascending axon network of the reticular formation is called the ascending reticular activating system (ARAS). Like the bell on a telephone, the ARAS acts as an alerting center for the rest of the brain. Any strong stimulation, light, sound, touch, or whatever, activates the ARAS, thereby sending impulses directly throughout the cerebral cortex (figure 7.2).

Descending axons of the reticular formation project into the lower brainstem and spinal cord. Some of these axons have a facilitating effect on spinal motoneurons, while others have an inhibitory effect. Descending reticular axons transmit many of the signals that modulate the basic pattern of spinal reflexes in accordance with postural needs as well as motor commands from the cortical center of motor programming.

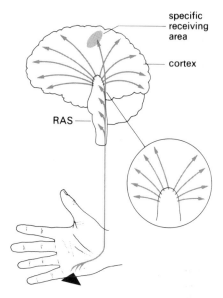

Figure 7.2 *Schematic drawing showing how a touch stimulus to the hand is relayed to a specific receiving area in the cerebral cortex. The sensory channel also sends collateral branches into the reticular activating system, which in turn projects alerting stimulation to many areas of the cerebral cortex. The inset shows the cortical projections arising from the forward end (thalamic section) of the reticular formation.*

From this description of the input and output sources of the reticular formation, we see that various feedback loops contribute to its functioning. For example, impulses from the sensory systems feed through the reticular formation, which then sends impulses to the cerebral cortex to increase its excitation; then the cortex sends back impulses to the cortex for further excitation. A second feedback loop exists whereby the reticular formation sends impulses to the spinal cord to increase muscle tone. The increased tone in turn excites receptors in muscles and joints that send impulses back to the reticular formation. The feedback loop can also be initiated at the cortical level. Cortical activity in the way of thoughts can produce collateral cortical impulses going to the reticular formation, stimulating neurons in this structure. The reticular neurons then feed back to the cortical neurons stimulating them, and they feed back further stimulation to the rectricular formation. Thus, thoughts can produce arousal and excitement.

One of the most striking differences between the brainstem reticular system and the diffuse thalamic reticular system is in the type of arousal response produced by each. When stimulated, the brainstem reticular system produces a widespread activation of the cortex that is prolonged and intense. On the other hand, stimulation of the diffuse thalamic system seems to produce a phasic, short-lived activation to specific areas of the cortex, especially the sensory projection areas. Thus, the general influence of the brainstem reticular system may provide a background of activation against which the specific activation of cortical areas by the thalamic mechanisms can occur.

The localized, phasic action of the diffuse thalamic system is blocked, or overshadowed, by intense stimulation of the brainstem system. The exact functional significance of this phenomenon has not been ascertained, but this overshadowing of the differential functions of the thalamic system by the brainstem system may be the cause of failures of discrimination that occur during periods of intense emotion.

Reticular Formation Functions

The reticular formation plays a critical role in three of the most important functions of human behavior: arousal, attention, and perception. At the most fundamental level, the brainstem reticular formation is essential to the maintenance of a wakeful state and arousal. Lesions that destroy the specific sensory pathways do not significantly alter the wakeful state, but lesions of the reticular formation greatly reduce the level of arousal,

rendering the individual unable to function normally. Without the reticular formation, the specific sensory signals can reach the cortical projection areas, but the sensory information cannot be fully processed because the background state of arousal is absent.

It also appears that the reticular formation is important in selective attention. Signals from some sensory systems appear to suppress those from others via the reticular formation by inhibiting reticular formation activity from some sensory systems. Also, the cortex may influence reticular formation activity by directing inhibition to some reticular formation neurons while simultaneously exciting others. Finally, the diffuse thalamic reticular system seems to be the source of selective activating influences on specific areas of the cortex. As such, the reticular formation may be a contributing factor in selective attention because the brief, phasic arousal mediated by this system may direct momentary attention to particular sensory inputs.

With regard to **perception,** in the absence of an activation of reticular formation, the specific sensory pathways cannot by themselves appreciably alter the activity of the brain outside the projection areas. Even though impulses from the specific sensory systems reach the projection areas, normal perception is difficult to sustain unless input from the reticular formation is discharged into the cortex at the same time. It appears that for the brain to perceive the meaning of the sensory information streaming in and to take action, if called for, the cerebral cortex must be activated not only at the projection areas, but totally. This is accomplished by the facilitating influence of reticular neurons on cortical neurons throughout the cortex, setting a background tone upon which specific projections can act and giving rise to a perception of the environment.

Arousal and Motor Behavior

We have convincing evidence that some amount of arousal is important for optimal performance, memory storage, and learning. There is also a good deal of evidence indicating that very high states of arousal cause a disorganization of behavior and a reduction in quality of performance. The notion of an optimum level of arousal for performance was first formulated over seventy years ago by two comparative psychologists and carries their names as the Yerkes-Dodson law (1908). The effects of arousal on motor learning and performance will be described in detail in chapter 20.

Selective Attention

Thousands of stimuli impinge upon us at any moment. Obviously, we cannot attend to all of them—our brains would be overloaded. To accommodate the awesome task of dealing with this deluge of stimuli bombarding our sensory systems, the nervous system has developed mechanisms to focus our reactivity to stimuli in accordance with our past experiences and current needs. This focusing process is called attention, or selective attention.

General Features of Attention

William James (1890), one of America's first psychologists, defined attention as "the taking possession by the mind, in clear and vivid form, of one out of what seems several simultaneously possible objects or trains of thought. . . . It implies withdrawal from some things in order to deal more effectively with others." Although psychologists and neuroscientists have extensively studied attention since James's time, **attention** is still viewed as a process that facilitates the selection of relevant stimuli from the environment (internal or external) to the exclusion of other stimuli and that results in a response to the relevant

stimuli. Attention is seen as an active, directional process that continues up until, and perhaps after, a response is made to a stimulus (Tecce 1972).

Both general and specific mechanisms underlie attention. The general mechanism underlies what is commonly called arousal (or activation), while the specific mechanism, **selective attention,** involves focusing on a particular part of the stimulus display. With respect to the first mechanism, effective and efficient processing of information demands an awake, alert individual. Although the brain continues to process information during sleep, its perceptual and learning capabilities are greatly diminished. Arousal was the subject of the previous section, so we shall not discuss this mechanism further here.

The specific mechanism for attention involves a choice from several simultaneous sensory inputs, a division of stimuli into relevant and irrelevant categories. The result is choice of one and neglect of the others. But how can stimuli be divided into relevant and irrelevant categories? It appears that a wide variety of factors govern the distribution of attention. First, physical properties of the stimuli that are important in attention are intensity (loud noise, bright light), size (large object), contrast (disparate stimuli), and movement (fast moving objects). Also in this class is the novelty of stimuli. Stimuli with these characteristics tend to capture the selective attention mechanisms.

Our past experiences, current motivational state, and expectations constitute a second set of attention-getting factors. Experience in an environment leads to an appreciation of which aspects of the environment convey little relevant information and which will be useful for appropriate responses or will require a response. In many cases attention is determined by the past experiences of the person or the person's memories of stimuli. Motivational states are an important determinant of what receives attention. The odor of cooking food will capture the attention of a hungry person, but will pass unnoticed to one who has recently eaten. When we have reason to expect a certain stimulus, it will more likely be attended to when it arrives.

A third attention-getting property is dependent upon current sensory input. Attention is determined to a large extent by the ongoing sensory information, especially the information that just preceded it. In other words, as one "chunk" of information is perceptually processed, feedback is sent to the selective attention mechanisms to regulate them to screen out information that the perceptual mechanisms have deemed irrelevant.

Finally, attentiveness is affected by the nature of the demands of a task. Many studies in which the task requires vigilance (monitoring an instrument, such as a radar screen, in which a significant event rarely and irregularly occurs) or repetitive performance have found a substantial decrement in performance over time periods of one-half hour or hour, with the most marked decrement occurring in the first fifteen minutes.

It must be emphasized that inattention to a stimulus does not mean that the brain has not processed that input. Stimuli to which we have not attended still register in some form in the brain, but the probability of noticing, storing, or responding to them is reduced. Much information appears to be registered in the brain without any attention on our part, and this information can enter memory and influence subsequent behavior.

When a stimulus attracts our attention, we typically perform orienting responses that enhance our reception of the stimulation. Some of these responses are voluntary and others involuntary—they are carried out automatically by the body. These bodily activities include changes in position (turning the head for visual focus or for better hearing), orienting toward the source of the stimulus, changes in sensitivity of the sensory system (widening of the pupils), modification in the ongoing electrical activity of the brain, and widespread changes in autonomic nervous system activity. These activities are accompanied by modification in arousal that produces a maximum receptivity and readiness to respond to the stimulus. These responses serve to facilitate the reception of stimuli and they prepare the individual to respond quickly in case action is called for.

Psychological Theories and Attention

In the past twenty-five years, concepts and theories that have been developed in the area of cybernetics and information theory for use with highly sophisticated electronic instruments, such as computers, have come into use by those who are attempting to discover how humans process information. Although the human information processing system, namely the nervous system, is vastly more complex than any computer, in many respects it has functions analogous to those of the computer. Concepts and theories developed for designing and perfecting computers have some relevance for explaining neural function.

Information theory in the service of electronic instrumentation suggests that the chain of processes from input to output involves the channeling of information from one point in the system to another. (For complete descriptions of these theories, see Broadbent 1958; Deutsch and Deutsch 1963; Neisser 1967; Norman 1968; and Kahneman 1973.) With any information system there is a finite capacity to channel the information in any X time period. When the channel capacity is overloaded, several mechanisms can be brought into play to accommodate the situation (omission, queuing, filtering, and approximating).

That the human nervous system possesses a limited channel capacity for attention is confirmed by everyday observation as well as by experimental research. For example, when we attend to one set of stimuli, we have to ignore others. Anyone who has tried to attend selectively to one person's speech in the presence of competing conversations has experienced the "cocktail party phenomenon." Cherry's (1953) research technique of presenting different information to the two ears and having subjects shadow one (repeat back) showed that subjects could not report about information coming to the opposite ear (except for their name or changes from verbal to music). These findings suggest that attended messages have passed through the information channels, while unattended messages are blocked before they gained access to the conscious perception mechanisms.

More recent research has led to a modification of this interpretation. The unattended messages are now believed to be attenuated rather than completely blocked, and though they are not attended to, they are subject to quite a high level of analysis. In recent years ideas that selective attention serves a single-channel central processor have been replaced with proposals that selective attention is a function of the differential allocation of information processing capacity to different channels carrying simultaneous information (see, for example, Kahneman 1973; Norman 1976; and Schneider and Shiffrin 1977).

While the nervous system possesses limited capacity for consciously perceiving input, input that is unattended is still processed and analyzed by the brain. Indeed, the allocation of attention to certain input does not seem to affect the acquisition of information about simultaneous unattended input, but it does reduce the likelihood that unattended input will interrupt the attended task (Klein 1976).

Neural Mechanisms for Attention

How the nervous system carries out the enormously complex task of ascertaining the significance of billions of stimuli each day with such amazing speed and accuracy is one of the unsolved mysteries of human behavior. Neuroscientists have just begun to unravel the mechanisms involved and at present they can only present a provisional and qualified scheme for the neural systems that subserve attention.

The general and specific components of attention have their neural substrates. The general component, which brings about the orienting response and increased arousal, is mediated by the ARAS part of the reticular formation. The specific component, which involves analysis and decisions about what stimuli are to be attended and what ignored, probably includes sensory processing at all levels, from the receptor to the cerebral cortex.

There is considerable controversy in the neurophysiological literature as to whether attention involves a peripheral filtering, or gating, of sensory inputs or CNS mechanisms. It is well known that impulses transmitted through the ascending afferent pathways do not maintain constant strength from reception at the sense organ to arrival in the cortex. We have evidence of regulation of afferent input at several levels in the nervous system. Hence, interference with afferent impulses, other than those pertaining to the subject of attention, is an obvious possibility. This afferent blockage could occur any place along the sensory pathways, from receptors to the sensory projection areas. It might also occur in the collateral paths that are found in the reticular formation.

Research on this topic suggests that the selective attention mechanisms may have two components, one that may not utilize the cerebral cortex and a second part that does involve the cortex. There is considerable anatomical and electrophysiological evidence for pathways originating in the brain and descending to the various synaptic relays of the specific afferent systems that could exercise an inhibitory control over sensory input (see review by Hernandez-Peon 1967). Research by Hernandez-Peon and his colleagues in the mid-1950s led to the position that afferent impulses can be blocked in the lower pathways, thus providing a mechanism whereby some sensory messages are selectively excluded from access to mechanisms of attention and conscious perception.

Recent research has thrown doubt on the early evidence that unattended input is blocked at the periphery or at central subcortical levels. Electrophysiological evidence suggests that all sensory input reaches the cortical projection areas over the specific afferent pathways. Further, it is at this point that input is subject to classification for attention or inattention. Much of this evidence comes from highly sophisticated techniques for recording electrical activity of the brain that have been developed in the past twenty years.

As we noted in chapter 2, the brain continuously emits brain waves. These spontaneous waves reveal little about sensory input because usually they are not correlated with specific stimuli. However, localized populations of neurons in the brain can be recorded during the processing of specific sensory stimuli. This is accomplished with either implanted or scalp electrodes and a specialized computerized summing technique that extracts the effects of this input from the EEG records. The combined neuronal activity in response to some specific stimulus generates what is called an **evoked potential** (EP) (because it is evoked by a stimulus rather than occurring spontaneously). The EP has advanced our understanding of the locations of neuronal populations that respond selectively to different stimuli. Much of what is now known about the locations of brain regions that process sensory input was first determined by mapping the brain systematically to determine where evoked potentials occur in response to particular types of stimuli. An EP in response to a bright flash of light as it might look when recorded from the visual projection area is shown in figure 7.3.

The EP reflects the pattern and intensity of neural activity elicited by external stimuli and thus constitutes one physiological basis of information processing. It is, therefore, an important index in determining how the nervous system achieves selective processing of information. Early

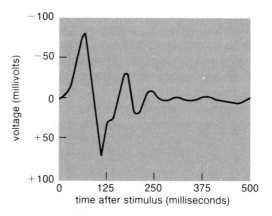

Figure 7.3   A hypothetical evoked potential to a flash of light. The stimulus was delivered at time zero on the graph. Note that the EP has several components. Shortly after the flash of light, the EP reaches a negative peak and then becomes positive, with several subsequent oscillations. Approximately the first 100 msec. represents a primary response. The following sequence of waves represents a secondary response that is associated with conscious perception.

EP experiments by Hernandez-Peon and his colleagues (1967) suggested that selective attention was achieved by a sensory filter that selectively blocked input in the sensory pathways leading to the cortex. These experiments subsequently attracted considerable criticism because of methodological problems (Moray 1969), but there is still the possibility that some form of input gating or filtering mechanism exists in the sensory pathways.

While some peripheral and subcortical filtering is still likely, recent neurophysiological interest has turned to the cortex as the site for selective attention. Experimentors have recorded EPs simultaneously from peripheral sites and from the cortex. In one condition subjects were asked to focus attention on a test stimulus (such as a click), while in another condition they were asked to perform some distracting task (such as reading a book) and ignore the test stimulus. No difference was found in amplitudes of peripheral EPs to the attended and unattended test stimulus. Moreover, there was no attenuation of the early specific components of the cortical EPs amplitude when attention was focused on the distracting task rather than the test stimulus; but the late secondary components of the EP varied with attention and were attenuated when attention was focused on the distracting task rather than the test stimulus (Picton et al. 1971; Picton and Hillyard 1974). These findings have been interpreted as follows: The early components of the EPs are localized in the cortex and are the specific response of the cortical projection area to input from the specific sensory system. The secondary components of the EPs are widely spread over the cortex and are a product of the nonspecific projections via the reticular formation as well as interaction of the cortical association areas. In this view, input arriving at the sensory projection area, and even its analysis, does not necessarily mean that it will be attended to. As noted above, it appears that attention to stimuli is contingent on the mechanisms mediating the secondary components of the EP. The secondary EP components contain the information processing that gives rise to selective attention.

One of the important factors in selective attention is expectancy. EEG and EP correlates to expectancy are well documented. When a person is asked to prepare to process an incoming stimulus—to expect to have to attend to something—the EEG shows a temporary blocking of rhythmic alpha brain waves. They are replaced by fast, desynchronized waves. There is a slow negative drift in the EEG, the **contingent negative variation** (CNV), which is terminated by an abrupt positive deflection, part of the EP, when the imperative stimulus occurs (figure 7.4). The CNV reflects a state of expectancy and it is accomplished by a variety of changes in autonomic activity, many of which are related to an enhanced arousal that precedes most difficult tasks. There is considerable evidence that the CNV, or expectancy wave, is a sign of selective attention.

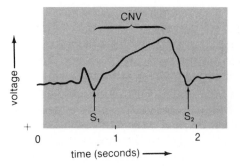

Figure 7.4 *A hypothetical contingent negative variation. The CNV is a slow negative potential that develops over the cerebral cortex in persons who "expect" some event to occur. In the illustration, presentation of a warning stimulus, S_1, signals that another stimulus, S_2, is going to occur. During the period between S_1 and S_2, a CNV develops that terminates abruptly when S_2 does occur.*

Attention and Motor Behavior

The use of the word *attention* implies that when people are attending to one thing they cannot simultaneously perform something else, but this is, of course, not true. Tasks can be performed simultaneously if one of them does not require too great attention. Walking, for example, requires very little attention (once learned), and other tasks can be performed simultaneously, such as talking or thinking.

Through early practice experiences, motor learners develop an ability to attend selectively to certain aspects of the stimulus display, and it is only after they can do this that they are able to develop an effective movement response. As motor skill learning proceeds to advanced levels, performing a task demands less and less active attention. A person highly skilled in a sport can perform quite well while devoting attention to other matters, such as tactics and surveying the playing conditions. Various types of motor tasks demand quite different intensities of attention. Less complicated tasks require less attention since, presumably, fewer control mechanisms are needed for their execution.

People are most likely to remember information to which they have given their fullest attention, and anything that assists learners to attend to the information they are to retain can improve their subsequent performance. The educator can influence skill learning and performance by instructions to the learner on how to allocate attention capacities. The important role of the teacher-coach with regard to selective attention is described by Whiting (1972):

One of the criteria on which a teacher . . . or coach might be judged successful is his ability to make his trainee's attention selective by pointing out toward what part of the display his perceptual systems need to be oriented and the information he is to try to abstract. Unsophisticated teachers may fail to appreciate that the beginner in a skill may not be utilizing the same information as the expert.

To the extent that instructors are aware of this aspect of developing skill, they may be able to find more effective means of directing the attention of learners.

Perception

The topic of perception has a vast and complex literature. Entire books are devoted to such topics as theories of perception, perceptual learning, perceptual development, and the physiology of perception. In this book only selected aspects of perception are discussed. This section is a general introduction to perception and its neural mechanisms. In subsequent chapters specific considerations in visual and kinesthetic perception will be examined.

Perception is the process of organizing and giving meaning to sensory input, and therefore serves a useful function as a guide to behavior. Indeed, our behavior depends largely on how we perceive the world about us. Perception helps to determine what responses we will make. Effective and efficient motor behavior is highly dependent upon it.

General Features of Perception

Physical energy impinging upon an individual's sensory receptors provides the raw data out of which meanings arise. Activation of the senses can be viewed as the first stage in a multi-stage process for bringing order and organization out of the kaleidoscopic environment. The process by which sensory input is organized and formulated into meaningful experiences is called **perception.**

As you sit reading this book, if you were to hear a sudden squealing sound followed by crashing noises on the street outside, you might guess that an automobile accident had occurred. But why would you surmise this? There is nothing about the sounds that enter your ear that requires such an interpretation. No. Instead, the sounds provide only the sound waves that are translated into spatiotemporal nerve impulses that are then combined with memories about streets, automobiles, and tires for an interpretation, or perception, of what has happened.

In addition to making present information meaningful, perception is a basic process in the acquisition and performance of motor skills. Stimuli possess information that is extracted by the individual as learning; that is, information is acquired through experience and becomes part of the individual's store of memories. This learning modifies the individual so that subsequent perception of the same stimuli will be different. Different people perceive the same stimulus in different ways because the stimulus activates different contents in their memory. Learning may also lead to thinking, which can be viewed as a manipulation of previous learning. The consequences of thinking modify the individual because new learning occurs, and in this way the perception of new stimuli is modified.

Percepton is influenced by many factors, including learning, and its relation to stimulating events is variable. The same stimulus can produce different perceptions and different stimuli can produce the same perception. Evidence that

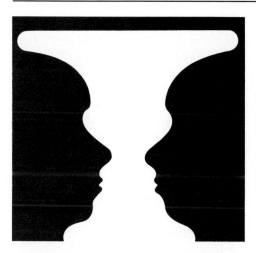

Figure 7.5 *A reversible figure. You can see either a vase or two faces in profile. The stimulus is not changing, one's perceptions are.*

perception is more than sensation is clearly demonstrated in viewing ambiguous or reversible figures. The same stimulus results in variability of perception (figure 7.5). The significance of these figures is that two different perceptions can occur with the same sensory stimulation for the same individual. There is also the related phenomenon that stimulus objects and their relationships to one another can be perceived differently by different people. There are, for example, notoriously wide variations in eyewitness accounts of accidents or crimes. Teachers are frequently appalled at the various perceptions that students have obtained from hearing exactly the same lecture.

One rather bizarre form of perceptual experience that illustrates quite dramatically the individual differences in perception is **synesthesia,** meaning perceptions that intermingle different sensory modalities. For example, some people see each of the days of the week as a color, a smell, or as being spatially arranged in a complex order. Others experience letters and numbers in terms of colors and sounds, and there are people to whom music brings vivid perceptions of color (Marks 1975).

Basic Types of Perception

The basic types of perception are detection, discrimination, recognition, and identification of incoming information for interpretation. The simplest perceptual type is detection. **Detection** requires the individual merely to indicate when a predefined stimulus event has occurred. The lowest stimulus intensity that can be detected is called the threshold. (For example, Do you see this light, sound, etc: yes or no?) There is no fixed threshold. Rather, the threshold varies with the type of stimulus, level of the subject's motivation, quality of instruction, and other variables. As perception develops, the individual comes to detect properties of stimulation not previously detected, even though thay may have been present all along. Through growth and experience with the world of stimulation, detection becomes more sensitive and precise.

Another type of perception is discrimination. **Discrimination** occurs when a stimulus event is defined as a difference between two separate stimuli on some attribute. (For example, Do these two stimuli seem different: yes or no? Are these two baseball pitches different? Are these football offensive maneuvers different?) Improvement in perceptual skill through discrimination seems to be closely related to selective use of stimulus cues. With experience, there is a greater noticing of the critical differences with less noticing of irrelevancies. For example, experienced athletes are not as easily fooled by fakes and deception used by opponents. Experienced baseball and softball players are not as easily fooled by a curve ball.

Recognition is a higher order type of perception. **Recognition** is an awareness that an object, person, or event is familiar; the individual can choose an item previously learned from among several items.

Finally, **identification** is an even higher order perception that is exhibited when an individual is given minimal information about the stimuli under consideration and can provide a personal response. (For example, What is this word? What defense is the opponent using? What kind of serve did the tennis opponent just make?) As these abilities become precise for each task, the individual improves in ability to deal with environmental stimulation.

Neural Mechanisms of Perception

Perception is not the direct end product of a relatively simple transducer process at the receptor, followed by undistorted transmission of impulses to the sensory projection areas, initiating cortical activity proportional to the physical stimulus. The various stimuli that impinge upon the individual are processed by a complex coding and recoding system at various levels of the nervous system, from the sense organs to the highest centers in the brain. The elementary processes of perception begin at the sensory receptors. Other mechanisms responsible for perceptual activities are located in the brainstem, thalamus, and in various regions of the cortex. They all play decisive roles in the recoding, analysis, and storing of information.

Perception has both neuroanatomical and electrophysiological bases. As noted above, various peripheral and subcortical structures take part in the initial stages of processing input. Each sensory modality has sensory projection areas into which input is directed as it reaches the cortex (see figure 6.1). The pattern of connections for each sensory modality culminates in columns of simple and complex arrangements of neurons that serve as "feature analyzer" units in the sensory projection areas. Moreover, neurons in the projection areas are arranged in such a way that they represent the whole receptor field to which they are connected. For example, in the somatosensory[1]

projection area the entire body surface is represented, but in proportion to receptor density. Since the lips and fingers have a high density of receptors, they are represented by large areas in the somatosensory projection area.

Within each projection area a complex organization of neurons forms the structural basis for the localization of stimulation and preliminary analysis of the simple features of input. Electrical stimulation of the visual projection area, for example, causes the individual to report seeing brief flashes of light, moving lights, colors, or simple forms, but not complex visual patterns or recognizable objects.

The feature analyzers of the sensory projection areas transmit messages on to higher level mechanisms for a synthesis of the current input with stored information. These mechanisms are made up of widely spread cortical areas, the association areas, working in conjunction with lower centers of the nervous system and the cortical projection areas. It is, then, the association areas that provide the crucial link between current stimulation and perception. The activation of these mechanisms is responsible for the richness of conscious perception. To illustrate, when projection areas are destroyed, the ability of the individual to utilize stimuli suffers greatly. Loss of the visual projection areas causes a person to become blind. However, if the visual projection areas are functional and visual association areas are damaged, blindness does not occur—but the individual's ability to interpret what is seen is diminished. Similar perceptual deficiencies occur with destruction of other association areas. Destruction of the association areas, then, tends to reduce the ability of the brain to analyze and synthesize the different characteristics of sensory input.

The electrophysiological correlates of perception are indicated by the evoked potential patterns. As previously suggested, the primary components of cortical EPs to sensory stimuli, whose

---

[1] Somatosensory refers to sensations arising from the body, that is, skin, joints, muscles, etc.

duration is 60–100 msec, seem to be largely the specific response of projection areas to impulses arriving via the specific sensory pathways. Several neuroscientists have suggested that these primary EP components represent the sum of responses of the feature analyzers of the projection area (Campbell and Maffei 1970; Regan 1972). The primary EP, as represented by the discharge of the cortical feature analyzers, does not underlie conscious perception: The EP is no different in conditions in which a stimulus is consciously perceived and conditions in which it is not. It is, instead, the secondary components of the EP, which follow the primary components and last for some 300–500 msec, that appear to underlie conscious perception. The secondary components emanate from widely spread locations in the cortex and are the product of interaction between the specific sensory pathways and diffuse projection pathways. They "reflect a process of synthesis by which percepts are constructed from the products of feature analysis and stored information," according to psychologist John Boddy (1978). A similar point is made by neuroscientists E. Roy John and his colleagues (John et al. 1973), who suggest that the secondary EP reflects "neural readout from memory . . . related to cognitive decision about the meaning for an afferent input." In both cases, what is being suggested is that the secondary EP components seem to reflect the processes underlying perception—that they are the neurophysiological correlate of perception.

Perceptual Styles

No two people perceive an object or an event in exactly the same way. Differences in sensory system proficiency and stored memories will produce differences in perception. Furthermore, such factors as set (a temporary condition of individuals that makes them ready to respond in a certain manner), motivation, and even personality influence perception. The famous linguist Benjamin Whorf (1961), after careful study of the Hopi and Shawnee languages, concluded that people in different cultures categorize the world of sensations in different ways, and these categories are reflected in the language of the culture. The categorizations, then, determine what is perceived.

There appear to be characteristic ways in which individuals structure their world and thus perceive objects and events. It is possible to speak of **perceptual styles** of people. One dimension of individual perception classifies people as analytic, flexible, or synthetic, depending on how they perceive stimuli. George (1952) differentiated among the analytic, flexible, and the synthetic. The first type of individual tends to perceive discrete parts of objects and breaks down complex stimuli, seeming to pull apart and isolate for perceptual purposes. At the other extreme, the synthesizer tends to see the whole rather than minute parts, tends to generalize and synthesize objects and events, and attempts to combine and relate stimuli. The flexible perceiver employs a changing perceptual style, depending on the nature of the stimuli and the particular situation. The perceptually flexible person has the ability to switch attitudes about a stimulus situation. Tasks that test the resistance to one form in order to visualize a second or third, or tests requiring the location of pictures of geometric design in more complex pictures, evaluate perceptual flexibility.

Another perceptual classification is visual versus haptic,[2] and refers to the prominence given to vision or somatosensory stimulation. Although both visual and somatosensory systems are used in perception of the environment, some individuals characteristically appear to give preference

---

[2] The word *haptic* comes from a Greek word meaning "to lay hold of" and applies when humans or animals feel objects with their bodies or extremities.

to visual impressions, while others are more perceptually adept for somatosensory input. For the latter, tactual, manipulative, or movement experience richly supplements perception. For example, teaching letter and word shapes by providing manual inspection of the configurations, such as running the hand and fingers over the words, has been found to be effective with some children but not for others.

People also vary in their perception of objects within a stimulus array. Those who are adept at distinguishing the figure from the background are said to be "field-independent," while those who are poor are said to be "field-dependent." Witkin and his colleagues (Witkin et al. 1954) placed subjects in a darkened room, facing a luminous frame that surrounded a moveable luminous rod. When the frame was tilted at various angles, the subject was required to bring the moveable rod to an upright position, in line with the pull of gravity. This required that the subject isolate the rod from its tilted background by relying on gravitational cues. Witkin found reliable individual differences in perception on this task. He describes subjects who are free of error on this task as field-independent, meaning that they have the ability to differentiate themselves from the environment. Tasks that require subjects to select an embedded figure in a picture that has been constructed to mask or camouflage it have also demonstrated that people vary in this perceptual ability.

Some people tend to accentuate differences between stimuli, while others tend to minimize the differences. Holzman and Klein (1954) labeled the former "sharpeners" and the latter "levelers." This classification was based on their findings from having subjects judge the size of objects projected onto a screen. Although not directly comparable, the research of Petrie (1967) has identified two related kinds of people, the "reducer" and the "augmenter," who differ from one another in the ways of processing their experience of the environment. Using tests of pain

tolerance and kinesthetic aftereffect, Petrie reported that reducers tend subjectively to decrease what is perceived, whereas the augmenter increases what is perceived.

To summarize, people perceive objects and events quite differently. Moreover, a variety of factors influence perception. But more significant, people perceive in reliably consistent ways, and various perceptual styles have emerged from the extensive research on perception.

Perception and Motor Behavior

The fact that there are individually preferred forms of perceptual style and that specific experiences affect perception suggests that environmental influences, such as sports experiences, can affect hierarchical modes of perception. Thus, the athlete may become more perceptually adaptive with experience. Some athletes, of course, may have innately superior perceptual modes for sports.

In motor performances the perceptual aspects of the tasks are sometimes quite important and other times not too important. In basketball, football, and baseball, performers must not only execute certain movement patterns, but they must perceptually organize a great deal of information about their own locations, the positions of their teammates and opponents, the score, the time period of the game, and other factors so that the most effective movements can be selected for that situation. In other sports, such as shot putting, gymnastics, and diving, a minimum of perceptual data is necessary for carrying out the task. In these latter sports, perceptual data are used in learning the task, but not so much in performance. Current information does not greatly affect the performance because the movement pattern tends to be basically preprogrammed.

Since people behave in relation to their perceptions, motor learning and performance is dependent to a great extent on the kind and amount of sensory information and the perceptions which this sensory input produces after being integrated and interpreted in the brain. Theoretically, the more proficient the sensory systems, the richer the information stored in memory about similar stimuli, the more likely the individual is to make effective and efficient movements. A substantial body of literature demonstrates that perceptual mechanisms are intricately related to the execution of skilled motor behavior.

In recent years scholars from several academic fields have begun extensive study of the relationships between perceptual abilities and motor behavior. The term *perceptual-motor behavior* is now frequently used by these scholars to indicate their focus on the interaction of input and output on motor behavior. The concept of perceptual-motor behavior, then, refers to the extracting of increasingly refined information to produce greater control over one's overt motor behavior. Research from this work has offered pertinent guidelines for improving instruction in motor skills of all types as well as advancing basic knowledge about human behavior. More detailed discussions about visual perceptions and motor behavior and kinesthetic perceptions and motor behavior will be presented in chapters 9 and 11.

Summary

Within the brain is a kind of inner brain that monitors all incoming sensory information and that is primarily responsible for controlling the general activiation of the brain. The integrated activity of this structure is called the arousal system. The neuroanatomical basis of arousal is the reticular formation. All sensory systems supply collateral axons to the reticular formation neurons. In addition to this input, the cerebral cortex and certain hormones also influence reticular activity.

The reticular formation plays a critical role in arousal, selective attention, and perception. We have convincing evidence that some amount of arousal is important for optimal performance, memory storage, and learning.

To cope with the awesome task of dealing with thousands of stimuli simultaneously impinging on an individual, the nervous system has developed mechanisms to focus attention upon a very limited number of these stimuli. This focusing process is called selective attention. Numerous factors determine which stimuli will be attended to and which will be ignored. It was once believed that irrelevant stimuli were filtered out by subcortical structures. However, more recent research with evoked potentials suggests that most sensory signals reach the sensory projection areas of the cortex, and it is between the projection and association areas where input is separated into conscious perception or irrelevant information.

Through practice experiences, learners develop the ability to attend selectively to certain aspects of the stimulus display. As they are able to do this, learners become more proficient in performing a motor skill. As motor skill learning proceeds to advanced levels, performing the task demands less and less active attention.

Perception is the process of organizing and giving meaning to sensory input. It is influenced by many factors. The basic types of perception are detection, discrimination, recognition, and identification.

There are both neuroanatomical and electrophysiological bases for perception. Feature analyzers in the cortical projection areas discern the simple features of input. The messages are transmitted to higher level mechanisms for a synthesis of the current input with stored information. The electrophysiological correlates of perception are believed to be represented in the secondary components of evoked potentials.

No two people perceive an object or an event in exactly the same way. Various perceptual styles characterize individuals.

Perceptual style and perceptual ability are highly related to motor learning and performance.

8

The Visual System

We live primarily in a visual world. Vision dominates our lives and is the richest source of information about our environment. During motor behavior humans depend heavily on the visual system. It is an important source of information about appropriate movements for performing a particular task. Indeed, the observation of others performing a task usually precedes our own efforts to perform. Vision is one of the primary monitors of movement. During the performance of a task, if it is done slowly enough, vision can be used to make movement corrections to bring the performance to the intended goal. The consequences of employing a certain movement pattern are also conveyed via the visual system—we see what we have done. Visual information is such a dominant source of information that, when vision is available, people tend to rely on it even though some other sensory system may provide more useful information for appropriate behavior.

In order to understand how light energy can be detected and processed into meaningful perceptual information for the guidance and control of motor behavior, we must first examine how light energy from stimuli enters the eye and is focused so as to cast an image on visual receptors, which, when stimulated, transmit impulses to central processing centers where visual perception occurs. In this chapter our concern will be with the basic structure and function of the visual system. In the next chapter we shall examine visual perception and motor behavior.

Figure 8.1   *The distance between a and b is wavelength. The visible spectrum is between the wavelengths of 400 and 750 nanometers.*

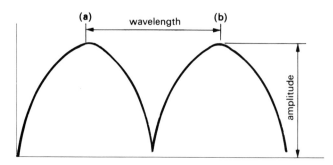

Radiant Energy

The light that stimulates the eye is a form of electromagnetic radiation. It belongs in the same class of phenomena as radio waves, X-rays, and cosmic rays. This radiation is energy traveling in the form of waves at 186 thousand miles per second, the speed of light. The distance between the peaks of two light waves is called **wavelength,** and wavelength is the only basic feature of visible light (that which the human eye can process) that differentiates it from X-rays, ultraviolet waves, and radio waves. The quantity of **radiant energy** in light that falls on a unit area of the visual receptors in a defined unit of time can be specified in terms of the height or amplitude of the wave and is subjectively interpreted as some degree of brightness (figure 8.1).

The part of the **electromagnetic spectrum,** or range, of wavelengths that humans can actually see is called the visible spectrum. It is only a tiny portion of the total electromagnetic spectrum. Wavelengths extend from radio waves, with wavelengths of many miles, to cosmic rays, with wavelengths of 0.00005 nanometers (one nanometer = one-billionth of a meter). The wavelength limits of the light visible to humans extend from about 400 nanometers, which is perceived as violet light, to about 750 nanometers, which is perceived as red light. Radiations of wavelengths beyond these limits are not visible and, therefore, are not considered to be light (figure 8.2). The various wavelengths are the basis of color discrimination, and the colors of the visible spectrum are the subjective interpretation of certain wavelengths.

Light waves are produced by objects that give off radiant energy. A light bulb, the sun, a match, are examples of stimulus objects that emit radiant energy. Some stimulus objects do not produce radiant energy, but rather reflect radiant energy. For example, a light bulb in a room produces radiant energy that strikes the wall. That radiant energy is then reflected from the wall to the individual's receptors in the eye. A desk or chair are other examples of objects that reflect, rather than emit, radiant energy. The human eye can, of course, be excited by light waves that are emitted or reflected.

Anatomy of the Eye

The visual process comprises five basic components: (1) refraction of light rays and the focusing of images on the sensory receptors of the eye; (2) transduction of light energy by photochemical activity into nerve impulses; (3) processing of neural activity at the receptors and the transmission of impulses through the optic nerve; (4) processing in the brain, culminating in perception; (5) reflexes associated with the visual system.

Several structures exist in the eyeball to carry out the eye's mechanical tasks. The light first passes through the cornea, the pupil, and lens, and then finally falls on the retina of the eye. At the retina, light is transduced into nerve impulses that are then projected into the cerebral cortex, where visual perception occurs (figure 8.3).

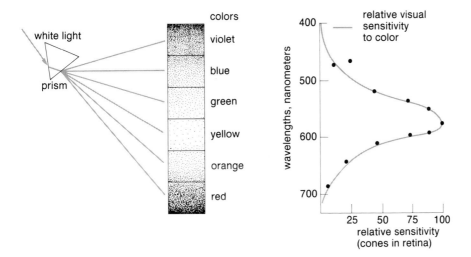

Figure 8.2 *The visible colors of light and their wavelengths. The chart shows the relative sensitivity of the human eye to color. The eye is most sensitive to orange-green-yellow. The dots on the curve indicate relative absorption of light energy by chemicals in the cones of the eye.*

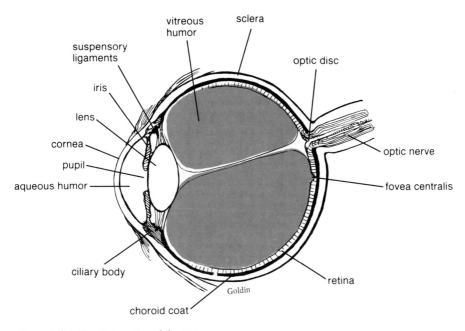

Figure 8.3 *Sagittal section of the eye.*

The Cornea and Sclera

The **cornea** is a transparent structure forming the anterior one-sixth of the fibrous tunic of the eye. It is an important part of the refractory system of the eye. The **sclera** is the white coat of the eye that makes up the posterior five-sixths of the eyeball and contains a hard, unyielding membrane that serves to maintain the form of the eyeball. At the posterior of the eyeball, the sclera is punctured by the fibers of the optic nerve.

The Pupil and Iris

The **iris** is a pigmented membrane located between the cornea and the lens. The central opening of the iris, the **pupil,** has a varying diameter. The size of the pupil, and therefore the amount of light entering the eye, is controlled by two muscles in the iris. When too much light enters the eye, one group of muscles contracts, reducing the size of the pupil. In dim light, another group of muscles contracts, enlarging the size of the pupil. This mechanism of pupillary reaction is triggered by the reflex reactions to visual input.

The Lens

The **lens** is a clear transparent tissue that lies just behind the iris and has a convex shape. It is held in place by suspensory ligaments and is innervated by the ciliary muscle. The suspensory ligaments ordinarily are tight and keep the lens flattened, but when the ciliary muscle contracts it pulls the ends of the suspensory ligaments forward, causing the lens to assume a more convex shape. By changing its shape, the lens ensures that a sharp image of the stimulus object falls on the sensory receptors at the back of the eyeball.

As the distance of objects changes, the muscles of the lens contract and relax. This adjustment in focusing power, enabling the eye to focus at various distances, is called accommodation. Without this lens accommodation mechanism, visual stimuli would be fuzzy and unclear rather than sharp and clear. This action of the ciliary muscle is, of course, a reflex response to excitation of visual receptors.

Chambers of the Eye

Structurally, the eyeball can be divided into two chambers, with the lens separating the chambers. Both chambers are filled with fluids that serve to maintain the shape of the eyeball and support structures within the eyeball. The anterior chamber is filled with aqueous humor, and the large chamber posterior to the lens is filled with vitreous humor.

The Retina

The **retina** is a complex structure consisting of the photosensitive receptors and other layers of cells that give support to the receptors or assist in the transmission of impulses. This structure lines about 180 degrees of the eyeball on its inner posterior surface. It is here that the photochemical process of transducing light energy into nerve impulses begins.

Although the retina is very thin, several distinct layers of cells can be differentiated (figure 8.4). At the back of the retina is a dark vascular coat, which lines the inner part of the eyeball, called the choroid. Associated with the choroid is a black pigment layer of cells that darkens the interior of the eye and absorbs the light rays that are not successful in activating the visual receptors. (If excess light were not absorbed, it would be reflected and would activate photoreceptors throughout the retina, thus blurring sharp resolution.) The next layer of cells in the retina contains the visual receptor cells that are sensitive to light, the rods and cones. **Rods** and **cones** make synaptic connections with **bipolar cells,** which form the middle cellular lamina in the retina. They serve mainly to relay stimulus information from the rods and cones to the final major retinal layer, where ganglion cells are located. The **ganglion cells** give rise to the nerve fibers forming the optic nerve.

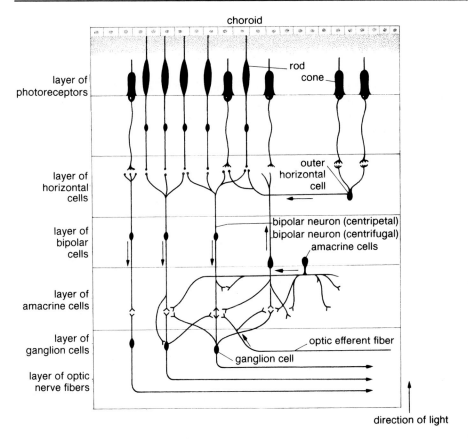

choroid

layer of photoreceptors

rod
cone

layer of horizontal cells

outer horizontal cell

layer of bipolar cells

bipolar neuron (centripetal)
bipolar neuron (centrifugal)
amacrine cells

layer of amacrine cells

layer of ganglion cells

optic efferent fiber
ganglion cell

layer of optic nerve fibers

direction of light

Figure 8.4 *The retina and cells of the eye structure.*

The Visual Receptors

The visual receptors are so named because of their shape, the rods being long and narrow while the cones are slightly shorter and have a bulblike appearance (figure 8.5). They actually constitute about 70 percent of all of the sensory receptors of the entire body, so perhaps it is understandable that we depend so much upon vision.

Although the rods and cones are the photosensitive sense organs for vision, they are located, paradoxically, in the back portion of the retina and actually face away from the front of the eye. Light must travel through all of the layers of the

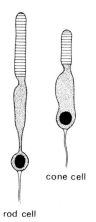

cone cell

rod cell

Figure 8.5 *Sensory receptor cells of the retina. On the left, a rod cell; on the right, a cone cell.*

Figure 8.6 *Fovea of the retina in a horizontal view.*

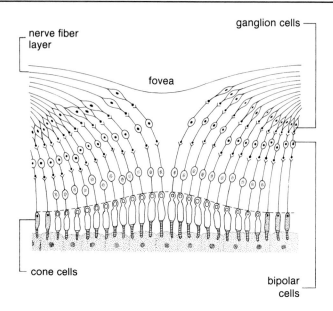

retina before reaching the visual receptors. Photosensitive chemicals peculiar to rods and cones are excited by light. When light energy impinges on these receptors, depolarization of the receptor cells occurs, which is analogous to the generator potential described in chapter 6.

In addition to being different in appearance, the rods and cones are responsible for different kinds of vision. Rods are the photoreceptors most sensitive to light and are, therefore, the primary receptors for night vision. Rod vision, at threshold, is about a thousand times more sensitive than cone vision. Rods are used primarily in black-white vision and so are called achromatic (absence of color vision). Conversely, cones function best at a high intensity of illumination and so are considered the day photoreceptors. In addition, cones contain special photochemicals that enable us to have color vision.

The Fovea

In the center of the posterior part of the retina is a small depression, about the size of the head of a pin, in which the retinal layers are exceedingly thin and which has only cone cells. This area of

the retina is called the **fovea.** The image of an object at the center of vision is formed on the fovea (figure 8.6). The fovea is the region of greatest visual acuity (clearness of vision) because the cones in this area of the retina are packed closely together and have a one-to-one connection with bipolar and ganglion cells. Moving outward from the fovea, there is a rapid decrease in the density of cones and a rapid increase in the number of rods. At the periphery of the retina there are very few cones. A pure cone fovea, such as humans have, is characteristic of all animals with a high degree of visual acuity.

Other Cells of the Retina

There are about 125 million rods and 6.5 million cones in the human retina, but only about one million ganglion cells whose nerve fibers form the optic nerve. Single ganglion cells connect, by way of bipolar cells, to numerous receptor cells. There are three major types of connections between the ganglion cells and the rods and cones. The first and most direct transmission network is found only among some cones in the fovea and consists of a single cone, a single bipolar cell, and a single ganglion cell. A second transmission network consists of several rods or several cones that feed into a common bipolar cell, which then connects with a ganglion cell. Third, there are transmission systems in which rods and cones share a common bipolar cell that connects with several ganglion cells.

In addition to these synaptic connections between the rods and cones, bipolar cells, and ganglion cells, another important type of synaptic connection in the retina allows for impulses to be carried laterally within the retina itself.

Horizontal cells are located between the receptor cell and bipolar cell levels, and amacrine cells between the bipolar and ganglion cell levels. The axons of both of these types of cells are oriented parallel to the retinal surface and at right angles to the axis of the other axons of the retina. These laterally oriented cells carry information across the retina at two distinct levels to relate activity in different parts of the visual field. They serve facilitation, inhibition, and other neuronal associations within the retina.

The Optic Disk

Axons of the ganglion neurons follow a course parallel to the surface of the retina and merge to the nasal side of the fovea, where they exit the eye at the optic disk. Here they become myelinated and form the optic nerve. Ganglion cells are comparable to the ascending tracts in the spinal cord.

The **optic disk** is also called the blind spot since this part of the retina has no rods or cones. Under normal viewing conditions we are not aware of the blind spot—our brain perceptually "fills in" the empty spot in our visual world.

Before describing the transmission network from the retina to the cerebral cortex, it is necessary to examine the process by which light energy is converted to nerve impulses. Light energy cannot be transmitted over nerve cells, so it must be transduced to nerve impulses.

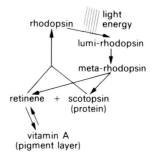

Figure 8.7 *The chemical sequence in rod function that is responsible for light sensitivity of rods.*

From *Physiology of the Human Body* 5th Ed. by Arthur C. Guyton, M.D. Copyright © 1979 by W. B. Saunders Company. Reprinted by permission of Holt, Rinehart and Winston, CBS College Publishing.

Transduction of Light Energy in the Retina

The first step in the process of vision is the conversion of light energy into electrical energy by photosensitive substances located in the outer segments of the rod and cone cells.

The Photosensitive Pigments

Within the outermost segment of the rods and cones are thin membraneous sacs that contain photosensitive pigments: **rhodopsin** in the case of rods and three kinds of iodopsin in the case of cones. These pigments are responsible for the transduction of light energy into neural activity. Exposure of the pigments to light cause some kind of change in the receptor membrane, and this change gives rise to a generator potential.

Light energy reaching the rods is absorbed by rhodopsin, which is bleached in the process. It is first converted into a substance called lumi-rhodopsin, but the energy absorbed from the light gives the lumi-rhodopsin a large amount of free energy. This is a very unstable compound and decays almost immediately into meta-rhodopsin, which is also an unstable compound; hence it splits rapidly into two additional substances, retinene and a protein opsin called scotopsin. During this decomposition of rhodopsin, the rods produce a generator potential that triggers nerve impulses in the ganglion cells. The exact manner by which the nerve impulse is generated by these chemical processes is unknown (figure 8.7).

After rhodopsin has been decomposed in the process of converting light energy into an electric current, the two remaining substances are re-synthesized into rhodopsin, with vitamin A playing an important role in the reconversion. This, then, is a continuous cycle, with rhodopsin being broken down by light energy and re-formed by chemical synthesis.

In the case of the cones of the retina, there are three types of pigment, each of which contains specific pigments that absorb light maximally at different wavelengths. The chemical process of converting light energy into a generator potential in the cones is very similar to that of the rods, except that the three types of pigment, the iodopsins, in the cones are different from the rhodopsin of the rods.

Color Vision

As noted previously, various wavelengths are the basis of color discrimination, and the colors of the visible spectrum are the subjective interpretation of certain wavelengths. One type of cone pigment is sensitive to wavelengths around 400 to 450 nanometers and gives rise to the color sensation of violet, or dark blue; a second type is sensitive to light around 500 to 550 nanometers and gives rise to the color sensation of green; a third type is sensitive to wavelengths around 750 nanometers, interpreted as red. Other colors are perceived as a result of the blending of impulses from the three cone types. All colors of the visible spectrum can be formed from these three basic colors, red, green, and blue. Color vision is said to be trichromatic because only three variables are needed to produce all color perceptions.

Optic Transmission

Until the ganglion cells of the retina are reached, information is transmitted through the receptor and bipolar cells by the electronic conduction of graded generator potentials that are able to initiate action potentials only in the ganglion cells.

These cells receive their input from bipolar cells and amacrine cells and project their output to the midbrain and thalamus.

The axons of the ganglion cells merge at the optic disk and form the optic nerve as they leave the eyeball. The optic nerves from the two eyes pass backward to unite in an X-shaped structure, the optic chiasma. Here the nerve fibers from the nasal portions of each retina, about 50 percent of all optic nerve fibers in humans, cross over to intermingle with the uncrossed fibers from the temporal portion of the opposite eye. From the optic chiasma, the optic nerves separate and project posteriorly as the **optic tracts.**

As a consequence of the crossing of fibers at the optic chiasma, the fibers from the nasal half of the retina in one eye and those from the temporal half of the other eye proceed together in the optic tracts. Therefore, objects in the left half of the visual field are represented by impulses projecting to the right hemisphere, and those in the right visual field are sent to the left hemisphere (figure 8.8). The optic nerves and tracts are the photoconductive counterparts of sensory tracts within the spinal cord and brainstem; the receptor and bipolar cells of the retina are, collectively, the first-order neuron and the ganglion cells are the second-order neuron.

Optic tract fibers make synaptic connections with several structures in the subcortical areas of the brain. About 70–80 percent of the fibers terminate in a part of the thalamus called the lateral geniculate bodies. The remainder terminate mainly in a midbrain structure, the superior colliculus.

The cells of the **lateral geniculate body** project their axons to the visual projection area located in the most posterior portion of the occipital lobes, just as the sensory fibers from the other sense modalities project to other sensory projection areas; this constitutes the third-order neuron for the visual system. Hence there are three orders of neurons from the eye to the cortex: the

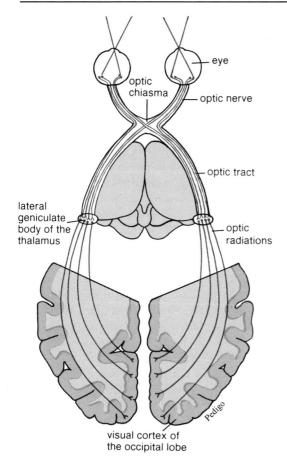

Figure 8.8 *The visual pathway includes the optic nerve, optic chiasma, optic tract, and optic radiations.*

dots, and circles, and detect the orientation of objects in space. Finally, sudden changes in light intensity, movement of an image across the retina, and detection of color are all important functions of this area of the cortex.

The feature analyzer cells of the visual projection area transmit impulses anteriorly and laterally to a whole series of association areas where a perceptual interpretation of the input is made. At present it is not possible to describe specifically how the data in the various cortical areas interact to produce visual perception, but electrophysiological and clinical studies have implicated the entire cerebral cortex in the visual process.

Destruction of certain cortical areas results in particular visual dysfunctions. Bilateral destruction of the visual projection area results in complete blindness. One with this condition would not see a table. In contrast, one who had a functional visual projection area but had no visual association areas would see the table, but would not be able to say that it was a table or explain its function. Such an individual would have difficulty determining the function or appreciating the significance of objects from cues without intact visual association areas. Neuroscientist Stuart J. Dimond (1978) articulately describes the syndrome of visual association dysfunction:

When damage occurs to the secondary visual areas, the patient's approach to the visual world undergoes characteristic changes. The capacity for acute visual perception is diminished. The patient may be unable to combine individual features into complete forms. Perception regresses to a primitive searching and the patient, far from being able to grasp the significance of a picture or a scene in one glance, finds himself forced to scan each of the elements of the picture in turn in order to reconstruct, in the absence of immediate perceptual grasp, the nature of the object or the scene from its elements. In other words, there is a defect in the more advanced capacities of perception which can be described as the insightful synthesis of vision.

retinal transmission, the optic nerve and tract to the thalamus, and the thalamus to the cortex (figure 8.8).

Throughout the visual pathways and into the visual projection area, rigid topographical organization is found. Moreover, cells in the visual projection area are hierarchically organized into simple, complex, and lower and higher order hyper-complex groups (Hubel and Wiesel 1968; 1979). They record light and darkness and analyze visual data into simple features, such as lines,

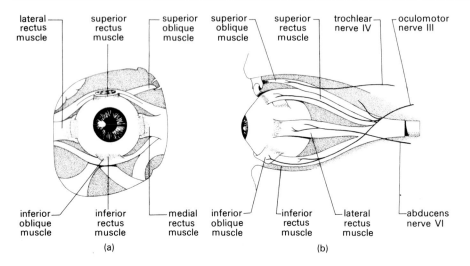

Figure 8.9   *The extraocular muscles. (a) an anterior view; (b) a lateral view.*

Transmission for Visual Reflexes

Some nerve fibers leave the optic tract and terminate in a midbrain structure, the superior colliculus. In addition to receiving nerve impulses directly from the optic tract, the **superior colliculus** receives input from the visual projection area and the auditory and somatosensory systems. This midbrain structure is believed to mediate purely reflex functions of the visual system because it projects fibers to various muscle groups of the eye. One example of a familiar type of visual reflex is blinking in response to an object that appears suddenly in the visual fields. Pupillary constriction in response to light and lens accommodation for proper focus are other types of visual reflexes.

The superior colliculus also projects fibers to the brainstem and spinal cord motor centers for control of head and eye movements. Orienting movements of the eyes and head are probably mediated by this structure. A great deal of the activity of the visual system is under the control of reflex mechanisms, and the superior colliculus is the center for mediating this activity.

Directional Properties of Vision

The eyeball is suspended in its orbit by **extraocular muscles** and a series of ligaments and connective tissue. The extraocular, or extrinsic, eye muscles control the position of each eye in its socket. They can be grouped into three pairs: the medial and lateral recti, the superior and inferior recti, and the superior and inferior obliques. Each pair of muscles forms an antagonistic pair (figure 8.9).

The extraocular muscles have the smallest ratio of motoneuron to muscle fiber of any place in the body, and the movements that these muscles control are the fastest, most accurate, and most complex in the body. Most eye movements are designed to maintain the retinal image in the same position on the retina. This is the basic task of the eye muscles.

An important function in three-dimensional space perception is also served by the extraocular muscles. These muscles control the convergence of the two eyes onto an object. As the eyes converge onto an object, each eye views the object from a slightly different direction and sees parts of the object that the other eye cannot see. When two slightly different images are focused on the sensory receptors of each eye, perception of a single three-dimensional object occurs.

Summary

Vision dominates our lives and is the richest source of information about our environment. The light that stimulates our eyes is a form of electromagnetic radiation, and the part of the electromagnetic spectrum of wavelengths that humans can see is called the visible spectrum.

The visual process includes the refraction of light rays and the focusing of images on the sensory receptors of the eyes, transduction of light energy into nerve impulses, transmission of impulses through the optic tract, and the processing of the input in the brain into perceptions. Also, a number of reflexes are associated with the visual system.

Light enters the eye through the pupil, passes through the lens and chambers of the eye, and terminates in the retina, a complex structure consisting of photosensitive receptors and other cells that assist in the transmission of visual nerve impulses. The photosensitive sense organs for vision are rods and cones. The former is used primarily in black-white vision, while cones enable us to have color vision.

After light energy is transduced into nerve impulses in the retina, the impulses are carried over the optic nerve. Optic nerves from the two eyes pass backward to unite at the optic chiasma. From the optic chiasma, optic nerves project posteriorly as the optic tracts. Optic tract fibers make synaptic connections with several subcortical structures in the brain. Visual signals enter the visual projection area located in the occipital lobes. From there, impulses disperse anteriorly and laterally to a whole series of association areas where perceptual interpretation of the input is made.

A great deal of visual system function is in the form of reflexes because visual stimuli must be tracked, focused, and the amount of light entering the eye regulated. Midbrain structures are responsible for much of the reflex activity. Extraocular eye muscles control the position of the eye in its socket.

9

Visual Perception and Motor Behavior

*V*isual perception is not just a copy of the image on the retina. Something more than reception of light stimuli by the eye must take place for the mass of sensory data to be organized into definite shapes, figures, and identifiable objects at variable distances from the body. In order to make effective use of visual information, an enormous amount of integration and interpretation must occur in the brain to give us visual perception. The image has only two dimensions, but our perceived visual world has three dimensions. We perceive our world as right side up, but the retinal image is upside down. Although there may be great disparities in the retinal image of an object when it is near or when it is far away, we usually perceive the actual size of the object quite accurately. Finally, we receive an image with millions of separate cells in the retina, but we perceive a unified object in space.

In order to perform many motor tasks effectively, it is necessary to make precise judgments about moving objects in space—catching and striking balls or the relationships of the body to other individuals or objects. These abilities depend upon visual perception. To take one example, depth perception is utilized extensively during motor performance. In all sports and games in which a ball is used, accuracy in judging the distance of the thrown or batted ball is necessary. Distance judgments about the location of teammates and opponents are essential for effective performance, and sports such as football, basketball, and baseball require simultaneous distance judgments about the location of the ball, teammates, and opponents. Because of the obvious importance of vision in the performance of motor tasks, researchers have attempted to correlate visual perceptual efficiency with motor behavior. In this chapter we review some of the salient information about visual perception and its relation to motor behavior.

Knowledge of the integrative activity of the nervous system has made remarkable progress in the past two decades, but we still have only a very sketchy understanding of the neurophysiology of the visual perceptual processes during complex motor behavior. More research on the integrative neural mechanisms will afford us a better understanding of these processes.

Focusing Properties of Vision

Objects in space must be located and brought into clear focus if the eyes are to serve as an effective sensory system. Several mechanisms are responsible for the accomplishment of these tasks. Objects are located as the eyes move around in their sockets, the extraocular muscles making this movement possible. Once an object has been located, reflex adjustments permit the object to be tracked if it moves or if the head is moved in relation to the object.

In order to form a clear image of an object on the retina, the eye must refract the light rays so that they come to focus at the retina. Light waves entering the eye are first refracted as they pass through the cornea. Then the waves are further refracted as they pass through the lens. The lens has the ability to change its convexity, which is even more important than just refraction with regard to focusing. The change in lens convexity is brought about when the image on the retina is out of focus. An out-of-focus image triggers impulses from the brain to initiate a change in the contraction of the ciliary muscle. A neuromuscular mechanism adjusts the convexity of the lens to keep a clear image on the retina.

Visual Acuity

Visual acuity is another term for sharpness of vision and refers to the degree of detail the eye can discern in a stimulus object. Good visual acuity means that a person can discriminate fine detail, while poor visual acuity implies that fine details are blurred and outlines and contours are indistinct.

An enormous number of physiological factors are involved in visual acuity. One of the most important factors seems to be the "graininess" of the retina. This refers to the density of receptors in the retina. It has been suggested that when visual receptors are relatively far apart, light falls on nonsensitive parts of the retina, thus diminishing its resolving power. This position is supported by reference to visual acuity in different parts of the visual field. It is a fact that visual acuity is highest in the center visual field, the fovea. Here the density of cones per square millimeter is greatest (about 147 thousand per square millimeter) and the one-to-one type of cone projections to ganglion cells allows separate paths for impulses due to light from different, small sources, such as two lines. Beyond the fovea the density of cones diminishes, as does visual acuity. This emphasizes the function of cones in visual acuity.

In addition to purely physiological properties of the eyes, visual acuity also depends upon various environmental factors: First, acuity becomes increasingly poor as the stimulus object moves away from the observer. Second, acuity improves with increased illumination. Third, acuity is better when the contrast between the object and its background is greater, but poorer if light of high intensity shines close to the line of vision.

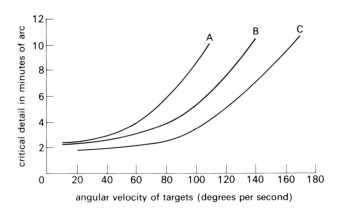

Figure 9.1 *Relation between visual acuity and the effective velocity of moving targets for each of three groups of observers A, B, and C.*

Dynamic Visual Acuity

Visual acuity for stationary objects more properly is called static visual acuity (SVA), and most acuity testing is for this type of visual efficiency. A second type of acuity, **dynamic visual acuity** (DVA), is the ability to discriminate an object where there is relative movement between the observer and the object. Dynamic visual acuity has interested researchers of motor behavior because the eyes have to be used most often to see moving objects rather than stationary ones. For example, the speed of a baseball thrown by a pitcher, and observed from first or third base, travels at an angular velocity of about 100 degrees per second.

Acuity for a moving target deteriorates markedly and progressively as the angular velocity of the target increases (figure 9.1). This finding applies substantially whether the target movement is horizontal or vertical, or whether the target is moving and the subject is stationary, or vice versa. DVA is, however, sensitive to illumination, and DVA performance can be improved through increasing target illumination.

There has been a continuing controversy about the relationship between SVA and DVA. Ludvigh and Miller (1958) found a very low correlation, but Burg (1966) reported a significant relationship between the two types of acuity. Weissman and Freeburne's study (1965) suggests a reconciliation of the previous findings.

They administered six speeds of DVA tests (20, 60, 90, 120, 150, and 180 degrees per second) and one static measure of visual acuity. DVA for the first four speeds showed a significant relationship with SVA, but the relationship disappeared at the two highest speeds. There appears to be a decreasing correlation between measures of SVA and DVA when the speed of the stimulus object in the latter tasks is increased.

Practice improves most perceptual skills and DVA is no exception. In general, the effects of practice are more pronounced when target speed is rather high, that is, 100 degrees per second, and slight or nonexistent at slower speeds. In addition, whatever learning takes place is largely confined to the early practice trials (Miller and Ludvigh 1962).

Measurement of Visual Acuity

The familiar Snellen eye chart is a frequently used method of testing SVA (figure 9.2). The chart comprises several lines of letters of different sizes, the smallest on the bottom line and the largest on the top. Subjects stand twenty feet from the chart. If they can read the letters of the size that they should be able to read at twenty feet, they are said to have 20/20 vision, which is normal. If they can read only the lines above the 20/20 line, their visual acuity is below normal. On the other hand, if they can read letters on lines below the 20/20 lines, they have superior visual acuity.

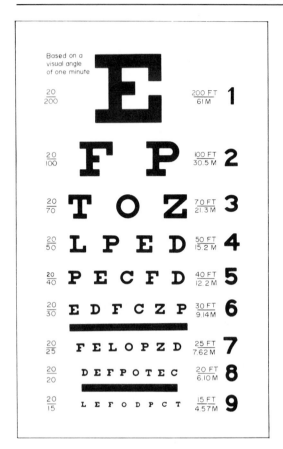

Figure 9.2 *A Snellen eye chart. With a full-sized chart, the subject with normal vision can read line 8 from a distance of 20 feet.*

More sophisticated instruments are used by optometrists and ophthalmologists, of course. The Keystone telebinocular has frequently been used by motor behavior investigators. This is a precision-built testing instrument used to assess various visual abilities in addition to SVA. It is commonly used by state automobile license bureaus.

Several techniques have been employed to test DVA. Two of the early researchers of DVA projected a C-shaped stimulus with a mirror arrangement so that the stimulus moved at various speeds across the subject's space field. The opening to the "C" was made to vary (left, right, up, down) and the subject's task was to indicate in which direction the opening appeared as it quickly traversed the field of vision (figure 9.3) (Ludvigh and Miller 1958).

Visual Acuity and Motor Behavior

Since deficiencies in visual acuity are so easily remedied with corrective lenses, very little investigation has gone into the effects of visual acuity on motor performance. Undoubtedly, poor visual acuity would adversely affect motor performance in many sports, especially the ones requiring tracking and intercepting balls and hitting a distant target, if performers did not have optical aids. Optometrists and ophthalmologists who have tested athletes for visual acuity have found that about 25 percent of them have uncorrected defective visual acuity (Garner 1977). They suggest that many coaches may unknowingly have top athletes sitting on the sidelines because of poor vision.

There is evidence that visual acuity can be temporarily modified as a result of vigorous exercise. Whiting and Sanderson (1972) utilized a simulated table-tennis task and reported improved visual acuity in a group of subjects after a playing period of ten minutes. The enhancement of visual acuity with exercise can be interpreted in terms of peripheral effects, such as increased blood supply to the retina, or attributed to a central effect of arousal. Exercise is accompanied by increased muscle tension, which is related to increased arousal levels because muscular activity stimulates the reticular formation. An increase in arousal enhances the efficiency of the sensory systems.

There is very little research on the relationship between visual acuity and motor performance, but what we have suggests that visual acuity does contribute to success in motor activities. One group of investigators studied field goal

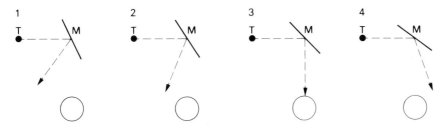

Figure 9.3 *A revolving mirror can pass the radiations from a target across the eye and thus produce the equivalent of a moving target. Each circle is the same eye but at a different instant. From left to right, the target is in effect approaching the eye. At third from left it is in full view; at the far right it has passed by. M is the revolving mirror, T is the target.*

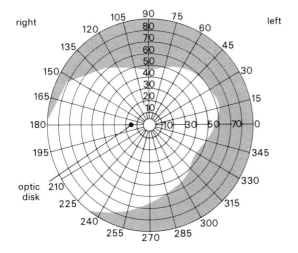

Figure 9.4 *A normal visual field of the right eye.*

From *Physiology of the Human Body* 5th Ed. by Arthur C. Guyton, M.D. Copyright © 1979 by W. B. Saunders Company. Reprinted by permission of Holt, Rinehart and Winston, CBS College Publishing.

and free throw shooting of collegiate basketball players. There was a correlation of .57 between SVA and field goal shooting and of .59 between SVA and free throw shooting (Beals et al. 1971). The group also reported a correlation of .76 between DVA and field goal shooting. A positive relationship between DVA and catching ability was reported by Sanderson and Whiting (1974), and Morris and Kreighbaum (1977) found a positive relationship between DVA and performance of female athletes in basketball and volleyball.

Field of Vision and Peripheral Vision

Field of vision refers to the entire extent of the environment that can be seen without a change in the fixation of the eye. Temporal field of vision is the area seen to the temporal, or lateral, side of the head. The more commonly used term for this latter aspect of vision is **peripheral vision.**

Measurement of Field of Vision and Peripheral Vision

A technique known as perimetry is used to measure the field of vision for each eye. The subject closes one eye and focuses the other eye on a small dot directly in front of the eye. Then a small dot (white or colored) or a light is moved inward along a meridian. Subjects indicate when they can see the dot or light and when they cannot. This is repeated for each meridian, and a chart is made showing the areas in which the subjects report seeing the dot or light and the areas in which they cannot (figure 9.4).

The perimeter, of course, can also be used for simple tests of peripheral vision, but psychologists, physical educators, and driver-education instructors have typically used instruments simpler than the field-of-vision perimetry tests.

Normal peripheral vision is about 170 degrees for the two eyes, while vertical vision is approximately 47 degrees above the midline and 65 degrees below the midline. Normally, peripheral vision fields are wider for white than for any other color. Blue is next, then red, and the smallest fields are measured for green. Detection of movement is more sensitive in the peripheral parts of the visual field than in the central portions. Since many animal species show this same characteristic, it has been suggested that it serves as a defensive mechanism to alert the individual to danger.

There is evidence that peripheral vision can be adversely affected by tasks in progress. Several investigators have reported that the detectability of a peripheral stimulus is reduced as the complexity or confusability of a central task being executed increases (Weltman and Egstrom 1966; Liebowitz and Appelle 1969).

Effects of Practice and Exercise on Peripheral Vision

Several rather old studies first indicated that peripheral visual acuity could be improved with systematic training (Holson and Henderson 1941; Low 1946). In his tests of peripheral acuity, Low found that peripheral acuity could be significantly improved with a twenty-five hour training program, and subsequent research has substantiated Low's findings (Johnson 1952). Although there is no direct evidence to explain the improvement in peripheral vision with practice, one might speculate that practice results in improvement in employing selective attention to stimuli in the periphery.

Research reported from the Soviet Union a generation ago (Graybiel et al. 1955) indicated that when peripheral vision was measured before and immediately after motor performances, there was a postexercise increase in peripheral vision. There was no mention of how long the improved visual efficiency persisted.

Peripheral Vision and Motor Behavior

Reaction time to a stimulus in the periphery has been studied by several investigators. Studies of reaction time in the peripheral field of vision require that the subject recognize an object accurately and indicate this recognition by some overt action. Slater-Hammel (1955) reported that reaction time increased (became slower) as the distance between the visual signal and the line of direct vision increased.

Looking directly at a target has obvious focusing advantages, but what are the effects of trying to hit a target when using peripheral vision? Sills and Troutman (1966) attempted to answer this question by having subjects shoot baskets using peripheral vision. They reported that as the number of degrees of peripheral sighting increased, accuracy in shooting decreased. The old coaching axiom "Keep your eye on the target" seems well founded.

The importance of peripheral vision to good performance in sports like basketball, football, and soccer is rather obvious. But apparently peripheral vision is important in sports in which this form of visual perception does not seem so obvious. In a study conducted in the Soviet Union, peripheral vision was excluded or the total vision was blocked on highly skilled javelin and discus throwers. It was reported that their performances were poorer under such conditions. The movements of javelin throwers with peripheral vision excluded became clumsy, and the distances of the throws were much shorter. Performances of discus throwers were very poor when their peripheral vision was blocked (Graybiel et al. 1955). Experimental study of the relationship of peripheral vision to performance of sport, dance, and industrial skills is very limited.

That athletes possess superior abilities over nonathletes has been reported for numerous perceptual abilities including peripheral vision. Ridini (1968) investigated the relationship between

Table 9.1   Horizontal, vertical, high vertical, and low vertical means for four groups.

Variable	Horizontal	Vertical	High vertical	Low vertical
Male athletes	186.55	119.90	50.11	69.79
Female athletes	182.83	126.93	57.31	69.62
Male nonathletes	167.32	108.36	47.36	61.00
Female nonathletes	169.32	114.76	52.04	62.72
Athletes	185.23	122.38	52.64	69.72
Nonathletes	168.32	111.56	49.70	61.86
Males	180.38	116.19	49.21	66.97
Females	176.57	121.29	54.87	66.42

Source: Based on Williams and Thirer 1975.

visual abilities and selected sports skills of junior high school boys. He employed three tests of peripheral vision, as well as other tests, and found that the athletic group was significantly better than the nonathletic group. Williams and Thirer (1975) investigated the differences between college athletes and nonathletes on vertical and horizontal vision. Both the vertical and horizontal fields of vision were superior for athletes as compared to nonathletes (table 9.1).

There is another way in which vision outside the center of focus may affect motor performance. Lee (1978) has noted that one of the functions of vision is to provide information about the positions of our limbs and body, even if we are not aware of such input. According to this view, spatial location of the limbs and body from peripheral vision is important for skillful motor control. Empirical support for this notion has been provided by Smyth and Marriott (1982) who demonstrated that visual information about the position of the hand is important for catching. Catching was much less accurate if the hand could not be seen.

Visual Perception of Depth

Our visual world is normally three-dimensional. This characteristic provides an aspect of vision that is at once richly aesthetic and critically functional. You need only to cover one eye to re-alize how different the world looks without three-dimensional sight. The ability of the visual system perceptually to organize depth is one of the wonders of nature. The retina does not have a structural means for achieving three-dimensional perception. Optically, the retina functions as a two-dimensional surface, but the visual world is perceived as three dimensional, not flat like a photograph. We are able to take the flat image from one eye, combine it with another flat image from the other eye, and construct a perception with the quality of depth.

Binocular Vision

Binocular vision, the coordinated employment of the two eyes in order to produce a single mental impression, provides the basis for depth perception. This ability to judge the distance of objects from the eye is one of the most critical functions of the eye. In spite of the impressive advances made in the study of visual perception over the past twenty years, there is still only fragmentary understanding of how three-dimensional space perception is achieved.

The cues on which depth perception is known to depend have provided considerable insight into depth perception. Recent research has begun to disclose the neurophysiological basis of these cues. Traditionally, the sources of cues for **depth perception** have been organized into two classifications: monocular cues and binocular cues.

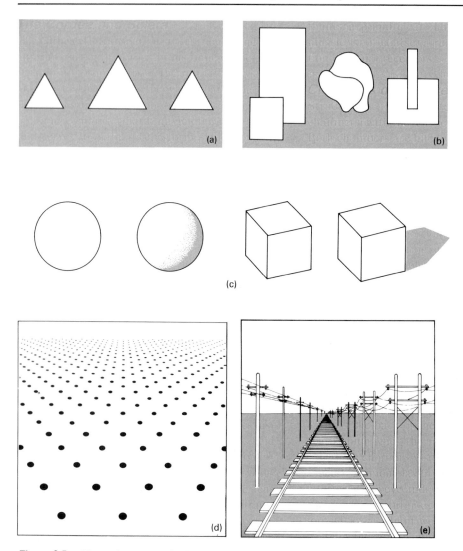

Figure 9.5 *Monocular cues to depth. (a) size of objects; (b) partial overlap; (c) shading; (d) texture; (e) linear perspective.*

Monocular Cues to Depth

Monocular cues are those available to a single eye, and binocular cues are those derived from the simultaneous activity of both eyes. Normally, both types of cues are used by the individual. Some of the more important monocular cues are proximal size, brightness, partial overlap, shading, texture, linear perspective, and movement parallax (figure 9.5).

When an object moves away from an individual, the image the object casts on the retina decreases in size. This proximal size of an object serves as a cue to its distance from the observer. Also, when the size of an object is known, the size of the image cast on the retina serves as a depth cue. Normally, the brighter the object, the closer it appears to be. As with size, this relation exists only when the object is identifiable. Partial overlap refers to two objects at a variable distance from the observer, and the view of one object is partially blocked by the other. Obviously the nearer object is the one blocking the view of the farther object. Shading provides an important cue to depth because shadows cast by objects can be used for depth perception. The distribution of light and shadow on two-dimensional pictures gives the appearance of depth.

All of the cues above apply to a single object or two overlapping objects without taking into account the other parts of the visual field. But surfaces and objects within the visual field have a powerful influence on depth perception. One powerful cue that is normally within the visual field but not the focal point is the texture of objects. Any regular marking or visible texture on surfaces within the visual field becomes gradually denser to the eye as the distance of the surface moves away from the observer. There is said to be a texture gradient that involves compression of the elements composing the surface of an object as it moves away. The grain and irregularities in near space are clear and large in the nearer parts and diminish proportionally with distance. The units into which the surface is divided become smaller with distance.

Linear perspective refers to the tendency of parallel objects to converge as they become more distant. A familiar example of this is railroad tracks when viewed from between the two tracks.

Parallax refers to the geometric fact that the direction of a stationary object from an observer changes if the observer changes locations, and that the direction of the object changes less for a distant than for a near object. In movement parallax, objects that are close to a moving observer seem to move faster because they appear to move farther than distant objects in the same time period. For example, when one is riding in a car, the fence posts beside the highway seem to be moving much faster than the fence posts in the distance. This phenomenon also causes the nearer

object to seem to be moving faster when two objects are moving in the same direction and at the same speed.

The entire visual system participates in depth perception. The lens of the eye focuses light rays coming from an object onto the retina. This *accommodation* for objects at various distances is accomplished by the contraction of the ciliary muscles. When focusing on a distant object, the lens is in its normal flattened state with little contraction of the ciliary muscles. But when focusing on a nearby object, the lens must be made more convex, which is accomplished by ciliary muscle contraction. Proprioceptive sensations from these muscles are believed to provide cues to the distance of objects. Since there are only slight changes in the amount of accommodation beyond a few feet from the observer, monocular accommodation cues to distance are effective only for short distances.

Hubel and Wiesel (1962) established that at the visual cortex there are classes of directionally specific neurons, that is, neurons that discharge when a stimulus moves across the visual field in one direction but fire at a reduced rate, or stop firing, when the stimulus moves in the opposite direction. The existence of such cortical neurons supports the notion that different features in a retinal image are processed separately by visual analyzer neurons that are sensitive to one type of stimulus and comparatively insensitive to other types.

In recent research, Regan and his colleagues, (Beverley and Regan 1973; Cynader and Regan 1978; Regan and Beverley 1978) have discovered cortical mechanisms for the processing of monocular and binocular cues to motion in depth. With respect to proximal size, these investigators and others (Zeki 1974) have found that as the size of a retinal image changes (as an object moves toward or away from an observer), directionally selective motion filters are activated that in turn activate a neural mechanism sensitive to changing size. Thus, underlying perception of motion in depth are cortical neurons that respond preferentially to the monocularly available cue of changing image size.

Binocular Cues to Depth

The functioning of two eyes rather than just one adds several significant sources of information about depth. The first binocular cue is binocular disparity, the second binocular parallax.

Binocular disparity refers to the fact that each eye provides a slightly different angle of view of our visual world. The image of an object on each retina is slightly different. The bilateral projection of nerve fibers to each hemisphere in the visual projection area and the presence of an interhemispheric link through the corpus callosum produce a binocular disparity between the two hemispheres. The impression that we receive from binocular disparity is that objects in space have roundness or depth.

Similar to binocular disparity is a phenomenon known as binocular parallax, which provides another cue for depth perception. Images of objects closer than the point of focus are seen as crossed, while those beyond the focus point are seen as uncrossed. If the eyes are focused on a near object, a far object is seen on the right by the right eye and on the left by the left eye. However, if the focus is moved to the far object, the near object is seen on the left by the right eye and on the right by the left eye (figure 9.6). These crossed and uncrossed images are normally suppressed and we are not conscious of them. One can become aware of this, though, by holding up an index finger about one foot from the eyes. Then, by placing the other index finger between the eye and the first index finger and shifting the focus back and forth between the two fingers, one gets an idea of this phenomenon.

As noted in the previous section, the entire visual apparatus is involved in depth perception, and binocular vision brings into play mechanisms

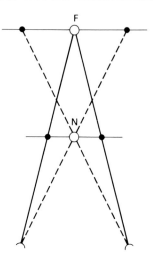

Figure 9.6   *Binocular parallax. When the eyes are focused on N, F is seen on the right by the right eye and on the left by the left eye. When focus is changed to F, N is seen on the left by the right eye and on the right by the left eye.*

that supplement those employed in monocular vision. Accommodation by the lens of the eye operates in binocular vision essentially the same way it functions in monocular vision. As with monocular vision, accommodation is one of the least effective of the binocular cues. The convergence of the two eyes that is necessary to bring the focused image of an object onto the retina is brought about by the extraocular muscles. Their contraction due to variation in the distance of a stimulus serves as a cue to depth and is much more effective than accommodation; but convergence is most effective only at short distance, just as with accommodation. An object that is far away causes the line of sight to become almost parallel and there is, consequently, insignificant convergence. For judging the distance of objects beyond twenty yards or so, convergence is not very effective as a depth perception cue.

There appear to be different, but not unrelated, cortical mechanisms for processing monocular and binocular cues to depth. Barlow and

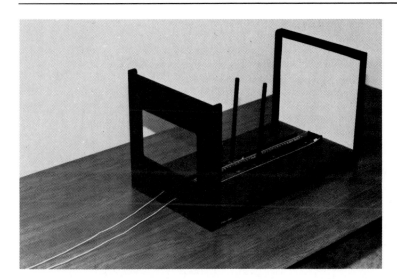

Figure 9.7   *Depth perception apparatus; the two rods are controlled by the string.*

his colleagues (Barlow, Blakemore, and Petti-grew 1967) reported that cortical cells that mediate the perception of depth respond strongly to the stimulus of binocular disparity. By recording the activity of single nerve cells in the visual projection area, they discovered groups of binocularly driven neurons that responded most strongly to pairs of optically fused stimulus bars with a specific binocular disparity. These findings suggest that binocular disparity is an adequate stimulus for binocularly driven stereoscopic, position-in-depth cortical analyzers.

More recently, Regan and his colleagues (Beverley and Regan 1973; Cynader and Regan 1978) have sought to determine whether disparity-sensitive neurons mediate the perception of motion-in-depth as well as the perception of position-in-depth. They found that, indeed, there are stereoscopic-motion analyzers sensitive to a particular direction of motion-in-depth. Moreover, the motion-in-depth mechanism and position-in-depth mechanism are more or less independent of each other.

The research on motion-in-depth perception suggests that information concerning motion-in-depth is processed by two distinct cortical mechanisms: a changing-size analyzer (described in the previous section) and a stereoscopic-motion analyzer that converges on the same motion-depth stage of the visual-perceptual system.

Measurement of Depth Perception

Two general types of depth perception tests exist, one measuring real depth and the other apparent depth. The Howard-Dolman apparatus has been the most commonly used test for real depth perception. The subject attempts to line up two black rods from a distance of twenty feet. One rod is stationary and the other is mounted on a moveable track. By pulling on a cord attached to the moveable rod, the subject attempts to bring this rod exactly beside the stationary rod (figure 9.7).

More sophisticated instruments are used by optometrists and opthalmologists, but the instruments usually measure apparent depth perception. These instruments have been devised on the same basis as the stereoscope. On a picture viewed through a stereoscope, surfaces and elements stand out, as do figures—the consciousness of three-dimensionality of space is greatly enhanced. The observer views stereographic cards and indicates perceived distances.

Development of Depth Perception

Whether depth perception exists as an inherent ability or whether it is developed through learning experiences has interested scholars for many years. Although we have evidence on both sides of this question, there is mounting evidence that some depth perceptual ability is inherited. Fantz (1961) reported that one-month-old infants could discriminate between solid and flat objects, even when the objects were viewed monocularly. Experiments by Gibson and Walk (1960) and Campos (1979) with a "visual cliff" show that young infants display depth perception.[1] Bower (1966) found that infants as young as six to eight weeks are able to make gross distinctions between objects that are nearer versus those that are farther away.

Effects of Practice and Exercise on Depth Perception

Depth perception, as measured by laboratory and clinical instruments, does not seem to be amenable to improvement through visually directed training programs. Although there is a paucity of research on this topic, the few studies that have been done have reported that training programs do not enhance depth perception (Newmeister 1977). On the other hand, empirical evidence

shows that the ability to judge distances in specific situations can be improved (Gibson and Bergman 1954). This, of course, is a specific response to a situation and not an improvement in depth perception ability. An improvement in certain types of visual perception (visual acuity and peripheral vision) has been reported during and immediately after exercise, but apparently exercise does not affect depth perception (Drowatsky and Schwartz 1971).

Depth Perception and Motor Behavior

In many motor activities the ability to make distance judgments is essential to effective and efficient performance. Virtually all athletes must make important depth discriminations to perform well. It is not surprising, then, that studies that have compared the depth perception of athletic and nonathletic groups have usually found that athletes involved in sports in which balls are thrown, hit, and caught possess better depth perception than nonathletic groups (Montebello 1953; Olsen 1956; Miller 1960; Ridini 1968). What is not clear from this research is whether the superior depth perception displayed by athletes is a result of innate visual abilities or whether depth perceptual abilities were enhanced via the sports experiences. Based on the findings that depth perception is not improved through training programs, one can speculate that persons with better depth perception are attracted and remain in sports because of this ability.

One aspect of depth perception and motor behavior for which there is little research is the possible relationship between learning motor skills and depth perception. One study suggests the existence of such a relationship. Mail (1965) found that some aspects of depth perception are positively related to proficiency in learning tennis.

---

[1] A visual cliff consists of a transparent surface of glass under which is a solid center support surrounded by an illusion of nonsupport. The "cliffs" on either side of the support are of different depths, one high and the other low. A subject (usually a child in the early stages of crawling) is placed on the center support and encouraged to move toward one of the sides. Typically, children at this age cannot be induced to move toward the high cliff side.

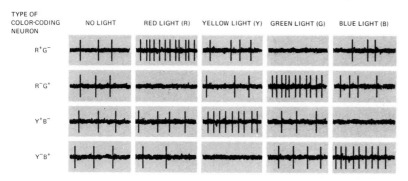

| TYPE OF COLOR-CODING NEURON | NO LIGHT | RED LIGHT (R) | YELLOW LIGHT (Y) | GREEN LIGHT (G) | BLUE LIGHT (B) |

Figure 9.8 *Patterns of response of the four types of color-coding neurons in the visual thalamus. The excitatory stimulus causes an increase in the number of spike discharges of the cell, and the inhibitory stimulus causes a decrease; for example, the red⁺green⁻ cell has a given rate of spontaneous discharging that increases when red light is presented but decreases to no discharges when green is presented.*

Color Vision

The visual system reacts to specific wavelengths of radiant energy, and we process this information into the subjective experience of color. As noted in the previous chapter, the phenomenon of color is very complex and will not be given more than a limited treatment here. Almost three centuries have passed since Isaac Newton speculated on how colors are perceived, and yet the process of seeing color is still not clearly understood.

In the human retina there are three light-sensitive pigments that are found in three different kinds of cones. One pigment has its greatest sensitivity in the wavelength for blue light and is called cyanolabe (the blue catcher); one in the spectrum for green light, called chlorolabe (the green catcher); and one for sensing red light waves, called erythrolabe (the red catcher). This arrangement of cones provides strong support to the component theory of **trichromatic** (three-color) vision.

All of the colors of the visible spectrum can be formed from three basic colors, red, green, and blue (or violet). If two or more wavelengths fall upon the retina simultaneously, the result is a color fusion, and the sensation is a color different from that of any single wavelength. For example, wavelengths for red and green give rise to the color sensation of yellow or orange; the fusion of blue and red produces a perception of purple.

While chemicals in the cones of the eye respond to the three primary colors, these receptors do not produce sensations directly. Instead, the color receptors feed into a set of neurons in the optic nerve and geniculate body of the thalamus that code colors in the form of opponent functions. In brief, color sensitive neurons in these parts of the visual system respond in an opponent way to red-green and to yellow-blue. For example, in the geniculate body one red-green neuron might be excited by red and inhibited by green, while another might be excited by green and inhibited by red. The same is true for yellow-blue neurons. The visual projection area begins to interpret color by noting how the four categories of opponent color neurons are firing. Changes in color will be interpreted in the brain by the relative activity of these four types of color neurons. Thus, it is the patterns of these opponent cells that seem to underlie the perception of color (MacNichol 1964; DeValois 1965) (figure 9.8).

The perception of color possesses three important qualities:

1. Hue, or tone, is a function of the wavelength of the radiant energy. Wavelengths of about 750 nanometers are seen as red, and those of about 400 nanometers are seen as dark blue (or violet). Each of the other hues of the visual spectrum has its own wavelength located somewhere between these two extremes.
2. Brightness depends upon the intensity of the light energy. Therefore, any particular hue can have a wide range of brightness. The human eye is most sensitive to the orange-yellow-green sections of the spectrum presumably because wavelengths in the center of the visible spectrum stimulate a greater number of receptors, producing a greater overall input. Thus, when the amount of radiant energy is equal, the human eye sees orange-yellow-green as much brighter than either red or blue.
3. Saturation, or purity, of a color depends upon the white light that is combined with the color. The less white light that is combined with a hue, the greater the saturation, or purity, of that hue. Conversely, the degree of saturation decreases as white light is combined with a hue.

Measurement of Color Perception

We have several methods of testing for color perception, but they tend to have certain limitations. Some limitations are due to the tests' length, some to their inability to deal with the various kinds of defects, and some to the differences between them and the everyday conditions in which color deficiency is significant.

One form of test is the pseudoisochromatic plate test. The plates are covered with various colored dots arranged at random, except for certain dots that form figures within the dot field. Subjects with normal color vision see the figures. People with certain color defects see the figures in some plates but not in others. There are several tests of this type.

Another type of test uses Munsell colored chips arranged in order of hue and is called the 100-hue test. It is somewhat similar to the old Holmgren yarn test, which consisted of sorting yarn strips into groups according to hue. Of course, more precise color discrimination can be determined by instrumentation. Optometrists and opthalmologists have rather elaborate means of assessing color perception.

Color Perception and Motor Behavior

The effects of color perception on motor behavior have attracted very few investigators. Cobb (1969) assessed color recognition in the peripheral vision of athletes in several sports and reported that there were significant differences with regard to color: Red and blue were recognized more readily than green or white. He suggested that it may be more beneficial for a team to wear blue or red uniforms if it is desirable to have the team members easily recognized as they compete. Unfortunately, very few coaches have an opportunity to select colors for their teams since color combinations are part of an institution's tradition. Morris (1976) studied the effect of three ball colors and two background colors upon the catching performance of elementary school children. He found that ball color affected their performance. Blue and yellow balls produced significantly higher catching scores than did white balls, and blue balls against white backgrounds and yellow balls against black backgrounds seemed to influence positively the catching performance. Manipulation of both ball color and background color may be one means of improving ball-catching performance.

Isaacs (1980) allowed seven- and eight-year-old children to indicate their choice for a favorite colored ball. Their ball-catching performance was then assessed with three balls of different color, one of which was their preferred color. He reported that children caught their preferred-color ball significantly better than the nonpreferred-color balls. He speculated that since color may serve as a selective attentional cue, children attended to the ball more intently when catching their preferred ball. He recommended that teachers allow children to choose the color of the ball with which they play.

Few people today remember that basketball rims used to be black and tennis balls white. Research conducted in the early 1950s by the National Basketball Coaches Association found that field goal and free throw shooting were better with an orange rim than with a black rim, and a rule was made that basketball rims had to be painted bright orange. The rule has been in effect over thirty years. Capitalizing on the fact that the color receptors are most sensitive to wavelengths in the orange-yellow-green portion of the visible spectrum, tennis ball manufacturers stopped making white balls and began making "optic yellow" tennis balls several years ago. Golf has been the most recent sport to convert to the colored ball.

Figure-Ground Perception

Perception is characterized by organization. People exhibit several fundamental visual-space organization characteristics with regard to organizing figures in space, but here we shall be concerned with only one: **figure-ground perception.**

The figure-ground phenomenon is considered to be one of the basic spatial organizing components of perception. The visible environment is more than an array of unrelated bits of sensory data. Instead, it consists of figures separated from their backgrounds. This is referred to as the figure-ground principle (see figure 7.5). Several of the most important differences between figure and ground are:

- If two fields have a common border, the figure seems to have shape while the ground does not.
- The figure appears to be a "thing," to be objectlike (even though it may be an abstract form), while the ground seems like unformed material.
- The color of the figure seems brighter and more solid than that of the ground.
- The figure tends to be perceived as closer to the observer than the ground, even though both are at the same distance.

Measurement of Figure-Ground Perception

The two principal methods for assessing figure-ground ability are the rod and frame test (RFT) and embedded figures tests. The RFT consists of a luminous square frame on which a luminous straight rod is suspended. Both the rod and the frame can be rotated independently. The apparatus must be placed in a completely darkened room while a subject is being tested. The subject stands fifteen to twenty feet away from the rod and frame with a remote switch for controlling the position of the rod. During testing the frame is rotated so that it is not upright, then the rod is rotated so that it is not vertical. The object for the subject is to return the rod to a perfectly vertical position. This is done by remote electrical control of the rod. The subject's response is recorded in degrees of deviation from the vertical (figure 9.9).

Some subjects are able to make accurate adjustments of the rod, others are not. In other words, some subjects seem to have a perceptual style that is influenced most by context (the ground represented by the luminous frame),

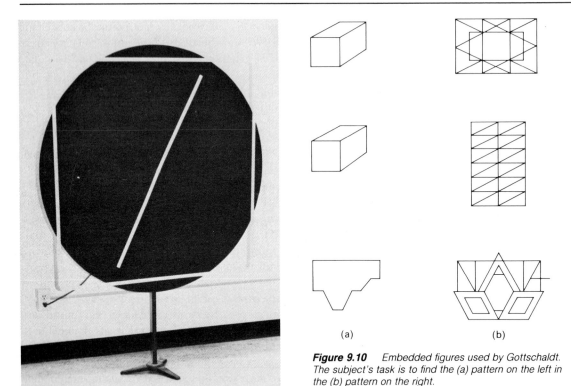

Figure 9.10   *Embedded figures used by Gottschaldt. The subject's task is to find the (a) pattern on the left in the (b) pattern on the right.*

Figure 9.9   *Rod and frame apparatus.*

whereas others are influenced most by figure (the luminous rod) when making judgments about verticality. The perceptual style of the former is said to be field-dependent, while the latter is said to be field-independent.

We have several embedded figures tests, but they are very similar, consisting of a series of pairs of figures. The subject's task is to find the simple figure of each pair within the much more complex figure of the two (figure 9.10). People who are adept at identifying the embedded figures are said to be field-independent, while those who are poor are referred to as field-dependent.

Effects of Practice on Figure-Ground Perception

We have little information about the effects of practice or specific experiences on figure-ground perception. Movement training of a very general nature, such as practicing ballet or modern dance, does not appear to alter field dependence/independence (Gruen 1955). Elliott and McMichael (1963) gave a relatively field-dependent group of people a training program specifically designed to improve field independence on the rod-and-frame test and reported that performance on this test was not noticeably amenable to training.

Figure-Ground Perception and Motor Behavior

Perhaps one of the most important and persistent figure-ground problems occurs in motor activities in which there is a ball or other object that must be tracked and hit or caught. In these situations, the ball must be identified quickly and accurately as the figure, with the rest of the visual array perceived as the ground. Due to the color of the balls and the backgrounds on which they are superimposed, it is frequently difficult to differentiate the figure from the background. Thus, in sports like baseball, football, and soccer, the ball may be visually "lost" in the background of the crowd, and sometimes even highly skilled athletes miss the ball because it cannot be differentiated from the background.

Although there is little empirical support, it would appear that people who tend to be field-dependent might have more difficulty performing and learning motor tasks. When people have been classified as highly skilled or poorly skilled on motor tasks, highly skilled performers tend to be more field independent than the poorly skilled (Meek and Skubic 1971). Also, when people are grouped into high field-independent and field-dependent groups, the field-independent group tends to perform motor tasks significantly better (Kreiger 1962; Shugart, Souder, and Bunker 1972). Finally, field dependence/independence has been found to be related to learning a ball catching task, with field-independent subjects showing a more rapid learning rate than field-dependent subjects (Jorgensen 1972; MacGillivary 1979).

When groups of athletes have been used as subjects, little in the way of differences in field dependence/independence has been found across sports (Pargman, Schreiber, and Stein 1974), nor have consistent relationships between field dependence/independence and athletic performance been found within sports teams (Pargman, Bender, and Deshaies 1975; Williams 1975).

Perhaps the homogeneity of athletes as a group reduces the likelihood of differences in field dependence/independence.

Familiarity with the background seems to aid figure-ground perception at a given site. Guidance cues seem to arise from the background, helping the performers even though they are not consciously aware of them. Perhaps one of the advantages of a day or two of practice at an unfamiliar sports site is the improved figure-ground perception for that environment.

Visual Tracking

While seeing a stationary object clearly and judging its distance are important factors in motor activities, in many motor tasks objects are moving and must be caught or hit for appropriate task performance. There are many sports and games where performance proficiency depends to a large extent upon catching and striking ability. One of the universal axioms in these activities is "Keep your eyes on the ball."

The main purpose of watching the ball is to know its flight characteristics so that appropriate responses can be made. Information about the position, direction, and velocity of a ball is necessary to predict future flight. The objective of a performer of a **visual tracking** task is to gain enough information about the characteristics of the ball in its initial flight to be able to predict when it will be within hitting or catching range and where it will be in space at that moment.

Monitoring an object in flight and then intercepting it is a complex perceptual-motor task. First, the object must be seen. The eyes obtain information that will enable the performer to anticipate future flight. Second, anticipation and prediction must occur, and these are complex functions based upon current information and stored memories about flight characteristics. Finally, appropriate motor responses must be mobilized to bring about accurate movements for

Table 9.2 *Component analysis of the task of catching or hitting a ball in flight*

1	2	3
Pursuit tracking task	Prediction of where the ball will be in a reaction time + a movement time	Catching or striking movement
Predominantly perceptual analysis	Central decision	Predominantly motor response
Covert processes		Overt response

Source: Based on Alderson 1972.

interception to be made. A component analysis of the task of catching or striking objects in flight is illustrated in table 9.2.

Eye Movements

Movements of the eyes are exquisitely coordinated when tracking a moving object. The system regulating eye movements consists of a complex of brain pathways and motoneurons of cranial nerves innervating the extraocular muscles. This is the oculomotor system. Each of the three sets of extraocular muscles is reciprocally innervated so that contraction of each pair synchronizes with relaxation of the other muscles.

The oculomotor system has important subsystems. One is the saccadic system that regulates saccadic movements, which the eyes use to fixate on new objects. Saccadic movements are the quick flicks of eye shifts as they move from one point to another. Saccadic eye movements serve to place the small area at the center of the retina, the fovea, on different parts of the visual field. These flicks are so fast that vision is momentarily suppressed while the movement takes place. A second subsystem is the smooth pursuit system, which is used in pursuing a moving object. The smooth pursuit system attempts to maintain a clear image of the moving object by matching target velocity with eye velocity. The purpose of smooth eye movement is to permit the visual system to maintain the moving object in a

stationary position on the retina in order to make perception of the object easier. The cerebral cortex and the superior colliculi are intimately integrated in function in order to make the pursuit system work. A third system, the vestibular system, monitors and evaluates the movements of the head and then, via a complex network of reflexes, stimulates the extraocular muscles to move the eyes to compensate for head movements.

The eyes can follow a moving object with no volitional effort. This involuntary fixation mechanism is involved with locking the eyes upon an object once it is located, and the automatic movements are mediated by reflex pathways from retina to visual projection area to association areas and then to the superior colliculus, from which motor signals are relayed over the cranial nerves back to the eye.

Highly specialized neural circuits in the visual system enable the human viewer to perceive information about the direction in which an object is moving. In addition to the visual mechanisms for perceiving motion-in-depth that were described in a previous section, the human visual system makes use of mechanisms that are directionally selective. Direction-specific cells are present in the visual cortex and presumably they provide the basis for the ability to see moving targets (Sekuler and Levinson 1977).

Measurement of Visual Tracking

Techniques for assessing saccadic eye movement speed have been developed by reading specialists (Frackenpohl and McCarthy 1969), but visual pursuit tracking is rarely tested in motor behavior laboratories. Professional eye care specialists must use refined instrumentation to make assessments of this type. When pursuit tracking is measured in motor behavior laboratories, it is typically done in conjunction with a catching or striking task. The subject must visually track and intercept an object. Of course, many factors influence the ability to intercept balls in flight, only one of which is eye movement in tracking the ball.

Effects of Practice on Visual Tracking

Perceptual processing of the flight characteristics of an object so that a person anticipates both its spatial and temporal future location prior to accurately catching or hitting it improves with practice (Burrows and Murdock 1969; Graboi 1971). One factor that may contribute to the improvement is saccadic eye movement speed. Specific saccadic eye movement training programs and programs in which subjects practice hitting thrown balls have been found to increase saccadic eye movement speed as well as efficiency of response execution (Williams and Helfrich 1977).

Visual Tracking and Motor Behavior

Traditionally, it has been assumed that keeping the eyes on the ball is essential for effective performance in ball skills, but a number of issues about this dictum might be raised: Why is it necessary? How long can visual information be useful? Is that what skilled performers do?

If a performer is to intercept a ball in flight by either catching or hitting it, it is necessary to begin to position the hands or striking implement (bat or racket) before the ball arrives. Otherwise the performer will be like the young child who lets the ball hit him on the chest before any hand movements are made. The purpose of watching the flight of the ball is to use this information for anticipating and predicting the future flight, thereby beginning interception responses well before the ball arrives. Kay (1957) discusses this function in watching the ball.

We may compare this situation with the case of someone trying to estimate the future position of a moving object say . . . the trajectory of a ball from a limited observation of its initial stages. . . . Let us imagine the situation is such that our . . . subject's head is fixed and he can only observe the trajectory of the ball by successive fixation. Thus we have the trajectory divided into a series of segments which one might think of as events a, b, c, and so on. An individual through his experience of watching how objects travel in space learns about the probable order and temporal relations of these events. Thus, given events a, b, c, he predicts the future position: and the skilled person is the one who can predict accurately on the fewest possible initial events. Once this is achieved the remaining events in the series are redundant or at the most confirmatory. So much for the popular dictum about "keeping your eye on the ball"!

Kay makes two salient points: First, with experience performers become very accurate at predicting future flight from initial flight information, and second, it may not be necessary to watch the ball up to the point of interception. With regard to these two points, we have both informal observational as well as empirical data that are confirmatory. Casual observation of skilled performers in ball sports verifies that they seem to need to watch less of the ball flight than beginners in making their responses to the ball. They seem to be able to take their eyes off the ball and observe teammates or opponents while the ball is in flight and they seem to have "all the time in the world" to organize their response.

Some years ago Hubbard and Seng (1954) photographed over twenty-five professional baseball players in batting practice to ascertain their visual habits while batting. The evidence conclusively showed that eye movements did not continue up to the point of bat contact with the ball, indicating that either the hitters were unable visually to track the ball as it approached the plate or that tracking stopped at a point where it could contribute no additional data that could be used for the swing. The investigators had this to say about the fact that eye focus did not continue up to contact:

Either the tracking was broken off at some point beyond which the additional information would have been superfluous since the bat was on its way, or was broken off because the visual apparatus broke down—became incapable of tracking at the very high relative velocity of a pitched ball near the plate—or both.

Although there was evidence that the batters' eyes were not focused on the ball at contact, some of the batters stated that they saw the bat meet the ball. Of course, just because the eyes are not focused on the ball does not mean that it was out of the field of vision; the ball and bat may have been seen with peripheral vision. A stimulus image need not be focused on the retinal fovea for the performer to extract information about the ball and respond accurately. Furthermore, there seems to be no simple relation between eye tracking of an object and accuracy of anticipatory motor performance (Haywood 1977).

Whiting and his colleagues in England have conducted a series of investigations designed to study the ability to intercept balls in flight. In one study, Whiting (1968) constructed an instrument that consisted of a miniature tetherball, which enabled a ball to be swung around a pole. The ball could be lit in various quadrants of its flight by a light within a metal screen while remaining in darkness for the remainder of its trajectory. Thus, the ball could be illuminated during parts

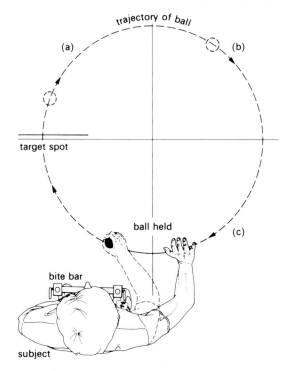

Figure 9.11   *Apparatus table showing quadrants in which ball could be illuminated, (a), (b), and (c).*

of its trajectory or during its entire course. The amount of visual information necessary for ball catching was studied as well as the effects of practice (figure 9.11).

Subjects were trained first in full light so that they could see the ball during its entire trajectory. Then they were required to perform the task under a series of restricted viewing conditions, including total darkness. The results showed that once having had the opportunity to see the ball throughout its flight, similar performance could be maintained when opportunity to see the ball was restricted. Of course, the total darkness condition produced a significant decrement in performance compared with the restricted light conditions.

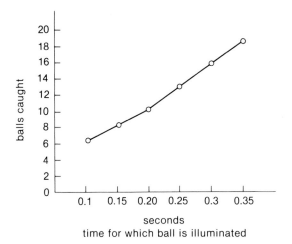

Figure 9.12   *Number of balls caught (out of 20) under differing periods of illumination.*

Whiting's results indicate that the subjects learned to anticipate and predict the flight of the ball from information received near the beginning of the ball's flight. He suggested that this learning effect occurs during the acquisition of ball skills in sports—the experienced performers have developed excellent anticipatory and judgment skills, and can predict ball trajectory from very brief inspection of the flight. Indeed, differences have been demonstrated in the dimensions of information extracted from a visual display by novice performers in a sport in comparison to that extracted by experts. Experts are able to make accurate discriminations about flight direction and trajectory sooner than novices (Ryan 1969; Tyldesley 1978).

Although it may be unnecessary to view a ball over its entire flight in order to intercept it successfully, there is a positive relationship between catching or hitting success and the length of time the ball is viewed by a performer. Several studies have been done wherein a ball was projected through a trajectory in which it was visible to subjects for only part of its flight (figure 9.12).

The subjects' job was to catch the ball (Whiting, Gill, and Stephenson 1970; Nessler 1973; Whiting, Alderson, and Sanderson 1973). The consistent finding in these studies was that opportunity to watch the ball for longer periods of time resulted in increased catching success.

These studies suggest that an advantage is to be gained from watching a ball for as long as possible because this information provides useful data for predicting future flight pattern. This information is useful at least up to the point in flight after which central nervous system processing time and movement time preclude the use of further information for the organization of the appropriate response. For example, it appears that a baseball batter must make a swing on the basis of information that is available to the hitter prior to the last 300 msec or so before the ball meets the bat. This estimate is based on the fact that visual reaction time is about 190 to 200 msec and the swing takes about 100 msec to bring the bat into the hitting zone. Assuming the ball is traveling at 10 feet per 100 msec, which is quite possible for a good baseball pitcher, the batter must initiate the swing while the ball is still 30 feet away. Since the distance between the baseball pitcher's rubber and home plate is 60′ 6″, the batter can gain useful information about its flight only during the first 30 feet.

There is some controversy in the literature as to whether reaction time is faster to a stimulus that is always present, such as a thrown ball, or to a stimulus that is suddenly presented, such as in a typical laboratory reaction-time (RT) study. Conceding that differences exist between a moving object that serves as a stimulus and a suddenly appearing stimulus, still there is an instant when the information about the flight pattern of the ball becomes a stimulus for a reaction and movement to intercept it. When that instant occurs, the processes that produce reaction latencies in laboratory RT work undoubtedly occur here too. A latency of about 190 msec presumably occurs between the time a batter decides to swing and the initiation of the movement.

Once initiated, how useful is visual information for altering the pattern of a ballistic movement, such as a bat swing? Recent evidence suggests that the time needed to process visual feedback information and use this information for motor control is about 100 to 135 msec (Smith and Bowen 1980; Carlton 1981; Zelaznik, Hawkins, and Kisselburgh 1983). Thus, since an alteration cannot be made to an unexpected movement error before some 100 to 135 msec, visual information about a moving object, such as a ball, is of little use during the last 100 to 135 msec. Watching the ball at this point would seem to make little difference. However, the delay in reacting to an unexpected movement error obtained via visual feedback might be slightly reduced if the performer could accurately anticipate the temporal occurrence of the error, the type of error, and the corrective movement that must be made to amend the error.

Another reason for watching the ball is that eye direction may be effective because of its effect on bodily position or posture. When the eyes are turned away, the shoulders and body tend to follow. Moreover, since there is no precise way of knowing when visual information becomes useless in a given sports situation, the instructional cue to "keep your eyes on the ball" seems appropriate.

Eye Dominance

The human is a bilateral creature, and many structures come in twos, such as arms, legs, eyes, and brain hemispheres. As the individual grows and uses these structures, typically one of each pair comes to play a dominant role. In dexterity, a person is left-handed or right-handed. In the case of the brain's hemispheres, since the left hemisphere has unique speech and language functions for over 90 percent of the population,

it has become known as the dominant hemisphere. As with other structures, the eyes display a characteristic called **eye dominance.** The dominant eye is the one that leads the other both in fixation and in attentive or perceptive function. It is the eye that is unconsciously and preferentially chosen to guide decision and action.

Although there is some tendency of dominance for individuals (right-handedness), patterns are not necessarily fixed. Some people are left-handed and right-footed, and vice versa; some are right-eyed and left-handed; and some people show right-handedness for some tasks and left-handedness for others.

Measurement of Eye Dominance

The two most commonly used eye dominance tests are the alignment test and the hole-in-card test. For the alignment test, the subject is given a pencil, asked to hold it up at arm's length, and, with both eyes open, to line it up with a black dot on a wall seven feet away. Subjects actually see two images of the pencil, but they automatically disregard one and bring the pencil, the dot, and one of their eyes into a straight line. Subjects are asked to close each eye and then asked if the pencil is still lined up. The eye used to sight with (the eye that sees the pencil directly lined up with the dot) is considered the subject's dominant eye.

To administer the hole-in-card test, a piece of cardboard, eleven inches square, with a small hole (one-fourth inch in diameter) in the center is held by the subject at arm's length with both hands directly in front of the body. The subject is asked to use both eyes and to look through the peephole at a white dot (one-half inch in diameter) on a blackboard seven feet away. After the object has been located, the subject is asked to close each eye and asked if the dot is still visible. The eye that sees the dot when the other is closed in considered the dominant eye.

Eye Dominance and Motor Behavior

In one of the pioneer studies of eye dominance, Lund (1932) reported superior performance on a target-aiming task when subjects used their dominant eye. Since then the majority of studies has indicated that unilaterals, meaning right-eyed and right-handed or left-eyed and left-handed, are better performers on a variety of motor activities than crossed-laterals, left-eyed and right-handed or vice versa. This has been demonstrated for sports skills such as bowling, swimming, baseball, and shooting (rifle, pistol, trap, skeet) (Fox 1957; Sinclair and Smith 1957; Adams 1965; Christina et al. 1981). However, no significant differences were found in basketball free throw shooting between unilaterals and crossed-laterals (Shick 1971).

Adams (1965) indicated that there is a strong belief among baseball coaches that the batter of the crossed-lateral type has a definite advantage over the unilateral batter. The advantage, some claim, is due to the position of the batter's dominant eye in relation to the pitcher and the pitched ball. This notion claims that most right-handed batters cannot view the pitcher and pitched ball as well with their dominant eye if it is located on the right side due to the unilateral's position in the batter's box. Often the batting stance is such that the right and dominant eye is partly obstructed from seeing the pitched ball by the bridge of the batter's nose. On the other hand, crossed-lateral batters do not have this problem regardless of the type of batting stance they use.

To test this hypothesis, Adams determined the effect of eye dominance on batting with collegiate baseball players. Comparisons were made on on-base average, batting average, strikeouts, called strikeouts, and missed swings. The unilaterals scored better than the crossed-laterals in most batting categories, contradicting the notion that crossed-laterals should be better.

In a similar study, Lakatos (1968) found that unilateral batters hit better against pitchers who threw with the same hand as the batters' batting hand than against pitchers who threw with the opposite hand. But crossed-lateral batters hit better against pitchers who threw with the hand opposite the batters' batting hand than against pitchers who threw with the same hand. More recently Llewellyn (1972), also using college baseball players, reported that handedness had a greater effect on hitting performance than whether the players were unilaterals or crossed-laterals. The right-handed batters were superior to the left-handed in his study.

The research on eye dominance and motor performance indicates that eye dominance seems to have some effect on certain aspects of motor behavior, and unilaterals tend to display superior performance on a variety of motor activities. However, there are crossed-laterals who perform quite well in these activities, and we have no compelling reason for switching a performer from a crossed-lateral to unilateral technique.

Motor Learning and Vision

A series of experiments over the past decade has shown rather decisively that vision tends to dominate other sensory modalities in a wide variety of perceptual-motor responses (for a review see Posner, Nissen, and Klein 1976). Visual feedback has been found to have a positive effect on learning to initiate a response and on movement extent performance during the early phase of motor learning (Newell and Chew 1975; Posner, Nissen, and Klein 1976; Adams, Gopher, and Lintern 1977; Christina and Anson 1981).

In what has become a classic study on the use of vision for motor learning and control, Pew (1966) showed that after a period of practice, subjects shifted from visual control of individual movements to the use of visual feedback for periodic correction or modulation of the movement pattern. In Pew's study, the subject controlled the horizontal position of a target on an oscilloscope by alternately switching between two keys. When the left control key was depressed, the target accelerated to the left, and when the right control key was depressed, the target accelerated to the right. The subject's task was to keep the target centered on the screen throughout each trial.

At first, subjects made individual movements, visually analyzed the outcome, made a correction movement, analyzed the outcome, and so on. This resulted in their being off target much of the time. As practice continued, however, the subjects changed their technique considerably. They began to make very rapid and regular alternating finger movements and then a single correction, or, as they began to drift off target, the alternating pattern was modulated so that one key was depressed slightly longer than the other during a series of movements. This finding suggests that with practice on a task, performers shift from visual control of component movements to the use of visual information for periodic modulation of the movement pattern.

The potency of visual feedback for the control of movement is illustrated by several studies that found that when vision is present, performers tend to rely on it as a source of information and ignore or suppress input from other sensory modalities—even though information from the other senses may be more relevant for making an efficient and effective response (Jordan 1972; Klein and Posner 1974; Klein 1977; Smyth 1978; Smyth and Marriott 1982). The preferential processing of visual input is shown by a study in which subjects were placed in a completely darkened room and told to swing one arm up and down at the elbow joint. Suddenly, a flash of light briefly illuminated the limb. Subjects reported that the limb felt as if it were at rest in the position in which it was caught by the flash (summarized by Granit 1977).

Several reasons have been proposed for visual dominance in motor learning and control. It has been suggested that vision is a source of concurrent feedback (feedback while the movement is being performed) as well as a potent source of terminal feedback (feedback after the performance is completed). Further, visual input is largely conscious input, whereas the proprioceptive information accompanying movement reaches consciousness to a much lesser degree (Granit 1977). Vision is also sensitive to detail, depth, and color, thus providing a resolution for the control of movement that is lacking with other sensory systems. Finally, it has been suggested that there is a bias or strategy to attend selectively to visual stimuli because when one is not attending vision, visual stimuli that are brief or weak will be missed altogether. A bias to attend selectively to visual stimuli may have evolved to overcome this deficiency in visual processing (Posner, Nissen, and Klein 1976).

Summary

In order to perform many motor tasks effectively, it is necessary to make precise judgments about moving objects in space and about spatial relationships of the body to other individuals or objects. These abilities depend upon visual perception.

Visual acuity is another term for sharpness of vision and implies the degree of detail the eye can discern in a stimulus object. Visual acuity for stationary objects is called static visual acuity, while the ability to discriminate objects that are moving or where there is movement between the observer and an object is called dynamic visual acuity. It has been found that many athletes perform with uncorrected visual acuity problems. In general, there is a relationship between visual acuity and motor behavior.

Field of vision and peripheral vision refer to parts of the environment one can see without a change in visual fixation. Several investigations have found that motor performance is impaired when field of vision and peripheral vision are restricted.

Depth perception is produced by the coordinated employment of the two eyes. Although there are many cues to depth that can be employed with monocular vision, it is the functioning of both eyes that gives accurate depth perception. Since many motor skills involve locating, tracking, and hitting or catching moving objects, depth perception plays a central role in effective motor behavior.

Color vision is possible because of three light-sensitive pigments found in three different kinds of cones in the retina. A recent trend in sports is to use yellow-orange objects, since the eyes are most sensitive to these colors.

Figure-ground perception is the separation of figures from their backgrounds. Figure-ground perceptual styles have been described as field-independent, which characterizes people who are efficient in discerning figures from the field, and field-dependent, which characterizes people who are inefficient in discerning figures from the field. People who are field-dependent tend to have more difficulty performing and learning many motor skills.

Movements of the eyes are exquisitely coordinated when tracking a moving object. Experiences with tracking moving objects enhances the acquisition of catching and hitting these objects. The longer a moving object is seen and the slower it is moving, the more readily it can be hit or caught.

As an individual grows and uses the eyes, one of them typically becomes the dominant eye. The effects of eye dominance on motor behavior indicates that eye dominance seems to have some effect on certain motor tasks, but the effects are very slight.

Vision is the dominant sensory-perceptual mode in the initial phases of motor learning. Visual input is such a potent source of information that a performer will ignore or suppress input from other sense modalities, even though information from other senses may be more relevant for efficient and effective performance. Visual input is largely conscious input, it is sensitive to detail, and there seems to be a bias to attend selectively to visual stimuli. These are some presumed reasons for visual dominance.

10

The Somatosensory System

*T*he word **somatosensory** (or just somatic) refers to sensations from the body, and somatosensory receptors are located in the skin, muscles, tendons, joints, and the vestibular apparatus of the inner ear. Collectively, somatosensory receptors are sensitive to stimuli that impinge on the skin and to stimuli arising from movement. Basically, each receptor is most sensitive to a particular form of stimulus. To organize these various receptors into some form of meaningful groups, neuroanatomists have divided them into two general categories: cutaneous receptors and proprioceptors. The **cutaneous receptors** are found near the skin and stimulation of them gives rise to four types of perception—touch-pressure, heat, cold, and pain. Receptors in the muscles, tendons, joints, and vestibular apparatus are collectively called **proprioceptors.** The impressions obtained from these receptors are known as kinesthetic perceptions (or kinesthesis). This chapter will describe the role of each of these somatosensory groups.

The cutaneous receptors do not play a primary role in motor behavior, but these receptors are usually considered together with the proprioceptors because many of them look and function like the proprioceptors. More important, information from both groups of receptors travels through the same spinal and brainstem routes, converge together on various subcortical neurons, and finally, convey their input to the same general projection area in the cortex. In these ways cutaneous input and proprioceptor input are integrated for kinesthetic perceptions.

Figure 10.1 *Sensory receptors in the skin.*

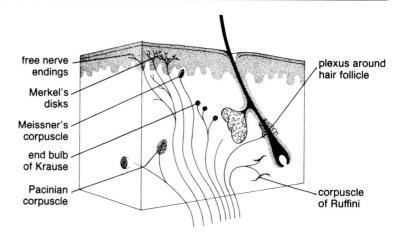

free nerve endings
Merkel's disks
Meissner's corpuscle
end bulb of Krause
Pacinian corpuscle
plexus around hair follicle
corpuscle of Ruffini

Cutaneous Receptors

With the exception of the distance receptors (visual, auditory, and olfactory), most of our sensory receptors that are responsive to changes in the outside world are located in the skin. These cutaneous receptors are closely grouped just under the skin in what is called the epidermis and in deeper layers under the skin, the dermis. They provide information about stimulation of the skin and deeper tissue and structures within the body. There is some ambiguity in the literature concerning the number and nomenclature of the cutaneous receptors, but touch-pressure, warmth, cold, and pain are commonly identified as the cutaneous sensory modalities.

Cutaneous receptors certainly contribute important information for keeping individuals apprised of their external environment, but they play a secondary role in motor control and learning. Hence we shall discuss only the cutaneous receptors for touch and pressure since they do provide important information for motor behavior, while other cutaneous receptors do not.

Touch and Pressure Sensations

The morphology (structure) of cutaneous receptors varies a great deal. Some are simple unmyelinated nerve endings, but others are much more complex, with the nerve ending covered by corpuscles. On the hairless parts of the body, such as the lips, palms, and bottoms of the feet, Meiss-

ner's corpuscles and Merkel's disks are very profuse. These appear to be receptors for light touch, but they also react to bending of hair or pressure on the skin (figure 10.1)

On the hairy parts of the body, free nerve endings wind themselves around the bulbous base of the hair follicles to form nerve baskets, and any deflection of the hair gives rise to a perception of touch. Free nerve endings exist in all parts of the skin and are activated by touch and probably by thermal stimuli.

Pacinian corpuscles are located in the dermis and are stimulated by deep compression of the skin. Structurally, the Pacinian corpuscle has an inner core of bare nerve filament surrounded by successive layers of tissue, giving it an appearance somewhat like that of a cross section of an onion. It responds to mechanical stimulation, but its axon sends impulses only at the onset and offset of stimulation and not during periods of prolonged skin displacement.

Cutaneous sensitivity is not uniformly distributed over the body surface. There is a relationship between density of receptors and sensitivity to stimuli. For example, density of touch-pressure receptors varies from an extremely high density in the fingertips to a low density in the back and thigh. As a result, two-point discrimination is quite different in these areas. On the fingertips, when the two points of a compass are placed together on the skin and gradually separated, a person will discriminate

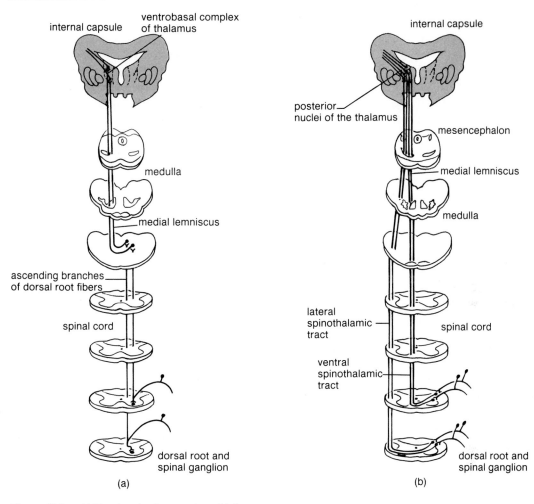

Figure 10.2 *(a) The dorsal column system; (b) the spinothalamic system.*

two points when only 2.3 millimeters (mm) separate the points. The distance increases to 67 mm when testing is on the thigh. The other cutaneous receptors have their unique distribution and sensitivity characteristics as well.

Transmission of Cutaneous Information to the Brain

Impulses that have been triggered by stimuli impinging on the cutaneous receptors travel over sensory neuron fibers in the peripheral nerves, enter the spinal cord (or brainstem in the case of cranial nerve transmission), and are transmitted by sensory pathways to the brain. Most of the cutaneous pathways ascend to the thalamus and terminate in the somatosensory projection area of the cortex.

The cutaneous and proprioceptive systems have very similar afferent transmission networks. We shall describe this network for cutaneous transmission now and add the details unique to the various proprioceptors later in the chapter.

The **dorsal column system** and the spinothalamic system are the two basic cutaneous nerve fiber pathways to the brain. As illustrated in figure 10.2, these two pathways are anatomically distinct and they have unique transmission characteristics. But it is important to note that in both systems, stimulation of somatosensory receptors evokes sensory effects mostly on the contralateral side of the cerebral cortex. Receptors in the left side of the body send impulses primarily to the somatosensory cortex in the right side of the brain, while receptors in the right side of the body send their messages to the left somatosensory cortex.

There are differences in transmission of these two systems. First-order nerve fibers of the dorsal column system enter the spinal cord and ascend in the dorsal column of the cord without synapse to the brainstem, where they synapse on the second-order neurons. The axons of the second-order neurons cross the midline and ascend to the thalamus. Third-order neurons ascend to the cerebral cortex. The dorsal column system tends to be composed of low-threshold, myelinated nerve fibers that transmit impulses at velocities of 80–100 meters per second. It is referred to as the fast-fiber network because transmission of information to the brain occurs within a small fraction of a second. Stimulation of sensory neurons in this system results in a very discrete signal being sent to a highly localized point in the thalamus and cortex.

By contrast, first-order fibers in the spinothalamic system enter the spinal cord and synapse immediately with second-order neurons located in the dorsal horns of the cord. The axons of the second-order neurons cross the midline of the cord and enter the **spinothalamic tract,** ascending directly to the thalamus. From the thalamus, the third-order neurons ascend to the cortex. The spinothalamic system tends to be made up of high-threshold, unmyelinated fibers that transmit signals at velocities of 1–40 meters per second, so this system is called the slow-fiber network. This slowness in transmission means that it can be used only for information that the brain can afford to have somewhat delayed. When a first-order neuron in this system is stimulated, the

signal is disbursed over a diffuse collateral network. As a result, stimulation of a sensory neuron causes stimulation of a widely dispersed area in the cortex.

The modalities of sensation transmitted by the two systems are listed by Guyton (1977):

The Dorsal Column System

1. Touch sensations having a high degree of localization of the stimulus and transmitting fine gradations of intensity.
2. Phasic sensations, such as vibratory sensations.
3. Kinesthetic sensations (sensations having to do with body movements).
4. Muscle sensations.
5. Pressure sensations having fine gradations of intensity.

The Spinothalamic System

1. Pain.
2. Thermal sensations, including both warmth and cold sensations.
3. Crude touch sensations capable of gross localization of the stimulus on the surface of the body.
4. Tickle and itch sensations.
5. Sexual sensations.

Somatosensory innervation of the face and much of the head is carried via the trigeminal nerve (cranial nerve V). First-order fibers enter the brainstem at the level of the pons and divide in a complex way to synapse on second-order neurons lying in various nuclei of the brainstem. Second-order neurons send their axons across the midline to ascend to the thalamus. Third-order neurons project to the cortex.

The Somatosensory Projection Area

The **somatosensory projection area** is that portion of the cerebral cortex to which all the cutaneous and proprioceptors send their messages. We shall, therefore, describe the functions of this area of the cortex at this time, adding information about its unique functions for proprioceptive input later in the chapter. The somatosensory projection area is located in the postcentral gyrus

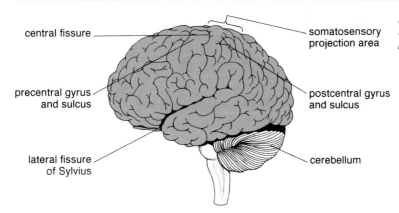

Figure 10.3 *Lateral surface of the brain showing the somatosensory projection area.*

central fissure

precentral gyrus and sulcus

lateral fissure of Sylvius

somatosensory projection area

postcentral gyrus and sulcus

cerebellum

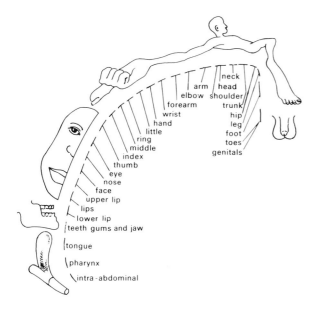

Figure 10.4 *The somatosensory homunculus (little man), showing the amount of somatosensory cortex devoted to a particular body organ.*

neck
arm head
elbow shoulder
forearm trunk
wrist hip
hand leg
little foot
ring toes
middle genitals
index
thumb
eye
nose
face
upper lip
lips
lower lip
teeth gums and jaw
tongue
pharynx
intra-abdominal

of the parietal lobe and extends from the longitudinal fissure into the lateral fissure (fissure of Sylvius) (figure 10.3). The precentral gyrus, or motor cortex, also receives some somatic projections. Indeed, it seems likely that most of the cerebral cortex receives some somatosensory projections.

The somatosensory projection area is mapped out in topographical manner, and the amount of this area of the cortex devoted to a given region of the body surface is directly proportional to the use and sensitivity of that region. In other words, the sizes of the various somatic projection areas are proportional to the number of specialized nerve endings in each peripheral area of the body. The lips, tongue, and thumb, for example, have a relatively large representation in the somatosensory projection area (figure 10.4).

Preliminary discrimination of location and modality of sensation occurs in the thalamus. Dull and poorly localized pain and intense temperature stimuli can be perceived even when fiber tracts from the thalamus to the cortex are cut. But exact localization or precise discrimination of somatosensory input depends upon a functional somatosensory projection area.

This localization ability of the somatic projection area is possible because of the organization of nerve fibers throughout the nervous system. Nerve fibers are spatially oriented in the nerve trunks, in the spinal cord, in the thalamus, and in the cerebral cortex. All the different nerve tracts of the CNS are spatially organized. This spatial organization is maintained with precision throughout the sensory pathway all the way from the receptor to the somatosensory projection area. Because of this organization, we can tell the difference between a song, a colorful sunset, or a slug on the arm only on the basis of the particular terminals in our brains to which the incoming nerve fibers are connected.

Nerve fibers of the somatosensory cortex and motor cortex are so intermingled that they can almost be considered a single mechanism. For example, electrical stimulation in the motor cortex has been found to elicit perceptions as well as movement. On the other hand, stimulation of the somatosensory projection area may cause movements, as well as somatic perceptions. The somatosensory cortex gives off fibers to motoneurons for cortical control of movement. At the same time, motor cortex fibers are known to descend to subcortical nuclei and synapse on neurons of the somatosensory system; as a result, signals from the motor cortex can modify input from the somatosensory system. This suggests that motor tracts may serve either a facilitative of inhibitory function for transmission of information through subcortical somatic nuclei, thus altering the input into the cortex.

Somatosensory signals pass from the somatosensory projection area into association areas in the parietal lobes, where the impulses are interpreted into the meaning of the input: Shape, form, roughness, smoothness, size, and texture of an object are ascertained. Quantities such as weight, temperature, and the degree of pressure are also interpreted. Here also is where the awareness of location of body parts, one to the other, and of one's self, is perceived. Destruction of association areas in the parietal lobe produces deficits in the sphere of somatic perception.

Damage to the somatosensory association areas may produce faulty of impaired recognition of various modality-specific stimuli. Disturbances of this type are called agnosias, the loss of the ability to recognize objects or symbols in one sensory modality. The recognition of an object through the somatic senses requires an intact parietal association area, whereas the awareness of simple aspects of somatic sensation, such as localization, can be brought into the conscious sphere through subcortical and somatosensory projection cortex functions. In addition to impaired recognition, a variety of distortion or disturbances of body image can accompany parietal lobe damage. The recognition of self is impaired. A person with such a condition may be unaware that his leg is his leg. Also, a variety of receptive language impairments arise from damage to the left parietal lobe. All these types of impairment entail a basic inability to synthesize the units of sensory input into coherent and meaningful wholes.

The Proprioceptors

In order to behave effectively, individuals must be able to monitor their own movements by knowing the relative position of the different parts of the body and by being able to maintain a particular orientation toward gravity. These functions are performed by complex sensory receptors, called proprioceptors, that are located in muscles, tendons, joints, and the labyrinth of the inner ear. The proprioceptors keep the brain apprised of the physical state of the body at all times.

The British neuroscientist and Nobel laureate Charles Sherrington (1906) introduced the word *proprioception* to include all those sensory systems that respond to stimuli arising in muscles, tendons, joints, and vestibular apparatus. The immediate stimuli arise from changes in length and from tension, compression, and the effects of gravity, from movement of parts of the body, and from muscular contraction. The receptor cells in these mechanisms require mechanical deformation for their activation and so are referred to as mechanoreceptors.

The Muscle Spindle

Muscle proprioceptors in skeletal muscles are of two types: the muscle spindle, which senses muscle length, and the Golgi tendon organ (GTO), which senses tension on the muscle. This section describes the muscle spindle; the GTO will be described in the following section.

The unique feature of the **muscle spindle** is that it contains both sensory receptors *and* muscle fibers. Therefore, it has both sensory *and* motor functions. Since our focus in this chapter is on somatosensory structures and functions, the sensory aspects of the muscle spindle will be emphasized. In chapter 12 its motor control functions will be examined. However, before turning to the sensory aspects of the muscle spindle, we must describe the muscle fiber and nerve innervation of the spindle; an understanding of these parts of the structure makes a description of muscle spindle receptor stimulation more meaningful.

Muscle Spindle Structure

Muscle spindles are found in all skelotomuscles. Small muscles that are used to regulate fine voluntary movements contain relatively large numbers of muscle spindles. The muscle spindle consists of a fluid-filled capsule tapering at both

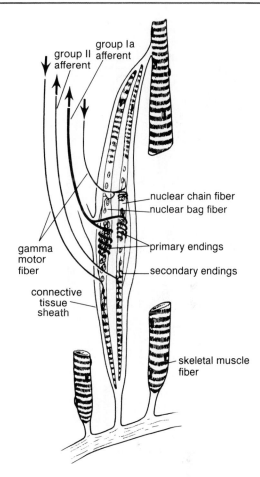

Figure 10.5 *Schematic representation of a muscle spindle.*

ends. The typical spindle is 4–7 mm long and 80–200 millimicrons (mμ) wide. In the equatorial region the capsule has a bulbous enlargement that gives the structure its spindlelike appearance. Within the capsule are specialized muscle fibers, called **intrafusal muscle fibers,**[1] and the spindle receptors (figure 10.5). We shall focus on the intrafusal muscle fibers first and then return to the spindle receptors.

---

[1] Since the muscle spindle contains a unique type of muscle fiber, the *intrafusal* muscle, to avoid confusion it will be necessary to refer to the main skeletal muscles as *extrafusal* muscles.

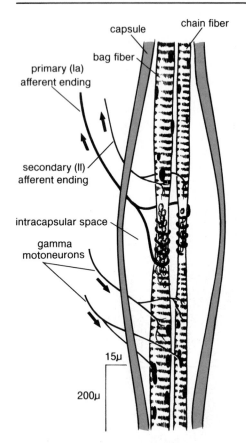

Figure 10.6 *Diagram of a muscle spindle showing afferents and efferents.*

The two types of intrafusal fibers are **nuclear bag fibers** and nuclear chain fibers. The former are longer and thicker and contain many centrally placed nuclei. They extend beyond the spindle capsule and attach to the connective tissue of the **extrafusal muscle fibers. Nuclear chain fibers** are shorter and thinner and have fewer nuclei within the central regions of the fiber. They are contained entirely within the capsule. A typical muscle spindle contains two nuclear bag fibers and four or five nuclear chain fibers (figure 10.6). The significance of these differences has not been entirely ascertained, but it appears that bag and chain fibers contract at different rates when stimulated by their gamma motoneurons.

(A description of these motoneurons is provided below.)

Intrafusal muscle fibers are thin, striated fibers about one-fifth the diameter of extrafusal muscle fibers and interrupted in their middle by a noncontractible region. The muscle spindle lies parallel with the extrafusal muscle fibers, so it is stretched or contracted in tandem with them.

Intrafusal muscle fibers receive their mot innervation from a specialized group of efferent nerve fibers called gamma motoneurons. **Gamma motoneurons** are to be distinguished from the other type of motoneurons in the nervous system—skeletomotor neurons. The cell bodies of both skeletomotor neurons and gamma motoneurons lie in the ventral horn of the spinal cord and their axons leave the cord via the ventral root to join the spinal nerve. But gamma motoneurons end on the polar ends of intrafusal muscle fibers and produce contraction at these sites, putting stretch on the central equatorial region of the muscle spindle. The skeletomotor neurons, on the other hand, end at the neuromuscular junction of extrafusal muscle fibers and produce contraction of these muscle fibers. Gamma motoneurons account for about 40 percent of the motor axons in spinal nerves.

Muscle Spindle Receptors and Their Stimulation

There are two types of sensory receptors (or spindle afferents) in the muscle spindle. The primary receptor is called the **annulospiral ending** (or Ia fibers[2]) and it is located centrally within the spindle capsule. It is derived from a large, myelinated sensory neuron that subdivides and sends spirals around each of the intrafusal muscle fibers. The

---

[2] In the neurophysiology literature, afferent fibers from the muscle receptors are labelled Group I and II fibers. Group I comprises two subgroups: Group Ia, from the annulospiral endings of the muscle spindle, and Group Ib from the Golgi tendon organs. Group II fibers arise from the flower spray endings of muscle spindles.

secondary sense receptors are located on either side of the central region of the spindle and they attach to the intrafusal fibers from small, sensory neurons. They are called **flower-spray endings** (or II fibers) and are more localized on nuclear chain fibers than on bag fibers. In general, group Ia fibers are part of large, low-threshold, fast-conducting sensory neurons that are particularly sensitive to dynamic stretch, while the group II fibers tend to be small, high-threshold, slow-conducting, and much less sensitive to dynamic stretch (see figures 10.5 and 10.6).

As previously noted, the muscle spindle lies parallel with the extrafusal muscles, with its ends attached to the sheaths of the extrafusal muscle fibers, so that its length varies in accord with those of extrafusal muscles. The contractile portions of the intrafusal muscles occupy the polar regions of the muscle spindle, while contractile elements are absent near the middle of these fibers. Both of the spindle afferent groups are stimulated when the noncontractile region of the intrafusal muscles is stretched, causing a mechanical displacement of the sense endings. Spindle afferents can be stimulated in three different ways: (1) by application of an external force that lengthens the whole extrafusal muscle; (2) by contraction of intrafusal muscle fibers; (3) by reduction in the firing of extrafusal fibers (so that they relax). When any of these events occurs, the noncontractile region of intrafusal muscle fibers is displaced, the sense endings are stretched, and nerve impulses are discharged toward the CNS. We shall examine the effects of these impulses and then return for a fuller description of the methods for stimulating the spindle receptors.

Impulses from the spindle afferents are transmitted over sensory neurons and enter the spinal cord (or brainstem if they are from cranial nerves), where many of the collateral axons synapse on skeletomotor neurons that supply the extrafusal muscles in which the spindle is located. Impulses transmitted over skeletomotor neurons produce contraction in extrafusal muscle fibers.

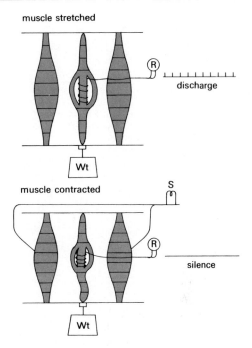

Figure 10.7 *Muscle spindle is arranged in parallel to muscle fibers. Thus muscle contraction slackens tension on the spindle.*

Other collateral fibers from the spindle afferents ascend the CNS pathways to end in the cerebellum and somatosensory projection area.

We can now return to a fuller discussion of methods by which the spindle afferents might be stimulated. As noted above, one means is the application of an external force that lengthens the whole muscle. Because muscle spindles are arranged in parallel with the extrafusal muscles, stretching of the extrafusal muscles (such as when an external force is applied) causes a stretch on the intrafusal fibers of the muscle spindle. This action displaces the spindle receptors, producing spindle afferent discharge. One of the effects of this spindle afferent discharge is to stimulate the skeletomotor neurons to produce contraction in the extrafusal fibers of that muscle, which reduces the stretch on the intrafusal muscle fibers, and the spindle afferents are silenced (figure 10.7).

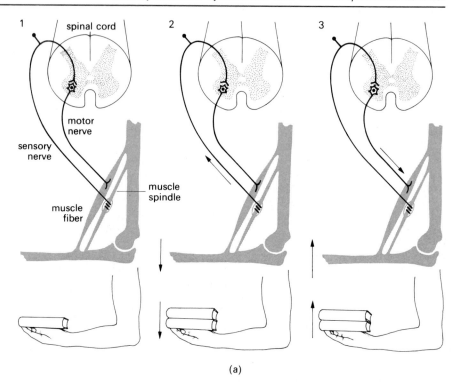

(a)

The knee jerk is an example of this phenomenon. When the patellar tendon is struck, the muscles in the thigh are stretched, including the muscle spindles. The spindle afferents discharge, transmitting their impulses to the spinal cord, where some synapse on skeletomotor neurons supplying the anterior thigh muscles. The skeletomotor neurons stimulate extrafusal muscles in the thigh, causing contraction of this muscle group, and lower-leg extension is the result.

Spindle afferents can be fired a second way and can indirectly control extrafusal muscle contraction without stretch stimuli being externally supplied. This is called the gamma loop and works in this way: Impulses transmitted over the gamma motoneurons produce intrafusal muscle contraction, which stretches the middle region of the intrafusals, stimulating spindle afferents, which in turn discharges impulses into the spinal cord (or brainstem). Many of these impulses synapse on

skeletomotor neurons that then send signals to the extrafusal fibers in the same muscles, producing extrafusal muscle contraction.

A third method for spindle afferent stimulation occurs through the coordination of both skeletomotor and gamma motoneurons. As previously noted, skeletomotor neuron discharge causes the extrafusal muscle fibers to contract, causing stretch to be taken off the muscle spindle that is in parallel with it; the result is that the spindle afferents will reduce or cease firing. However, if the gamma motoneurons cause intrafusal muscle contraction at the same time as the skeletomotor neurons cause extrafusal muscle contraction, the intrafusal muscle fibers will contract and "take up the slack" in the intrafusal fibers. Then, if there is a reduction in the firing of the skeletomotor neurons, the extrafusal muscle fibers begin to relax or lengthen. The result is that the spindle afferents are stimulated because the intrafusal fibers are stretched by the lengthening of the extrafusal fibers (figure 10.8).

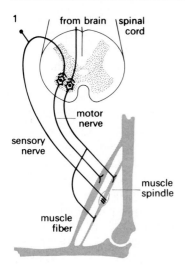

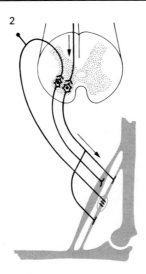

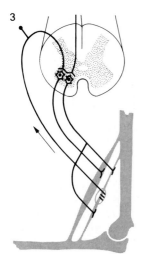

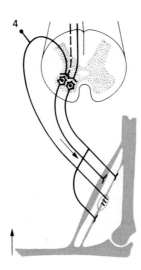

(b)

Figure 10.8 *In (a) the schematic illustration shows how the stretch reflex is mediated. A muscle is under the influence of the stretch reflex when it is engaged in a steady contraction of a voluntary nature, such as when a person's elbow is flexed steadily against a load (1). A sudden unexpected increase in the load (2) stretches the muscle, causing the sensory receptors in the muscle spindle to send nerve impulses to the spinal cord (upward arrow), where they impinge on a skeletomotor neuron at a synapse and excite it. As a result, motor impulses are sent to the extrafusal muscle (downward arrow), where they cause it to contract (3). More complicated nervous pathways than the one shown may also be involved in the stretch reflex. Any real muscle is, of course, supplied with many motoneuron fibers and spindles.*

In (b) the servomechanism involved in the control of voluntary muscle contractions is shown. The basic diagram (1) is the same as it is in the illustration of the stretch reflex, but with provision made for impulses from the brain to cause the intrafusal muscle fibers to contract by way of the gamma motoneurons. When a signal is transmitted along gamma motor fibers (2), the intrafusal muscle fibers contract, exciting the spindle sensory ending, just as if the spindle had been stretched. Consequently a contraction of the main muscle is excited by way of the gamma-loop (3, 4). In a real muscle this is further complicated by the existence of a direct pathway from the brain to the skeletomotor neurons.

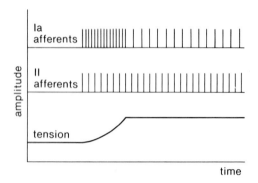

Figure 10.9   *Typical response patterns of (a) the Ia and (b) the II muscle spindle afferents to a single stretch (bottom trace). Note the Ia afferent adapts more rapidly than the II fiber.*

Static and Dynamic Responses of Muscle Spindle Receptors

Spindle afferent firing during stretch of a muscle is its dynamic response, while afferent firing at any constant length of the muscle is its static response. Both the group Ia and II spindle afferents are stimulated by stretching of the muscle, so they both give "length-sensitive" responses. However, they provide the CNS with different types of sensory information. The dynamic component of the signal predominates in the Ia afferents, meaning they respond extremely actively to a change in length, but a static component is also present, so the response to change of muscle length contains input relating to both the velocity of the stretch and its amplitude. Group II afferents provide primarily a static response to muscle length and give only a small dynamic response, so they function primarily as detectors of stretch amplitude, giving a regular, virtually nonadapting, firing pattern (figure 10.9).

Muscle Spindle Afferent Transmission in the CNS

For the past eighty years there has been a great deal of controversy about spindle afferent transmission within the CNS. While the transmission from spindle afferent to skeletomotor neurons for the production of reflex actions has been well documented for many years, this clearly is only a part of its central function. But whether the spindle afferent transmission also projected to higher centers has been unclear until rather recently.

Research over the past two decades indicates clearly that muscle afferents do in fact project to the somatosensory cortex, principally via the dorsal column system (Oscarsson and Rosen 1963; Phillips, Powell, and Wiesendanger 1971; Hore, et al. 1976). However, the fact that spindle afferent impulses project to the somatosensory projection area does not in itself confirm that the sensory information is consciously perceived. Indeed, there have been strong arguments that projections from muscle receptors do not subserve conscious awareness of position or movement. Instead, they are generally viewed as being used in the control of movement and posture without producing any conscious perception, in spite of projecting to the cerebral cortex. In rebuttal to these arguments, noted neurophysiologist D. I. McCloskey (1978, p. 777) said:

Of course, the sort of conscious experiences relevant in kinesthesia would not be sensations referable to the muscles themselves—for we are no more likely to feel kinesthetic sensations *in* our muscles or joints than we are to hear sounds *in* our heads or see objects *in* our retinas—but would be sensations of movement, or force, or tension, or of altered position in the parts moved *by* the muscles.

He concludes that the principal receptors subserving the senses of movement and position are the muscle receptors of the muscle spindles. The contribution of muscle receptors to kinesthesis will be taken up in more detail in the next chapter.

Muscle spindle afferent transmission to the cerebellum is carried over many fibers via the spinocerebellar tracts in the spinal cord, and over cranial nerves that synapse in the pons for spindle afferents from the head and neck muscles (figure 10.10). It has long been accepted that the cerebellum uses the spindle afferent information in

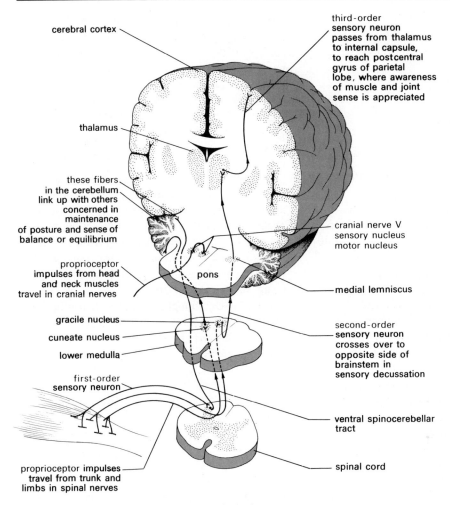

Figure 10.10   *Proprioceptive pathways to the brain.*

regulating muscle contraction because the effects of cerebellar damage show the great importance of this structure in motor regulation. However, precisely what it does, and how, remain mostly unknown. Knowledge about the use to which the cerebellum puts the input it receives from the spindle afferents is almost totally lacking.

The Golgi Tendon Organ

The **Golgi tendon organ** (GTO) (or group Ib fiber) is a muscle receptor concerned with detecting and signaling tension on a tendon. This receptor is usually found at the origin and insertion of a muscle, rather than in the tendon proper.

Figure 10.11   *Anatomy of the*
Golgi tendon apparatus.

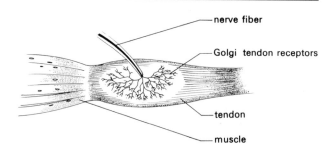

nerve fiber

Golgi tendon receptors

tendon

muscle

Golgi Tendon Organ Stimulation and Functions

The GTO is generally supplied by a single, myelinated axon of relatively large size (8–12 mμ). The main axon of each tendon organ divides into a series of nonmyelinated sprays, and each ending is enclosed in a delicate capsule that is closely applied to the surface of the musculotendon tissue. The GTO is arranged in series with muscle and tendon. When a muscle is stretched or when it contracts, it develops forces that are applied to GTOs, causing them to be stimulated. It is the distortion of the endings that results in the discharge of these receptors. The GTO acts, then, as a tension receptor, in contrast to the in-parallel length and velocity detection of the muscle spindle system (figure 10.11).

Simple passive stretch of a noncontracting muscle stimulates GTOs only when considerable tension has built up and the muscle stretched beyond its normal length. But the threshold to GTOs is very low for active muscle contractions. The adequate stimulus is the contraction of motor units with fibers directly in series with the GTO. This occurs because the force of muscle contraction is transferred more effectively to the GTO than is the force of muscle stretch (Houk and Henneman 1967; Proske 1979).

Since GTOs have a low threshold for tension produced by muscle contraction at the musculotendinous junction, they actually participate in the instantaneous movement of feedback of proprioception information to the CNS. The GTO, therefore, continuously provides information about the degree of active contraction in the muscle. Houk and Henneman (1967) note that "tendon organs continuously transmit to the spinal cord a filtered sample of the active forces being produced in the muscle." As a consequence, GTOs "can provide accurate feedback to the nervous system about the force being developed by individual muscles under both static and dynamic conditions" (Crago, Houk, and Rymer 1982).

Golgi Tendon Organ Transmission in the CNS

Golgi tendon fibers enter the CNS and some synapse on spinal neurons, while collateral fibers ascend the spinal cord and enter the brain. The latter have a fairly direct route via the spinocerebellar tract to the cerebellum, but the projection of tendon organ afferents to cortical projection areas is still unclear. If there are such projections, the receptive areas are most likely the same as for the spindle afferents.

The tendon organs appear not to have any part in the development of our immediate consciousness of the position of body parts, but they are important components of the proprioceptor system. They work cooperatively with other receptors in muscles and joints to signal forces acting in these structures during movement.

Joint Receptors

In the joints throughout the body are receptors that are stimulated when the bones move in any direction. Some authors call these kinesthetic receptors, but others refer to them as **joint receptors.** We shall use the latter term.

Joint Receptor Types and Stimulation

Three structurally different types of receptor groups are located in the tissue around joints. The first is a "spray"-type of ending, located in the joint capsule, which resembles those found in the GTO (Bannister 1976); the second is a modified Pacinian corpuscle found mostly near articular or ligamentous attachments; the third is a Golgi-type ending located in ligaments of the joint. There are also free nerve endings. The spray-type endings are *tonic,* or slowly adapting, while the Pacinian endings are *phasic,* or rapidly adapting receptors. The Golgi-type endings and free nerve endings are not clearly delineated in adaptation.

Joint Transmission in the CNS

Joint afferent fibers enter the CNS and ascend to the thalamus and somatosensory cortex in a manner similar to other somatosensory afferents. Joint afferents have a particularly diverse collateral system that, in addition to supplying a rich input to the cerebellum, actually reaches interneurons at all levels of the CNS. These interneurons typically receive convergent input from other somatosensory afferents, making it difficult to specify an exclusive perceptual role for joint receptors (Clark, Landgren, and Silfvenius 1973).

Joint Receptor Function

Until quite recently joint receptors were believed to supply the principal input for the perception of limb and body position during movement. Research over the past decade has shown that joint receptors alone do not signal steady joint angle over the entire range of limb movement (Matthews 1977; McCloskey 1978). Rapidly adapting

joint receptors fire during movement of the joint, but these receptors are unlikely to provide detailed information about joint position, velocity of joint movement, or even direction of movement. They may simply help to signal the occurance of movement without signaling details of its nature. Most slow adapting joint receptors have maximal firing rates at extreme flexion or extension of the joint. Thus they are unsuitable for supplying input about the entire range of steady joint positions. But, according to Tracey (1980), they could act as "limit detectors." According to him, joint receptors in the hip could "signal the end of the flexion phase of the step cycle; their reflex effect might help to terminate activity in the appropriate flexion muscles, and contribute to the initiation of the extension phase of the step cycle."

The Vestibular Apparatus

One important aspect of the proprioceptive sense is not obtained from muscle, tendon, or joint action, but takes place in the vestibular apparatus, located adjacent to the inner ear. The **vestibular apparatus** is a part of the membranous labyrinth inside the temporal lobe in the inner ear. One part of the bony membranous labyrinth is concerned with hearing. This part is contained in the cochlea. The other part, the vestibular apparatus, is made up of two kinds of receptors: semicircular canals, which respond to angular acceleration, and otolith organs, which respond to linear acceleration (figure 10.12).

The vestibular apparatus is sensitive to two kinds of information. It is sensitive to the position of the head in space, that is, it signals whether the head is upright, upside down, or in some other position. Second, it is sensitive to sudden changes in direction of movement of the body. The vestibular system is sometimes classified as part or the visual system because one of its functions is to assist in visual fixation during head and body

Figure 10.12   *The vestibular apparatus consists of a series of fluid-filled sacs and ducts. The three semicircular canals are at the left; they are oriented in the three planes of space and respond to angular accelerations of the head. In the center are the two otolith receptors: the utricle and saccule. Each semicircular canal has a bulge, the ampulla. At the lower right in the figure is the cochlea, the receptor for hearing.*

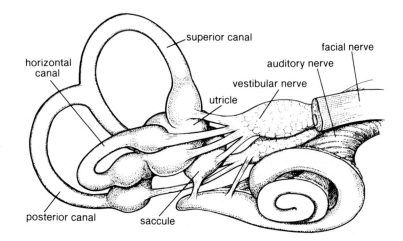

movements. At other times it is classified with the auditory system, presumably because it is in close proximity to the auditory system and both systems are connected to the CNS by the same cranial nerve. We have followed the example of most texts, placing this mechanism with the proprioceptors, since the underlying function of the vestibular apparatus is to maintain equilibrium and to preserve a constant plane of head position primarily by modifying muscle tone, in addition to directing the gaze of the eyes.

The Semicircular Canals

The **semicircular canals** can be viewed as angular accelerometers because they lie in planes at right angles to each other and are stimulated by rotations of the head in any one of three planes or in any combination of the three. Each canal is filled with fluid endolymph and has a bulge, the ampulla, which contains a patch of hair cells embedded in a crest-shaped surface, the crista. The hair cells project fingerlike processes upward into a gelatinous membrane called the cupula. The hair processes embedded in the cupula constitute the sense endings in the semicircular canals (figure 10.13).

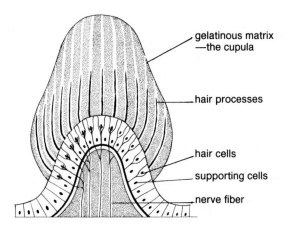

Figure 10.13   *The crista ampullaris and the cupula in which the hair processes are embedded.*

This arrangement of sensory receptors in the semicircular canals functions so that whenever the head undergoes angular or rotary acceleration or deceleration, the sense endings are mechanically displaced. The hair cells to which they are attached then transduce movement of the fluid into nerve impulses. If the head is moved, inertia causes the fluid to move in a direction opposite that of the movement. When the cupula bends to the side, it excites the hair cells to initiate nerve

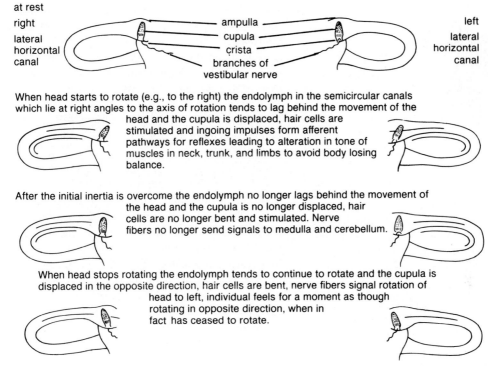

When head starts to rotate (e.g., to the right) the endolymph in the semicircular canals which lie at right angles to the axis of rotation tends to lag behind the movement of the head and the cupula is displaced, hair cells are stimulated and ingoing impulses form afferent pathways for reflexes leading to alteration in tone of muscles in neck, trunk, and limbs to avoid body losing balance.

After the initial inertia is overcome the endolymph no longer lags behind the movement of the head and the cupula is no longer displaced, hair cells are no longer bent and stimulated. Nerve fibers no longer send signals to medulla and cerebellum.

When head stops rotating the endolymph tends to continue to rotate and the cupula is displaced in the opposite direction, hair cells are bent, nerve fibers signal rotation of head to left, individual feels for a moment as though rotating in opposite direction, when in fact has ceased to rotate.

Figure 10.14   *Diagram of how movement stimulates receptors in the semicircular canals.*

impulses. If the movement stops, the fluid continues to flow momentarily and the cupula is bent in the opposite direction. So the maximum stimulation of the hair cells occurs when the inertia is greatest, that is, when motion is starting or ending. If motion is continued at a steady rate in the same direction, such as while riding in an automobile, then very little semicircular sensation occurs (figure 10.14).

Excitation of the semicircular canals occurs primarily from acceleration or deceleration and change of direction. These structures apprise the nervous system of sudden changes in movement. This information allows certain brain centers to make necessary balance adjustments, sometimes even before imbalance occurs. Such adjustments are essential in movement activities where direction changes occur rapidly.

Finally, since the semicircular canals achieve maximum sensitivity for rotary acceleration and deceleration, they sacrifice sensitivity to linear acceleration and deceleration. Other parts of the vestibular apparatus are maximally activated by linear movements.

The Otolith Organs

Otolith organs are two similar fluid-filled saclike structures, the **utricle** and the **saccule.** Each organ has a patch of hairs known as the macula. In the utricle the patch is approximately horizontal in the upright head, but in the saccule it is approximately vertical. In the utricle the hairs project upward into the gelatinous otalith membrane, while in the saccule they project sideways. Many tiny calcium carbonate crystals are embedded

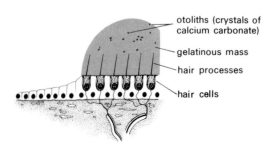

Figure 10.15   *The utricle and saccule structure.*

within the otolith membrane (figure 10.15). The density of the otolith membrane is about three times that of the canal fluid. When the head suddenly undergoes change, the otolith membrane, having greater inertia than the fluid in the canal, bends the hair tufts to one side—much as the bristles of a brush bend backward when the brush is moved across a surface. This bending initiates impulses in adjoining nerve cells that are then transmitted into the brain.

The utricle and saccule operate differently and give information different from that of the semicircular canals, although the receptor cells of these structures are very similar to those in the semicircular canals. The information signaled by these structures is mainly concerned with body position in relation to the force of gravity. They respond to linear acceleration, that is, movement of the head in a straight line: forward, backward, upward, downward, or tilting of the head. They do this by responding to changes in the position of the head in space.

Since the hair cells of the utricle are set on a horizontal plane (whereas those of the saccule lie on a vertical plane), the utricle is maximally stimulated when the head is bent either forward or backward, and is minimally excited when the the head is erect. The saccule appears to be maximally stimulated when the head is bent to the side and when the body is raised or lowered in space. So it is believed that the utricle supplies information about disturbances to equilibrium by shifting forward and back, while the saccule supplies such information by tilting laterally or by upward and downward motion.

Vestibular Transmission in the CNS

The movement of hairs in either the semicircular canals or otolith organs sets off afferent transmission that projects via the eighth cranial nerve into the CNS. First-order fibers leading from the hair cells of the semicircular canals, utricle, and saccule project into the medulla as the vestibular branch of the eighth cranial nerve just below the pons. The vestibular nerve on each side passes to four vestibular nuclei in the medulla and pons of the brainstem. The names of the four vestibular nuclei are superior, medial, lateral, and spinal vestibular nuclei. With one exception, the first-order fibers synapse in one of these four nuclei. The exception is that some first-order fibers lead directly to the cerebellum (figure 10.16). However, the widespread vestibular innervation with the cerebellum comes mostly through second-order neurons via the vestibular nuclei.

Second- and third-order nerve pathways that connect the vestibular apparatus with the brain and spinal cord are complex and not as well traced as those for the other somatosensory pathways. Moreover, since the nuclei that receive vestibular input are multimodal—meaning they also receive input from visual and other somatosensory sources—it is difficult to isolate a pure vestibular input beyond the first-order neurons.

At the present it does not appear that vestibular pathways mediate directly with the thalamus for cortical projection. There is evidence, though, that vestibular input does arrive indirectly in a limited area of the cerebral cortex that

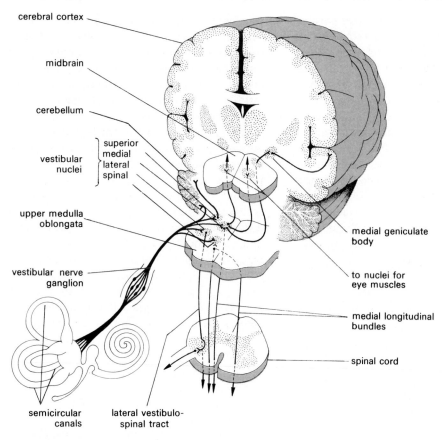

cerebral cortex

midbrain

cerebellum

vestibular
nuclei
{ superior
medial
lateral
spinal }

upper medulla
oblongata

vestibular nerve
ganglion

semicircular
canals

lateral vestibulo-
spinal tract

medial geniculate
body

to nuclei for
eye muscles

medial longitudinal
bundles

spinal cord

Figure 10.16   *The vestibular pathways of impulse
transmission.*

is contiguous with the somatosensory cortex. In contrast to the visual and auditory systems, the vestibular system does not appear to fit the scheme of sensory modality specificity because, in monkeys, some 80 percent of the vestibular cortex neurons are also influenced by muscle spindle and joint afferents. Central convergence of these two modalities of proprioceptive afferents is apparently essential not only for lower reflex mechanisms, but also for the conscious perception of position and movement (Abraham 1977).

Vestibular Function

Most vestibular apparatus input is used for reflex purposes. In most cases it is limited to reflex movements of the head and neck in coordination with eye-muscle movements. One of the simplest functions of vestibular input is its action to stabilize the eyes. When a person rotates about the body axis, the eyes perform a series of slow movements in a direction opposite to the rotation, with alternating, quick return sweeps. This is called the nystagnus reflex. The slow phase serves to retain a stationary image on the retina. The quick phase occurs when it becomes no longer possible to fixate on an object because of the rotation and the eyes' sweep forward to fixate on a new object.

Input from the vestibular apparatus also plays a critical part in the maintenance of our upright posture and equilibrium. Impulses from the vestibulospinal tract exert a strong tonic effect on the antigravity muscles. Damage to or severance of the fiber tracts above the vestibular nuclei has the effect of eliminating the central inhibitory control, which is normally maintained by cortical and subcortical mechanisms above the level of the vestibular nuclei. The result is an exaggerated extensor thrust (contraction of postural muscles). The individual becomes completely rigid, which is known as decerebrate rigidity.

Righting reflexes are primarily mediated by the vestibular apparatus. These righting reflexes dominate other sensory and motor systems and are a powerful force in maintaining the body in an upright position. The head takes the lead in the righting reflex. Once the head orientation occurs, reflexes for orienting neck, shoulders, and body follow in sequential order. The righting reflexes will be discussed in more detail in chapter 13.

Coordination of Other Proprioceptors with the Vestibular Apparatus

The specification of vestibular function is difficult because vestibular input is only one source of information for a multimodal system of balance and space orientation. For example, the detection of the position of the body in space is not just a function of the vestibular apparatus. One of the most important information mechanisms necessary for the maintenance of equilibrium is that derived from joint and muscle spindle receptors in the neck. These proprioceptors in the neck apprise the CNS of the orientation of the head with respect to the body. When the head is bent forward or backward, the vestibular system sends information on the position of the head. Simultaneously, proprioceptors in the neck send information that the head is angulating in relation to the rest of the body. The information is processed by the higher brain centers, and necessary muscular adjustments are made, after coordination of the two sets of data. Thus, while the vestibular apparatus detects head position, additional information is required because the relationship of the head to the body must be known. Proprioceptors in the neck supply this essential information and are, therefore, as necessary for regulating equilibrium as are the reflexes initiated in the vestibular apparatus. In addition, vision and pressure sensations from the footpads also play important roles in the orientation of the body in space. Indeed, it appears that vision normally provides the most sensitive information for balance control (Lee 1978).[3] However, the vestibular apparatus and other proprioceptors will bring about righting reflexes even if the visual receptors or pressure receptors in the feet are damaged or destroyed.

All of the proprioceptors provide sensory data that, when organized and combined with information mainly from the cerebellum (for equilibrium), provide the basis for movement patterns, muscle tone, and the stimulation of muscles for upright bodily posture.

---

[3] One can verify the contribution that vision makes to balance by standing on one leg, hands on hips, with eyes open, and then closing the eyes. Body sway increases and balance becomes unstable once the eyes are closed.

Summary

The word *somatosensory* refers to sensations from the body. Somatosensory receptors are found in the skin, tendons, muscles, joints, and vestibular apparatus. Somatosensory receptors are divided into two general categories, cutaneous receptors and proprioceptors. The former are found near the skin and stimulation of them produces sensations for touch-pressure, heat, cold, and pain. Proprioceptors are found in the muscles, tendons, joints, and vestibular apparatus, and the impressions from these receptors are known as kinesthetic perceptions.

Cutaneous sensitivity is not uniformly distributed over the body, so two-point discrimination is quite different in the various parts of the body.

There are two basic somatosensory pathways to the brain, the dorsal column system and the spinothalamic system. The part of the cerebral cortex to which somatosensory signals are transmitted is found in the parietal lobe and is called the somatosensory projection area. Somatosensory signals pass from the somatosensory projection area into association areas where the input is interpreted into the "meaning" of the sensations.

Muscle proprioceptors in skeletal muscles are the muscle spindles and Golgi tendon organs (GTO). The muscle spindle is a fluid-filled capsule containing specialized mechanoreceptors and intrafusal muscle fibers. Spindle receptors are sensitive to stretch on a muscle. Whenever the spindle receptors are displaced, they fire off and send spindle afferent information to the CNS. Since the muscle spindle lies in parallel with the extrafusal muscle fibers, any stretch on these fibers will fire the spindle afferents. A motor supply to the intrafusal muscle fibers via gamma motoneurons can cause intrafusal muscle contraction and thus produce spindle afferent firing.

The GTO is a muscle receptor concerned with detecting and signaling tension on a tendon. It was once believed that the only function of the GTO was as a reflex protective mechanism for the muscle. It is now known that this receptor contributes input for kinesthetic perception.

Joint receptors are found in all the joints of the body. Until recently, joint receptors were believed to supply the principal input for perception of limb and body position during movement. This view has been revised and it now appears that spindle afferents contribute significantly to kinesthesis, while joint receptors play only a supporting role.

The vestibular apparatus is part of the membranous labyrinth inside the temporal lobe of the inner ear. It is made up of two kinds of receptors, semicircular canals and otolith organs. The vestibular apparatus is sensitive to the position of the head in space and to sudden changes in direction of movement of the body. It functions to maintain equilibrium and to preserve a constant plane of head position.

11

Kinesthesis and Motor Behavior

*T*he perceptual experience that arises from stimulation of the proprioceptors is called kinesthesis. Motor skills instructors frequently assume that kinesthesis is an important sensory modality for motor learning and performance. They often attempt to induce learners to use kinesthesis as a cue while learning and performing motor tasks. Students may be asked to concentrate on "getting the feel" of the correct movements as they perform. Or they may be placed in correct beginning or terminal positions for a given task and asked to "sense" the limb positions and muscular contractions. In recent years various weighted objects have been used in motor skill instruction in the belief that the kinesthetic perceptual illusions that occur when the normal weight objects are subsequently used in performing the task will produce improved performances. These various methods are examples of attempts to utilize kinesthesis for learning and performance.

In this chapter we shall examine the various dimensions of kinesthesis and review the findings with respect to the relationship between kinesthesis and motor behavior.

Definition of Kinesthesis

The word *kinesthesis* was coined by Bastian (1888) and derives from the two Greek words meaning "to move" and "sensation." The word **proprioception** has often been used interchangeably with kinesthesis because Sherrington (1906) included the sense of movement along with the sensing of tensions, pressures, forces, and bodily orientation in space that might not involve any movement at all. There have been frequent attempts to redefine kinesthesis in more exact ways. Some have attempted to limit kinesthesis to information about the joint receptors (Smith 1969), while others have suggested an extension rather than a restriction of the concept. For example, Gibson (1966) argued that kinesthesis should be viewed as "the obtaining of information about one's own action" regardless of the sensory modalities involved. He suggested that it is a fallacy to ascribe kinesthesis to proprioceptors because information concerned with movement can be obtained through many sensory systems.

Given that some difference of opinion exists as to what constitutes kinesthesis, for our purposes **kinesthesis** is the discrimination of the positions and movements of body parts based on information other than visual or auditory. The immediate stimuli arise from changes in length and from tension, compression, and shear forces arising from the effects of gravity, from relative movement of body parts, and from muscular contraction. It includes the discrimination of the position of body parts and the discrimination of movement and amplitude of movement of body parts, both passively and actively produced (Howard and Templeton 1966).

Neural Mechanisms for Kinesthesis

In spite of years of study and research, kinesthesis is not fully understood either physiologically or psychologically. Although the classes of afferent receptors that are candidates for subserving

kinesthesis are those from the skin, muscles, tendons, joints, and vestibular apparatus, and although there is a fairly complete picture of their structures and transmission pathways, considerable confusion exists with regard to the exact role that each receptor type plays in kinesthesis.

As noted in the previous chapter, each of the somatosensory receptors is structurally different and responds to different types of stimuli. It is therefore rather obvious that each would have a different role in providing input to the brain for translation into perceptions.

Muscle Receptors and Kinesthesis

Muscle spindle afferents and Golgi tendon organs constitute the **muscle receptors.** The role of spindle afferents in kinesthesis has been quite controversial for the past century. Perhaps the first investigator to attempt to identify the sources of information for kinesthesis was Goldscheider (1889), who anesthetized the joints of the index finger and concluded that impulses arising from the joints were the most important, but that input from muscles and tendons also played a role. Similar experiments conducted in the 1950s and 60s downgraded the role of the muscle receptors and emphasized the importance of the joint receptors. Two neuroscientists stated: "There is . . . no evidence for and strong evidence against the notion that impulses provoked by stretch receptors in muscles provide information for perception of movement or position of the joints" (Rose and Mountcastle 1959). Other investigators came to the same conclusion. Gelfan and Carter (1967) stretched the muscles of subjects who were undergoing minor types of surgery by pulling on their exposed tendons with forceps, thus permitting activation of muscle stretch receptors and tendon end organs. Since none of the subjects experienced any sensation referable to the muscles, the investigators concluded that "there is no muscle sense in man," meaning that there is no conscious awareness of muscle length or change of muscle length as a result of muscle afferent discharges.

The case against the role of muscle receptors in kinesthesis was based on a variety of research findings in addition to those in which subjects failed to preceive when exposed muscles were pulled on during surgery. The strongest case against the muscle receptors subserving kinesthesis prior to 1970, however, was the failure to demonstrate cortical projections of muscle afferents. This served to bolster the view that these receptors did not provide input that gained access to consciousness.

At the same time, a primary role for **joint receptors** in kinesthesis was accumulating based on findings that joint receptors had the appropriate stimulation properties to signal joint movement or limb position over the whole range of movement (Andrew and Dodt 1953; Boyd and Roberts 1953; Skoglund 1956). By the end of the 1960s the view that kinesthesis was a function exclusively of the joint receptors had become a kind of dogma (Mountcastle and Darian-Smith 1968; Smith 1969).

Investigations over the past fifteen years, using new experimental techniques and more sophisticated equipment, have brought about a complete revision of the roles of muscle and joint receptors in kinesthesis. The result has been an upgrading of the role of the muscle receptors. We now have compelling evidence that muscle receptors contribute significantly to kinesthesis. So much evidence had accumulated by 1975 that noted neuroscientist Per Ebbe Roland (1975) could state that "during voluntary contractions we receive precise conscious information about applied force and angular movements from the musculo-tendinous receptors." More recently, in an exhaustive review of the literature concerning the role of the muscle receptors in kinesthesis, Matthews (1982) concluded that muscle "afferents are now reasonably established as contributing to muscle sense. . . . The spindle primaries (Ia fibers) probably contribute mainly movement information; the secondaries (II fibers) relatively

more of positional information . . . and the tendon organs, sensations of force." (In another review of kinesthesis in the same publication, Burgess et al. [1982] came to the same conclusion.)

One of the major breakthroughs responsible for the revision of the role of the muscle afferents in kinesthesis was the discovery of projections of muscle receptors to the deep folds of the somatosensory cortex in a number of related species, and undoubtedly in humans, that had not been located by earlier researchers (Phillips, Powell, and Wiesendanger 1971; Heath, Hore, and Phillips 1976; Hore et al. 1976). According to McCloskey (1978), "The signals of both velocity and position contained, but differently mixed, in the discharges of spindle primaries and secondaries can be processed to give, at a cortical level, a firing rate related only to velocity or only to position."

The contribution of Golgi tendon organs to kinesthesis is still uncertain, but the fact that tendon organ signals reach consciousness has recently been discovered (Roland and Ladegaard-Peterson 1977). Since it is now well established that muscle receptors not only provide kinesthetic perceptions of movement and positions and that they also provide signals perceived as intramuscular tension, the converging evidence suggests that force information is derived from tendon organs signaling the tension in the muscle (Crago, Houk, and Rymer 1982). In his review, Matthews (1982) concludes that "the awareness of 'force' must be attributed to muscle receptors and probably to the tendon organs." It appears, then, that tendon organs are important contributors to kinesthesis, working cooperatively with other proprioceptors in muscles and joints to signal the forces acting in these structures during motor activity.

Sensation of Weight

While sensations of force appear to be attributable to tendon organs, the discharges of these or other muscle and joint receptors are not used for the subjective estimation of the weight of lifted objects or for the perception of effort in the performance of a motor task (McCloskey, Ebeling, and Goodwin 1974; Matthews 1982). Instead, "corollary discharges" sent from motor centers to sensory centers at the time that centrally generated motor commands are sent to lower centers appear to produce perceptions of weight. Within the CNS it is known that axons from the motor cortex send collaterals to spinal neurons projecting to sensory centers—the dorsal column relay nuclei, various thalamic nuclei, and the somatosensory projection area itself (Wiesendanger 1969). This corollary transmission produces the judgments of muscular tensions and the weight of lifted objects (Gandevia and McCloskey 1977).

Joint Receptors and Kinesthesis

As noted in the previous section, during the 1950s and 60s many neuroscientists considered joint receptors the major input source for kinesthesis. Some claimed that they were the sole mechanism for this form of perception. The evidence for this view was derived from studies that appeared to show that during movement certain joint receptors fired over only a limited range of joint angle. These ranges overlapped in such a way that the whole extent of joint movement was covered, with at least one receptor firing at any given joint angle (Andrew and Dodt 1953; Boyd and Roberts 1953; Skoglund 1956).

The observations on coding of joint angle and acceleration by the joint receptors were challenged by Burgess and Clark (1969), who showed that in a sample of 209 joint receptors only four were specifically stimulated at intermediate joint positions. All the others were fired either at full flexion or full extension, and often at both. The investigators concluded that joint receptors "are

not capable of providing appreciable steady-state position information over most of the working range." These results have been confirmed by other investigators (Grigg 1975; Lundberg, Malmgren, and Schomburg 1975; Millar 1975; Grigg and Greenspan 1977). The discrepancy between the earlier findings and the more recent work is the result of different experimental preparations. The earlier preparations caused the firing of joint receptors at intermediate joint angles that would normally only be stimulated at extreme angles (Grigg 1975).

Other evidence has cast suspicion on the role of joint receptors in kinesthesis. Early researchers had reported that anesthetizing both joint and skin receptors diminished kinesthesis a great deal in the affected part. They concluded that joint receptors were therefore the most important receptors for kinesthesis. But recent findings demonstrate that skin receptors can signal joint position, so these receptors are now viewed as more important to kinesthesis than previously believed (Knibestol 1975). Perhaps the most damaging evidence to the role of joint receptors has been prosthetic surgery. Here the whole joint capsule, with its receptors, is often removed. Typically, total replacement of joints with prostheses causes only minimal kinesthetic dysfunction.

The recent findings that joint receptors alone cannot signal steady joint angle over the whole range of limb movement and that removal of joint receptors with prosthetic surgery does not impair greatly kinesthesis at a joint has resulted in a downgrading of the role of joint receptors in kinesthesis. This view does not preclude, however, the possibility—even the likelihood—that afferents from joints may contribute to position and movement sense. The receptors may be capable of signaling information on the velocity and acceleration of joint movement, or even the forces generated by muscles acting at the joint, rather than steady-state-joint angulation or position. However, we have little evidence of this at this time (McCloskey 1978).

Joint information reaches the somatosensory cortex and therefore has the potential to contribute to perception. What seems likely is that joint receptors activated by a particular movement are integrated in the CNS with signals from other somatosensory receptors. The exact process by which this occurs has not been determined, but recent "evidence excludes the possibility that the joint afferents can be allocated an exclusive role in kinesthesia" (Matthews 1982). Instead, the joint receptors "appear to contribute to the deep pressure sensations that occur toward the end of a joint's range" (Burgess et al. 1982).

Cutaneous Receptors and Kinesthesis

Very little is known about the contribution of the skin receptors to kinesthesis. But recent research suggests that these receptors may be more important than has traditionally been believed. Slowly adapting **cutaneous receptors** suitable for providing kinesthetic information have been identified in lower animals as well as humans (Knibestol and Vallbo 1970; Chambers et al. 1972). Knibestol (1975) has demonstrated that skin receptors in the human finger can signal joint angle over a wide range, suggesting a kinesthetic role for cutaneous receptors.

When both joints and skin are anesthetized, there is a pronounced impairment in the appreciation of position and movement (Provins 1958; Gandevia and McCloskey, 1976), but kinesthesis is preserved when joint receptors only are anesthetized (Cross and McCloskey 1973; Grigg, Finerman, and Riley 1973; Clark and Burgess 1975). These findings suggest that cutaneous receptors have a role in kinesthesis, but it is not yet clear whether the role is specific to joint position or movement or whether it is less specific and merely supports or facilitates the specific kinesthetic information from muscle receptors and joint receptors.

Vestibular Apparatus and Kinesthesis

In many respects the vestibular apparatus is a sensory system without a home. The receptors of this mechanism are usually not considered part of the exteroceptors (vision, hearing, taste, cutaneous), and many neuroscientists omit them from the proprioceptor category. Their major function, though, is concerned with sensing bodily position and movement. So we give them a home here, as do many other writers, with the receptors for position and movement sense.

The major functions of the vestibular receptors are carried out reflexively. But their signals indirectly project to the cerebral cortex, suggesting a potential role in perception. Interpretations of lateral, horizontal, and vertical movement as well as bodily orientation in space are the likely outcomes of vestibular afferent information, although postural orientation may not depend solely on vestibular input (Howard and Templeton 1966). Indeed, Lee (1978) has demonstrated that visual information appears to dominate vestibular function in the control of balance.

Integration of Receptor Inputs for Kinesthesis

Receptors in the skin, joints, muscles and tendons, and vestibular apparatus contribute to movement and position sense. Cutaneous receptors appear to support and facilitate signals from the muscle and joint receptors, and may even provide specific perceptions of joint position and movement, especially in distal joints. The role of joint receptors in kinesthesis is problematic, but they appear to provide some central facilitation for signals from muscle receptors. The muscle receptors appear to be the principal receptors for the sense of joint movement and position, with spindle Ia afferents concerned primarily with signaling movement, the group II afferents with position, and the GTOs with force. Bodily orientation and movement in space and posture are signaled by the vestibular apparatus.

Even though each receptor type is stimulated differently and presumably signals a distinct aspect of movement, position, and force, the similarity in structure of receptors in muscles, tendons, skin, and joints, together with the growing belief that input from all these receptor types are important to kinesthesis, suggests that input from all those receptors activated by a particular movement at a joint may be combined and integrated in the CNS. It has been demonstrated that skin, muscle, tendon, and joint signals do converge at the spinal level (Lundberg, Malmgren, and Schomburg 1975).

All of the mechanoreceptors project to the somatosensory cortex, and several of the afferent types also project to the motor cortex, particularly those from muscles and joints. But the way in which position and movement perception are represented by the firing of cells in various areas of the cortex is known only vaguely. Consequently, there is little understanding of how information from the different receptors is combined and integrated. But the importance of combined inputs from a number of different receptors has become increasingly clear (Marsden, Merton, and Morton 1972; Evarts and Tanji 1976). It appears that joint, muscle, and cutaneous afferents have separate but convergent projections to the somatosensory projection area. As one example, the somatosensory projection area that contains the richest input from joints appears also to receive input as a collateral from the projection area that receives mainly inputs from muscle afferents (Goodwin 1976).

It appears, then, that the CNS orchestrates the information from the skin and proprioceptors by combining and integrating the input in some way to resolve the ambiguity by any one set of receptors, thus providing very accurate perceptions about body position, movement, and force.

Measurement of Kinesthesis

The past century has witnessed varying degrees of scientific interest in kinesthesis. During the latter years of the nineteenth century and first few years of the twentieth, interest in this topic reached a peak, then waned for several years. Advancements in electrical instrumentation in the past twenty-five years have spurred electrophysiological studies, and a considerable body of information has been added to our understanding of kinesthesis.

In the peak period mentioned above, investigators of kinesthesis studied primarily the psychophysical dimensions of this phenomenon. They attempted to determine minimum angular displacement and minimum velocity of movement thresholds for various parts of the body. Traditionally, movements of constant angular velocity were imposed on a joint, and subjects were asked to indicate when they were confident that a movement had occurred. This method was introduced by Goldsheider (1889), who measured joint thresholds using himself as the subject. He reported that the shoulder and hip joints had the lowest thresholds for passive movements. Sensitivity in the proximal joints, such as the shoulder and hip, according to Goldscheider, exceeded that of the distal joints, such as the fingers and toes. Subsequent psychophysical studies on joint thresholds have fairly consistently replicated Goldscheider's results.

A weakness in the studies that have established movement thresholds using passive movements is that active, or voluntary, movement may create a different pattern of kinesthetic information because of the greater tension and stretch on the proprioceptors. Lloyd and Caldwell (1965) studied the difference between passive and active positioning movements on the lower leg. They found that active movements of the lower leg produced greater accuracy of positioning than passive movements in the middle ranges of movement

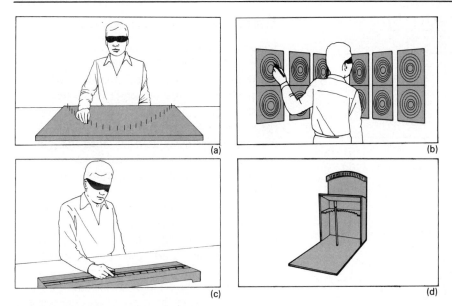

Figure 11.1 *Kinesthetic tests of accuracy of positioning movements. The tests require a blindfolded subject to (a) touch a certain peg or (b) mark a certain target, in response to verbal instructions. In tests (c) and (d), respectively, the subject reproduces certain movements with a knob or a stick control.*

(the full range was from full extension of the leg to 100 degrees of flexion), but not for the positioning near the extreme parts of the range.

In addition to the interest psychologists have shown in the psychophysical dimensions of kinesthesis, physical educators and human factors engineers have been quite interested in the precision with which individuals can position and move their bodies on the basis of proprioceptive information. They have developed tests that attempt to measure kinesthesis from dimensions other than its psychophysical properties.

Tests of kinesthesis most frequently used in investigations by physical educators have been composed of tasks requiring a blindfolded subject to assume or reproduce a prescribed arm or leg position in the vertical or horizontal planes, make discriminations of balance and orientation of the body and its parts in space, and make discriminations of force and extent of muscular contraction (figure 11.1). For example, Scott's (1955) tests of kinesthesis (all are done blindfolded) include:

1. **Lower leg flexion**
   Standing on one foot, knee pointing downward, flex lower leg of free foot until lower leg is horizontal (90 degrees).
   Score = deviation from 90 degrees.

2. **Wrist flexion**
   Forearm supported on table, hand relaxed over edge. Extend wrist according to model (20 degrees) flexion. Score = deviation from 20 degrees.

3. **Target pointing**
   Standing sideways to target, pointer in hand. Raise pointer to target.
   Score = deviation from center of target.

Table 11.1   Intercorrelations of Tests of Kinesthesis

	1	2	3	4	5	6
1		−04	−02	−09	19	−01
2			−13	02	02	02
3				−01	07	−08
4					04	08
5						07
6						

Activity
1. Shoulder-sagittal
2. Shoulder-horizontal
3. Knee
4. Veering
5. Balance-dynamic
6. Balance-static

Source: Adapted from Temple and Williams 1977.
Note: Decimal points have been omitted.

During the past decade researchers studying kinesthesis have frequently used a linear positioning task for joint position. This task was described in detail in chapter 2 (also see figure 2.10).

Efforts to find a general kinesthetic perceptual ability have been disappointing. Performance measures, such as the ability to direct a limb to a given point or maintain balance on a narrow support, tend to indicate little relationship among items on kinesthetic measures. In one of the earliest studies of the relationship between items on a kinesthetic test battery, Wiebe (1954) obtained low correlations on a twenty-one-item test battery, indicating that the various test items were not measuring the same quality. He concluded that there was no general kinesthetic sense. Rose and Glad (1974) also reported low intercorrelations among nine tests of kinesthesis. Recently, Temple and Williams (1977) correlated performances on several kinesthetic test items: three movement reproduction items, a veering item, and two balance items. The intercorrelations are shown in table 11.1. These findings suggest that kinesthesis is certainly not a general ability. Instead, it comprises a number of specific abilities.

Factors Affecting Kinesthesis

Kinesthetic detection thresholds are influenced by several variables. How the limbs are held during testing periods has been found to influence threshold. Sensitivity to weight is greatest when the shoulder is the fulcrum and is poorer when the weight is lifted from the wrist. Elbow-joint movement sensitivity is lower when the joint is extended than when it is flexed. Kinesthetic sensitivity to movement is better in the upper limbs than in the lower limbs.

Kinesthetic accuracy of positioning seems to be better for more familiar movements. Lloyd and Caldwell (1965) found that the greatest accuracy of positioning coincided with the normal walking arc of the lower leg. These investigators suggested that perception of the limb position seems to be best in the range of movement used more frequently in daily activities. Phillips and Summers (1954) found that people perform significantly better on tasks of kinesthesis with their preferred arm than they do with their nonpreferred arm.

Whether kinesthesis is improved with practice is still an open question. Meday (1952) found greater improvement for her experimental group following twelve practice periods on a scale press test and a target toss for direction than for the no-practice control group. Christina (1967) found that in most cases test performance on a side-arm positional test was more exact following practice. Several other investigators, on the other hand, have reported no significant improvement on various kinesthesis tests as a result of practice.

The question remains whether the improvement noted by some investigators is really an improvement in kinesthesis or whether improvement has occurred as a response to a specific situation. Practice certainly leads to more precise specific responses, but that does not establish improvement in kinesthesis of broad dimensions. Participation in a wide variety of motor activities will presumably result in some improved body positional control, balance, and movement control, but large general improvements in kinesthesis probably do not occur.

Kinesthesis and Motor Learning and Performance

The role that kinesthesis plays in motor learning and performance has generated a heated controversy over the past seventy-five years. The classic position is that proprioceptive information is critical to motor behavior; but a recently accelerating trend suggests that kinesthesis is important, but not essential, to both motor learning and performance.

Motor Control and Kinesthesis

An early theory of motor control suggested that each component of a movement pattern produces feedback via the proprioceptors. The feedback from one component of the movement was seen as being instrumental in triggering the next component in the pattern, and so on. This theory became known as the **S-R chaining hypothesis** (some authors refer to it as the peripheral hypothesis) because movement control was viewed as being a series of conditioned responses (Greenwald 1970).

In addition to its intuitive appeal, this theory also had empirical support from one of the most respected neurophysiologists of the early twentieth century, Charles Sherrington. In 1895 Mott and Sherrington (1895) carried out their classic experiment. They **deafferented**[1] a single limb in each of a series of monkeys and found that although some random movements of these limbs remained, no purposeful use was made of the limbs. From these results they concluded that proprioceptive information is necessary for the performance of voluntary movement. This study was replicated by others over the next twenty-five years and the conclusions were similar in each case. The notion that proprioceptive information was essential for movement evocation became an article of faith.

Over the past twenty years the notion that proprioceptive feedback is essential to motor control has come under increasing criticism. Motor control, independent of proprioceptive feedback, has been demonstrated in insects, amphibia, mammals, and humans (Lashley 1917; Nathan and Sears 1960; Wilson 1961; Szekely, Czech, and Voros 1969; Taub, Perrella, and Barro 1973). Taub and Berman (1968) carried out a series of studies to determine whether proprioceptive information is necessary for various types of learning and the performance of various categories of movement. They deafferented the limbs of monkeys and then tested for the amount of movement and learning that was possible afterward. With one limb deafferented, they found (as had Mott and Sherrington) that no purposeful use was made of that limb. However, when the intact limb was immobilized, leaving the deafferented limb free, the animals did make purposeful movements, demonstrating that purposeful movements could be made with deafferented limbs. Next they deafferented both forelimbs. After a recovery period of two to six months, the animals were able to use the limbs rhythmically and in excellent coordination with the hind limbs. Other workers, taking precautions to ensure that all proprioceptive feedback was eliminated, have confirmed Taub and Berman's studies (Bossom 1974). Taub and Berman summarize their findings in this way:

The most general conclusion that can be drawn from our research is that in mammals, once a motor program has been written into the CNS, the specified behavior, having been initiated, can be performed without any reference to or guidance from the periphery. Moreover, there does not appear to be any reason why the initiation, the trigger, cannot also be wholly central in nature.

---

[1] *Deafferent* means to remove or surgically interrupt sensory pathways, thus blocking certain afferent nerve impulses from reaching the brain.

So despite the early failures to retain purposeful movements after deafferentation of a limb, there is now general agreement that good recovery of voluntary movements can be obtained after deafferentation. This suggests that complex movements can occur in the absence of proprioceptive input, and that skilled movements do not completely depend on kinesthesis. This conclusion has additional support from research in which proprioceptive input was abolished through anesthetization or nerve block techniques. Kinesthetic perceptions were impaired by these techniques, but ability to duplicate voluntary movements was retained (Browne, Lee, and Ring 1954; Laszlo 1967).

Although we have rather compelling documentation that motor control can occur in the absence of proprioceptive information, there is, nevertheless, experimental and clinical evidence that proprioceptive information normally plays an important role during movement. While motor control of limb movements can be regained after deafferentation, the elegance of normal movements is lost. Regained movements are done clumsily and without the normal coordination of body segments (figure 11.2). After deafferentation, mechanical interference with a movement is not detected and is not, therefore, consciously corrected. Since normal movements are not affected this way, it appears that proprioceptive information is used in their execution (McCloskey 1978).

Another indication of the normal dependence on proprioceptive input during voluntary movement is the various constant errors that occur during the execution of movements that are obstructed or impeded while they are in progress (Granit 1972). Finally, postural stability is impaired when proprioceptive input is eliminated; swaying is exaggerated, sometimes to the point of falling. In the disease tabes dorsalis, the nerve pathways from the legs to the brain can be completely destroyed, while motor nerves from the brain to the legs remain intact. Tabes dorsalis

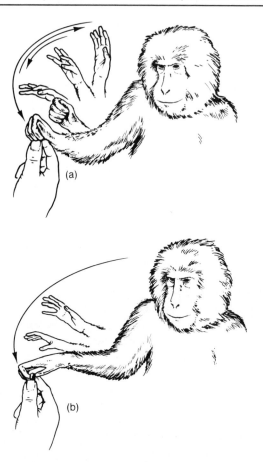

Figure 11.2 *(a) Shows shovel grasp in monkeys following motor recovery after deafferentation. The oscillation of the arm toward and away from food is seen only in some animals; (b) shows dexterity seen in a normal arm extension and grasp using finger and thumb opposition.*

victims will lack proprioceptive information from their legs, while retaining some motor control of them. But, in walking the gait is uncertain and the movements of the legs are poorly coordinated, which results in stumbling and staggering, unless compensated for by visual monitoring.

Traditionally, one of the strongest arguments that motor control does not depend on proprioceptive input is that some movements are executed so fast and are completed so quickly (for example, a golf swing) that there is no time for sensory input to play any basic controlling role. Indeed, angular velocities from 200 to 500 degrees per second have been recorded from hip and leg movements and up to 8000 degrees per second for joints in the upper limb, such as the wrist. Obviously, the components of such movements cannot be controlled by an S-R chaining procedure. Nevertheless, the time in which input could influence a movement in progress has been greatly reduced by recent research findings. Kinesthetic reaction time was taken to be 119 msec for many years, but more recent findings show it to be closer to 30–40 msec (Evarts 1973). Lemon and Porter (1978) reported that some cells in the motor cortex respond to peripheral inputs within 10–25 msec of a stimulus. It has been suggested that this might be part of a "long-loop" pathway mediating transcortical reflexes. It has also recently been suggested that some modification of rapid movements that are in progress may be possible on the basis of internal centrifugal[2] mechanisms (Angel 1976).

The issue of motor control during fast movements is still unresolved. Evidence is accumulating, though, showing that the potential for controlling fast movements in progress—even modifying them—is more likely than has been believed. Moreover, the proprioceptive afferent signals available prior to the execution of rapid movements are likely to have considerable importance in "framing" the appropriate motor commands.

To account for the evidence that proprioceptive input is not essential to motor control, two notions have traditionally been advanced: the "sense of innervation" idea and motor programming theory. According to the first, movements are controlled by reference to perceived sensations of innervation. The most direct approach to verifying sensations of innervation as sensations of movement has been to paralyze a body segment, ask the subject to attempt to move it, and then ask whether it is perceived to move (Goodwin, McCloskey, and Matthews 1972; McCloskey and Torda 1975). Typically, there is no perception of movement, suggesting that motor commands do not give sensations of movements and therefore that motor control is not performed by reference to perceived sensations of innervation.

Motor program theories of motor control have become increasingly popular in the past decade. The **motor program** notion proposes that when a movement pattern is to be executed, neural impulses are transmitted to the appropriate muscles with the exact temporal and force characteristics necessary to carry out the action, and the neural impulses are largely uninfluenced by the resultant peripheral feedback. Many years ago Woodworth (1899) suggested that programs for simple motor responses are set up in advance of their beginning and are uninfluenced during their execution by any feedback, while complex responses can be performed and initiated as a unit. His position has been revived with the current popularity of motor program theory.

The fact that voluntary motor control does not depend upon proprioceptive input does not diminish the role of the proprioceptors in unconscious reflex motor control. Two of the main functions of spindle activity appear to be those of contributing to the postural reflexes and the maintenance of muscle tone.

---

[2] *Centrifugal* refers to efferent signals within the central nervous system.

For posture, the muscle spindle intrafusal fibers "set" the spindle at a length compatible with appropriate upright posture. Slow stretching of muscles due to the shifting of the center of gravity causes afferent response in the spindles and a contraction of the stretched extrafusal muscles, which will correct the displacement. Postural adjustments mediated by the muscle spindle afferents go on continuously in the body.

The tonic function of spindle afferents has been mentioned by numerous neurophysiologists. Gamma motoneurons may be fired by stimulation of the reticular formation, indicating that the gamma system, including the spindle afferents that it stimulates, is suited for prolonged, tonic forms of activity. Thus, the gamma system is an important mechanism in the maintenance of muscle tone. Tonic discharges can be facilitated or inhibited from various central regions, including the cerebellum, known to be concerned with the regulation of muscle tonus.

Like the other proprioceptors, the joint receptors are involved with certain reflex activities. The head exerts important influences upon movements of the trunk and limbs, and neck reflexes arising from stimulation of joint receptors in the cervical spine are important in movement. The tonic neck reflex, present from birth, becomes subsumed under neck righting reflexes in infancy and produces suitable adjustments in body and limb muscles to ensure that the body follows the head. Recent data suggest that joint receptors probably cooperate with other receptor types in the reflex control of locomotion (Tracey 1980).

The major functions of the **vestibular apparatus** are carried out reflexively. The semicircular canals serve a major role in the maintenance of equilibrium during movement. Stimulation of the semicircular canals produces appropriate muscular responses for maintaining or regaining body balance, either by causing movements of body segments to keep the center of gravity over the base of support, or by changing the base of support to keep it under the center of gravity. The utricles are concerned with postural reflexes and in the differential distribution of muscle tone. Shortly after birth, reflexes arising from the utricles appear, called tonic labyrinthine reflexes (TLR) and tonic righting reflexes. Stimulation produced by head movement or body position produces stereotyped adjustments. These reflexes will be discussed in more detail in chapter 13.

As growth and development proceed, the labyrinthine reflexes as well as the tonic neck reflexes become subordinated, and voluntary motor control becomes more dominant. But these reflexes are not completely eradicated in the adult (Hellebrandt and Waterland 1962; Hellebrandt, Schade, and Carns 1962), and in fact may be used to facilitate muscular effort.

Kinesthesis and Motor Learning

Although motor performances and even motor learning are possible in the absence of proprioceptive input (providing vision is present), the incorporation of proprioceptive input as a source of movement-produced feedback has been found to be a powerful variable in motor skill acquisition. Any disturbance of proprioceptive input will potentially adversely affect motor learning. Indeed, most motor program theories of skill acquisition give a major role to feedback in the acquisition of motor programs. Keele (1973) emphasized that complete development of motor programs for complex human motor tasks is facilitated by feedback and that proprioceptive input plays an important role. According to Keele, normally, when developing a motor program a standard, or model, of the appropriate task performance is constantly being compared with feedback from the program that has just been employed. When there is a difference between the standard and the feedback, the motor program is updated. Eventually a motor program emerges that brings about the desired performance—there is a motor pro-gram-standard match. Movement-produced feedback in motor learning is an integral part of other recent models of motor learning (Adams 1971; Schmidt 1975). The topic of motor pro-grams will be described in more detail in chapter 14.

There does seem to be a general relationship between kinesthetic perceptual ability and motor skill learning, but considerable confusion exists in the literature with respect to this question. One of the sources of confusion is surely the tests and measurements that investigators have used to as-sess kinesthesis. This problem was discussed in an earlier section of this chapter.

Several investigators have reported a rela-tionship between kinesthesis and motor learning (Phillips and Summers 1954; Fleishman and Rich 1963). Phillips and Summers found that there is a greater relationship between kinesthesis and task performance during the early stages of the learning process and that the role of kinesthesis decreases during learning. However, most evi-dence appears to support the opposing point of view. As an example, Fleishman and Rich (1963) demonstrated that kinesthetic ability was of greater importance later in learning. They gave a kinesthetic sensitivity test to a large group of subjects, then divided them into groups high and low on kinesthetic sensitivity. Then subjects learned a two-hand coordination task. They at-tempted to keep a target follower on a moving target, with the left-right movement of the target follower controlled with one hand and movement toward and away from the body controlled with the other. The two kinesthetic groups began at the same level, but in the later stages, as kines-thetic ability apparently became more impor-tant, the kinesthetically superior group surpassed the other group (figure 11.3).

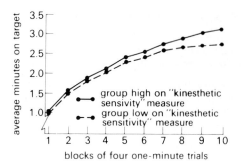

Figure 11.3 *The two kinesthetic groups begin at the same level but, in the later stages the kinesthetically more sensitive group surpasses the low sensitive group.*

Some people prefer to, or are more proficient in, processing information through the proprio-ceptive mechanisms. Temple and Williams (1977) identified subjects as high, moderate, or low in proprioceptive processing proficiency. They then selected motor tasks that were high in proprio-ceptive demands. High proprioceptive informa-tion processors exhibited more rapid skill acquisition than did low subjects, suggesting that differences in the level of mastery of a task with high proprioceptive demands may be a function of an individual's perceptual proficiency (figure 11.4).

Proprioceptive information is a source of feedback in motor behavior. But most research on the uses of vision and proprioception suggests that when these two sources of feedback are both available, vision tends to dominate and attention is primarily allocated to vision. As an example, Adams and his colleagues (Adams, Gopher, and Lintern 1977) examined the effects of visual or proprioceptive (or both) feedback on learning a positioning task. While proprioception was found to play a part in the regulation of the movements employed in their study, visual feedback was the

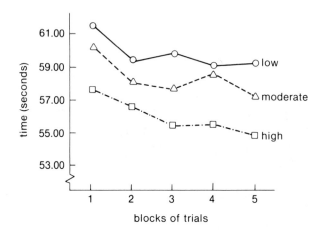

Figure 11.4 *Performance curves for high proprioceptive agility task: proprioceptive information processing preference groups. (Less time indicates better performance.)*

more powerful of the two. To the belief that proprioception is eminent in the regulation of movement, the investigators recommend a revision:

Proprioception has a role in the regulation of movement and its influence increases with training, but its role is smaller than vision's. When proprioception is combined with vision it continues to play a role but a minor one. . . . Vision overpowers proprioception when it is present and degrades proprioception's influence, but proprioception is not potent enough to work conversely and erode the influence of vision.

Others have found that vision tends to dominate proprioception when input from both modalities is available, and the dominance of vision occurs even when the visual information is irrelevant and could be ignored (Klein and Posner 1974; Smyth 1978).

Kinesthetic Aftereffects

Kinesthetic aftereffects refer to a perceived modification in the shape, size, or weight of an object or to perceptual distortion of limb position, of movement, or of intensity of muscular contraction as a result of experience with a previous object. For example, it is a common experience that

the perceived weight of a lifted object is biased by the weight of a previously lifted object. The batter who swings several bats just before stepping to the plate, so that one bat will seem lighter, exemplifies the use of kinesthetic aftereffect to produce an apparent change in weight of the bat. To use another example, running and jumping while wearing weighted shoes is usually followed by a perceived ability to run faster after the heavy shoes are removed.

Kinesthetic aftereffects were first experimentally studied by Gibson (1933) in the early 1930s. In his original study, the subject passed one hand over a curved surface. After this experience it was found that a straight surface felt curved in the direction opposite to that of the exposure object. Numerous investigators have confirmed the existence of this phenomenon, but the whole field of aftereffects is relatively unstudied in the field of psychology.

Most studies of kinesthetic aftereffects have used tactile-manipulative tasks or fine motor tasks. In kinesthetic aftereffects experiments, a stimulus object is first manipulated. This is called the I, or inspected object. Then a second stimulus object is presented, referred to as the T, or test object. In the case of Gibson's study referred to above, the curved surface was the I (inspection)

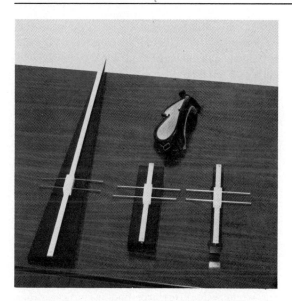

Figure 11.5 *Kinesthetic aftereffect equipment. A blindfold, inspection blocks, a long tapered block.*

object and the straight surface was the T (test) object. Petrie (1967) has developed a set of wood blocks that may be used to assess kinesthetic aftereffects. Several blocks of different sizes serve as inspection objects, and one long tapered block of wood (tapering from one-half inch at its narrow end to four inches at its wide end) serves as the test object. The blindfolded subject attempts to indicate the width of the inspection block, grasped in one hand, by moving the other hand to the same width on the test object, the tapered block (figure 11.5). These kinesthetic aftereffect blocks have been used in research on this modality of aftereffect.

Studies of kinesthetic aftereffect for gross motor movements are not plentiful, but a unique study by Cratty and Hutton (1964) demonstrated that locomotor activity under blindfolded conditions produced aftereffects. Subjects guided themselves ten times through pathways curved sharply to either the right or to the left. They were

then placed in a straight test pathway. Aftereffects were evidenced by reports that the straight pathway was curved opposite to the direction of the curved pathway to which the subjects had been exposed.

Several generalizations can be made about kinesthetic aftereffects: (1) There is a greater displacement, or aftereffect, with longer inspection time; (2) aftereffects are maximal immediately after experience with the inspection object and then diminish gradually, leaving slight aftereffects that may be of long duration; (3) the displacement tends to continue to diminish the longer the time delay between inspection and test; (4) displacement can occur in one of two forms, assimilation or contrast. In assimilation the displacement of the test object is toward the inspection object; contrast is displacement of the test object away from the inspection object. Kinesthetic aftereffects usually produce contrast, but Petrie (1967) reported that subjects displayed either contrast or assimilation in a consistent manner; (5) when attention is distracted during the inspection test, the resulting aftereffects are reduced.

No definitive explanation of the underlying neural mechanisms responsible for kinesthetic aftereffects has been formulated, but it seems that motor unit activity recruited for a given task, such as in manipulating a heavier-than-normal object, remains available and functioning when one performs with an object of normal weight. As we noted previously, judgments of weight or achieved muscular force are based on the magnitude of motor commands, while perceptions of movement arise primarily from the skin, muscle, and joint receptors. Presumably, some complex interplay of the motor commands and the afferent feedback from the movement produced by these commands produces the kinesthetic aftereffect when a performer switches from a heavy to a light object (Granit 1972; Gandevia and McCloskey 1977).

Kinesthetic Aftereffects and Weighted Objects

A considerable body of literature is concerned with kinesthetic aftereffects and motor performance after practice with weighted objects. As noted above, typically the perceived heaviness of an object (or the body) is biased by the weight of a previously used object. If the previously used object is heavier than the one subsequently used, the latter is perceived as lighter and therefore easier (or faster) to move. The major empirical question is whether the use of the weighted objects does in fact alter performance or whether it merely produces a perceptual illusion.

Nelson and Nofsinger (1965) measured the speed of elbow flexion just before and after applying various weights. They reported no significant difference between preoverload and postoverload speed, although the subjects reported "feeling faster" during the postoverload trials. Stockholm and Nelson (1965) investigated the immediate effects of the use of weighted vests on vertical jumping performance. Three different vest weights were used in the experiment. Subjects performed vertical jumps with the weighted vest, followed by jumps without the weights. No improvement in vertical jump performance occurred after the weighted practice. Boyd (1969) reported virtually identical results. Even prolonged practice with weighted objects does not result in improved performance, although people using the weighted objects invariably report a perception of improved performance (Lindeburg and Hewitt 1965; Winningham 1966; Straub 1968).

Most investigations, then, suggest that kinesthetic aftereffects are not accompanied by a measurable improvement in speed in moving objects (or the body) after practicing with weighted objects. Presumably, the reason that the weighted objects do not enhance speed of movement is that they do not bring about an increase in strength in the muscles involved. It is well established that strength development requires work against high resistance with few repetitions (Edington and Edgerton 1976). The overload provided by the weighted objects probably is not enough to achieve a threshold for strength development.

Using Kinesthetic Cues in Teaching

The employment of kinesthetic cues as a teaching technique poses some rather serious difficulties. First, it is not at all clear to what extent kinesthesis is used, or is capable of being used, by the learner. Second, such a bewildering number of proprioceptive signals impinge upon the learner prior to, during, and immediately after execution of a movement pattern that it is difficult to select the appropriate kinesthetic cues for attention during any of these periods. Third, no consistent body of research findings indicates that an emphasis on kinesthetic cue utilization is an effective instructional method.

Given these problems, some techniques have been tried in an effort to enhance motor learning through kinesthesis. In most cases they are intuitively appealing and none has proven to be detrimental to skill acquisition, so the enterprising instructor may wish to experiment with one or more of them.

One approach to enhancing skill acquisition through kinesthetic cue utilization has been to have learners practice the movement patterns with their eyes closed or while blindfolded. One assumption behind this method is that learners have the potential to be aware of their movements through proprioceptive input without the aid of visual cues. Another assumption is that concentration will be on the movement rather than its outcome, and stimuli in the environment, which may be distracting, will be eliminated, thus making the learner aware of normally ignored feedback.

Several investigators have reported that removing visual information during the learning process enhanced learning rate (Dickinson 1968). On the other hand, Durentini (1967) found no differences in improvement in basketball free throw shooting between a group of subjects who practiced shooting while blindfolded and a group who practiced in the usual manner. The lack of visual cues apparently did not improve kinesthesis for that task. From the scant literature currently available, the effectiveness of this method has not been verified as a means of promoting learning.

A second method of emphasizing kinesthesis in motor learning has been a manual manipulation technique in which learners relax as they are guided through the movement pattern. The assumption is that as learners are guided through the movement, the proprioceptors associated with the movement will be activated and will provide the learners with correct cues. Smith (1969) has suggested that manual assistance helps learners to "get the feeling of the proper movement," but we have little support for this claim and some reason to be suspicious of it, since the passive movement of body segments does not produce the same pattern of afferent impulses as active movement, and thus input is distorted. More research is needed to ascertain the effectiveness of this procedure.

A third technique employs an emphasis on "feel." The learner is repeatedly told to "feel the position" or "feel the movement." In his very popular instructional manual, *The Inner Game of Tennis,* Gallwey (1974) has a section on "feeling" in which he says:

It would be useful for all tennis players to undergo some "sensitivity training" with their bodies. The easiest way to get such training is simply to focus your attention on your body during practice. Ideally, someone should throw balls to you, or hit them so they bounce in approximately the same spot each time. Then, paying relatively little attention to the ball, you can experience what it feels like to hit balls the way you hit them. You should spend some time merely feeling the exact path of your racket on your backswing. The greatest attention should be placed on the feel of your arm and hand at the moment just before they swing forward to meet the ball. Also

become sensitive to how the handle feels in your hand. . . . When I hit my best backhands, I am aware that my shoulder muscle, rather than my forearm is pulling my arm through. By remembering the feel of that muscle before hitting a backhand, I program myself to attain the full benefit of the power it generates. Similarly, on my forehand I am particularly aware of my triceps when my racket is below the ball. By becoming sensitive to the feel of that muscle, I decrease my tendency to take my racket back too high. . . . In short, become aware of your body. Know what it feels like to move your body into position, as well as how it feels to swing your racket. . . . In tennis there are only one or two elements to be aware of visually, but there are many things to feel. Expanding sensory knowledge of your body will greatly speed the process of developing skill.

Unfortunately, there is very little experimental support for this teaching technique.

A few limited situations in teaching sports skills lend themselves to an emphasis on feel, such as the preliminary and terminal positions in the baseball, golf, and tennis swings, gymnastic stunts, and others. Since correct preliminary and terminal positions in these tasks are important to proper movement execution, it behooves learners to learn these positions. They may be aided by learning the "feel" of these positions. Learners can attempt to achieve the correct preliminary and terminal feel and thus perhaps execute the movement correctly.

Various instructional aids have been employed for directing attention to feel while practicing a task. For example, a "golfer's groove" was reported to be effective in driving golf balls (Yost, Strauss, and Davis 1976). The golfer's groove is a metal frame on which a moulded plastic tube is bolted. The learner stands within the frame, resting the golf club shaft on the plastic tube. Using the tube as a guide, the learner takes the proper backswing and foreswing at the angle and plane of the correct golf swing; the correct swing is "traced" by the device. After several practice swings using the golfer's groove, the learner steps out of the frame and practices hitting golf balls without the aid of the device. The notion behind the use of this aid is that the feel of the proper swing plane obtained while using the device will be used as feedback for structuring the correct motor commands when hitting balls without the device.

There are potential problems in asking either the novice or the expert to concentrate on feel. Beginners cannot benefit from the feel of a movement pattern because they cannot associate anything with a successful effort. To ask the highly skilled to experience the feel may result in "paralysis from analysis." This is exemplified in the following ditty:

A centipede was happy, quite
Until a frog in fun,
Said, "Pray which leg comes after which?"
Which raised her mind to such a pitch
She lay distracted in a ditch
Considering how to run!

Summary

The perceptual experience that arises from the stimulation of the proprioceptors is called kinesthesis, and it involves the discrimination of the positions and movements of the body parts, both passively and actively produced. The neural mechanisms that underlie kinesthesis are still not fully understood, but it is now fairly well established that the Ia spindle afferents contribute mainly movement information, the group II spindle afferents provide primarily positional information, and the tendon organs provide sensations of force. Corollary discharges produce subjective estimates of the weight of lifted objects and the perception of effort in the performance of motor tasks.

During the 1950s and 60s the joint receptors were considered the major input source for kinesthesis, but recent evidence excludes the possibility of an exclusive role in kinesthesis for the joint receptors. Very little is known about the contribution of skin receptors to kinesthesis, but it appears that skin receptors in some joints signal joint angle over a wide range. Vestibular afferent function is mostly reflexive, with interpretations of lateral, horizontal, and vertical movement, as well as bodily orientation in space, also likely outcomes of vestibular function.

There have been varying degrees of research emphasis in kinesthesis over the past century. The psychophysical dimensions of this phenomenon were studied extensively in the latter nineteenth century and early twentieth century. More recently tests have been developed to assess kinesthesis from dimensions other than its psychophysical properties. Efforts to find a general kinesthetic perceptual ability have been disappointing.

The dependence on kinesthesis for motor control has been called into question by studies showing movement and motor learning when kinesthetic input has been restricted or eliminated. Nevertheless, it appears that kinesthetic perceptions are normally employed during motor activities. There does seem to be a general relationship between kinesthetic perceptual ability and motor skill learning, but the issue is quite complex and considerable confusion exists in the literature on this question.

Kinesthetic aftereffects are perceptual distortions of shape, size, or weight of objects. Like other perceptual illusions, they are produced by exposure to certain types of stimuli. Practice with weighted objects typically produces the perception that normal weight objects are lighter and that performance is improved after experience with the weighted objects, but this is usually only a kinesthetic aftereffect.

Several instructional methods have been employed to enhance kinesthetic cue utilization, namely practicing with the eyes closed, manual manipulation of the learner, and emphasis on feel. These techniques, while intuitively appealing, have little empirical support for enhancing motor learning.

The Motor System and
Control of Movement

12

The Motor System

A perennial goal in the study of motor behavior is to infer function from structure—to relate behavior to the organization of the nervous system. The traditional view of the brain in regard to movement is that the highest level in its hierarchical organization is the cerebral cortex. Recent investigations seem to indicate that the structures participating in the integration and control of muscular movements include a complex of subcortical, as well as cortical, structures, each playing a highly specific role in the whole functional system that produces voluntary movement. In this chapter we describe the principal structures that make up the motor system, and in the next chapter we shall examine how the motor system functions to control and regulate motor behavior.

It is convenient to study the motor system by first identifying and describing the transmission network that carries motor impulses from their origins to the motoneurons that actually innervate muscle fibers, causing muscular contraction or relaxation. After we have done that, the structures responsible for the motor impulses can then be identified and discussed. These structures may be treated as though the nervous system were composed of a series of levels. Starting from the top, the levels are the cerebral cortex, the basal ganglia, the cerebellum, the brainstem, and the spinal cord.

Each of the structures that contribute to motor integration and control plays a unique role. It must be emphasized, however, that the functional parts of the motor system are intimately interrelated, and that in order to achieve almost any kind of complex motor behavior, the entire system contributes to some extent. So describing this system as a series of levels does not imply that the levels somehow function independently of one another. This description is merely a convenient method for writing about them.

Motor Pathways

Before we identify and discuss the various structures that control motor activity, it is necessary to describe the motor pathways over which impulses pass on their way to producing muscle contraction or relaxation. The sources of sensory information about the external world and our bodies are many and varied, but the means for control of voluntary movement are few. We have several different kinds of sensory receptors, with their various pathways to the brain, but only two major motor pathways. These two motor pathways from the cortex to the spinal cord and the motor nuclei of the cranial nerves are (1) the pyramidal system, also called the corticospinal tract, and (2) the extrapyramidal system. These descending cortical and subcortical pathways represent the main instrument by which the brain controls movement.

The Pyramidal System

This motor transmission network is made up of those neurons that originate in the cerebral cortex, the axons of which descend to the spinal cord. Hence it is also called the **corticospinal tract.** The axons of this system are some of the longest in the body. The name, **pyramidal system,** comes from the symmetrical, wedge-shaped bulges its fibers form on the ventral surface of the medulla, just below the pons. The neurons of the cortex that send their axons down the pyramidal tract provide a direct channel from the cortex to the spinal neurons, which in turn cause either muscle contraction or relaxation. This direct connection of the cortex with motoneurons ensures that the cortex very effectively and quickly brings about a desired movement (figure 12.1). These corticospinal neurons also receive collateral sensory input, which provides a means by which sensory information can be used to influence the control of movement (McGeer and McGeer 1980).

About 40 percent of the cell bodies of neurons that make up the pyramidal system are found in the motor cortex (a region just in front of the central fissure), about 20 percent originate in the somatosensory area in the parietal lobes, and the remainder originate in other parts of the cortex. Pyramidal system neurons are of two types. One is the huge neurons in the motor cortex called Betz cells, which are about sixteen microns in size. These large Betz cells of each hemisphere of the motor cortex contribute about 3 percent of the total axons of the system. The second type of pyramidal system neuron, and by far the most numerous, are small neurons distributed throughout the cortex and having both myelinated and unmyelinated axons. These small axons account for about 95 percent of the total corticospinal tract.

Pyramidal system axons leave the cortex, descend in the internal capsule, and pass through the pons, giving off collateral axons to the motor nuclei of the cranial nerves for the control of facial, eye, and glandular activity. When they reach the medulla, collateral axons innervate cranial motor nuclei for the control of the pharynx, larynx, neck, upper back, and tongue muscles.

In the medulla, the pyramidal tract axons organize into bundles of axons, the pyramids, one pyramid on each side of the midline fissure. In the medullary pyramids, about 80 percent of the one million axons of each of the bilateral pyramidal tracts cross over the pyramidal decussation and terminate mainly on spinal cord interneurons, which in turn synapse on the motoneurons that control muscle action. About 50 percent of the crossed pyramidal axons end in the cervical region of the spinal cord, while the other half end in lower parts of the cord. Uncrossed pyramidal axons continue through the pyramids and descend in the spinal cord. These axons then cross the midline of the cord a few at a time and synapse with motoneurons in the cord.

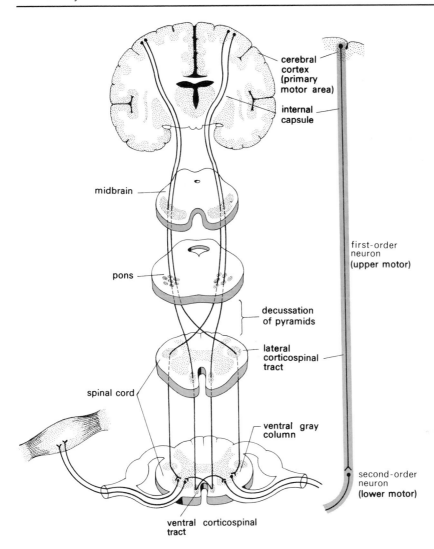

Figure 12.1 *The pyramidal motor pathways.*

Much descending transmission over the pyramidal tract does not go directly to the spinal motoneurons. Instead, impulses synapse on spinal interneurons, and these in turn relay impulses to the spinal motoneurons, whose axons project out to muscle fibers.

It appears that the muscles specifically controlled by the pyramidal system contain motor units with a relatively low ratio of muscle fibers.

We noted in chapter 5 that a low ratio of motoneuron innervation to muscle fibers permits smaller portions of the muscles to be independently controlled, which permits a pronounced precision and delicacy of movement. This aspect of pyramidal system control of delicate movement becomes evident when lesions are made in the pyramidal tract. Lesions produce a severe flaccid paralysis for a couple of weeks. Then the

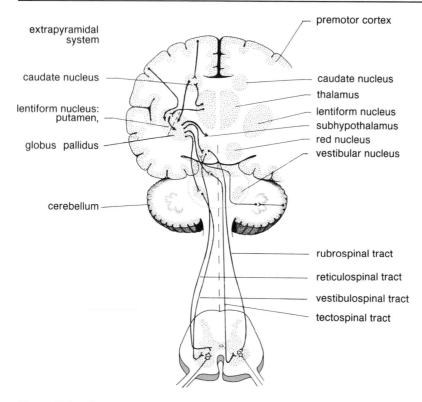

extrapyramidal system

caudate nucleus

lentiform nucleus:
putamen,

globus pallidus

cerebellum

premotor cortex

caudate nucleus

thalamus

lentiform nucleus

subhypothalamus

red nucleus

vestibular nucleus

rubrospinal tract

reticulospinal tract

vestibulospinal tract

tectospinal tract

Figure 12.2   *The extrapyramidal motor pathways.*

proximal muscles of the arms or legs begin to re-cover and the shoulder or hip joint can be moved. Later, more distal muscles in the limbs may improve, but the fingers or toes rarely recover their former dexterity.

The Extrapyramidal System

The second motor pathway is known as the **extrapyramidal system.** By definition, this tract includes all of the motor axons not included in the pyramidal tract. The extrapyramidal pathway differs from the pyramidal pathway in two ways:

1. The chains of axons are interrupted synaptically in the basal ganglia, the pons, the medulla, or the reticular formation.
2. The axons do not pass through the medullary pyramids.

The extrapyramidal pathway originates in the motor area of the cortex as well as in other cortical areas. Axons descend in the internal capsule and many terminate in various subcortical structures, especially the basal ganglia, cerebellum, and thalamus, and in nuclei of the brainstem. Each of these structures and nuclei in turn has direct or indirect connections with each other (figure 12.2).

Extrapyramidal neurons have connections with many subcortical parts of the brain. It is believed that these multiple connections serve to modify some of the operations of the pyramidal system, perhaps helping to refine and smooth out movements. Moreover, extrapyramidal neurons carry a large portion of the impulses for postural adjustment and reflexive movements. Disorders in the extrapyramidal system lead to difficulties in walking, turning, and standing up.

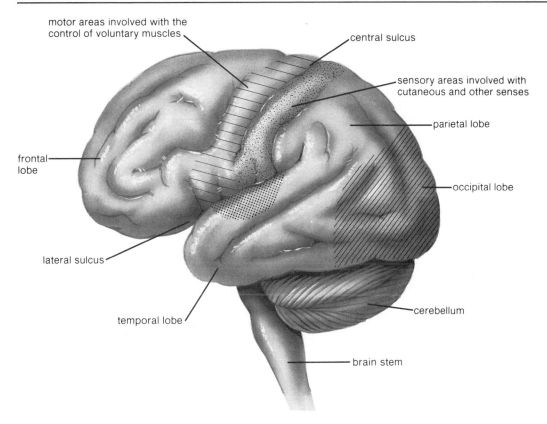

Figure 12.3 *Motor areas of the cortex.*

Pathways to Cranial Nerves

Since motor activity of the head and neck is carried out by the muscles supplied by cranial nerves, the pathways that innervate the cranial nerves are not separated anatomically into pyramidal and extrapyramidal. The reason is that most of these descending pathways terminate before reaching the medullary pyramids.

The Motor Cortex

The region of cerebral cortex from which most neurons arise for motor integration and control is called the **motor cortex** area. This part of the cortex has a primary area that lies immediately anterior to the central fissure and a secondary area, known as the **premotor cortex** area, that lies just anterior to the primary area, about 1 to 3 cm in width (figure 12.3).

The motor cortex area contains about thirty-four thousand giant Betz cells and millions of smaller neurons. It projects fibers to all association areas of the cerebral cortex, and many descending fibers lead out of the motor cortex. Axons of these descending neurons pass from the cortex and descend through the internal capsule. Impulses from the motor cortex reach spinal cord motoneurons either by relaying in various subcortical levels or by projecting through the direct motor pathway to the brainstem and spinal cord. More of the axons arising from neurons in the premotor cortex terminate in the subcortical structures and nuclei of the brain instead of projecting directly to the spinal cord.

The motor cortex is somatotopically organized, that is, each part controls specific muscle groups of the body. However, the different muscle groups of the body are not represented equally

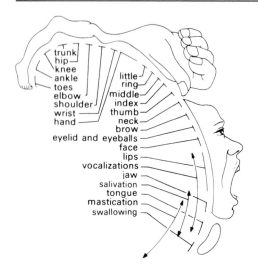

Figure 12.4 *The motor homunculus (little man) showing the extent of representation of the various body muscles in the motor cortex.*

in the motor cortex area (figure 12.4). As a rule, the degree of representation is proportional to the precision of movement required of a given part of the body. The hand and the mouth muscles have almost two-thirds of the total representation in the motor cortex area. The large number of motor cortex neurons for innervation of the hand and face is one of the factors responsible for the fine degree of motor control humans have over these structures and reflects the importance of these parts.

The "mapping out" of the human motor cortex was done by electrically stimulating the motor cortex during brain surgery on unanesthetized patients. Movements elicited by electrical stimulation of the motor cortex consist largely of flexion and extension of the arms and legs, opening and closing of the fists, and vocalization. The limb movements are typically expressed on the side of the body opposite the stimulation, but some ipsilateral activity may also occur. This technique gives an indication of what each portion of a part of the cortex might be used for. The technique does not use the motor cortex as it is employed by the stream of impulses that produces a voluntary movement. Thus, movements elicited by

electrical stimulation of the motor cortex do not necessarily by themselves tell us the complete story about the role of the motor cortex in the control of movement.

The motor cortex receives its main direct input from other cortical areas and from subcortical areas via the thalamus. An example of the former is found in the close functional interrelationship between the motor cortex and the somatosensory areas of the cortex; the two areas may be said to fade into each other. Many of the cells of the motor cortex extend back into the somatosensory areas, and cells of the somatosensory areas extend forward into the motor area. Electrical stimulation of the anterior parts of the somatosensory cortex often evokes muscle contractions, while stimulation of certain parts of the motor cortex evokes sensory experience. In addition to the motor-somatosensory relationships, numerous association fibers from diverse areas throughout the cortex are major sources of input to the motor cortex.

Subcortical influences to the motor area come from feedback circuits involving the basal ganglia, cerebellum, brainstem, and even the spinal cord, as well as from peripheral afferent sources through subcortical nuclei. For example, the strongest sensory input to a particular portion of the motor cortex arises from the body part whose movements it controls. The motor cortex hand area receives its strongest input from sensory receptors in the hand.

The motor cortex serves to coordinate the complex innervations on the motor area from other parts of the CNS. As Eccles (1977) says, "The motor cortex . . . is not the prime initiator of a movement. . . . It is only the final relay station of what has been going on in widely dispersed areas in your cerebral cortex."

Damage or destruction of the motor cortex evokes a loss of the fine voluntary movements, particularly of the fingers and feet. Effects are more prominent in the distal muscles than in the proximal muscles of a limb. A small lesion in the motor cortex does not always paralyze particular muscles. Rather, it prevents the use of the muscles in connection with certain movements.

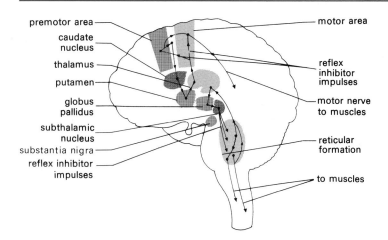

premotor area
caudate nucleus
thalamus
putamen
globus pallidus
subthalamic nucleus
substantia nigra
reflex inhibitor impulses

motor area
reflex inhibitor impulses
motor nerve to muscles
reticular formation
to muscles

Figure 12.5 *The basal ganglia, showing their innervations with the cerebral cortex and various structures in the brainstem.*

The Prefrontal Cortex

The cortex anterior to the central fissure is comprised exclusively of the frontal lobes, which can be subdivided into three major areas: the motor cortex, the premotor cortex, and the prefrontal cortex. The first two have been described in the previous section.

Occupying the most anterior region of the cortex is the **prefrontal cortex,** which is also important in the control of movement. This area has many complex reciprocal connections with other cortical regions. It also has rich reciprocal connections with the thalamus, hypothalamus, and other subcortical areas that appear to mediate emotion and motivation.

For many psychologists and neurologists, the prefrontal cortex area is the most fascinating part of the brain, probably because it embodies the unique difference between the brains of other animals and of humans. Experimental and clinical evidence suggests that it must be included in the cortical areas responsible for motor behavior because numerous studies on this part of the brain demonstrate that it plays an important role in the integration of motor behavior. These will be taken up in the next chapter.

The Basal Ganglia

We are now ready to examine the lower levels of the motor system, that is, below the level of the cerebral cortex. One of the most important subcortical levels for coordinated movement is called the **basal ganglia.** The basal ganglia are the highest centers for motor control in birds and the lower animals that have little cerebral cortex (figure 12.5).

Basal ganglia have two major inputs, the ascending reticular formation and the motor areas of the cerebral cortex. The latter represents the highest and most important portion of the extrapyramidal system. Basal ganglia also have two primary output pathways. The first pathway descends through the thalamus and makes connections with various subcortical structures throughout the diencephalon, the midbrain, and the brainstem. The second output pathway ends in a part of the thalamus that projects fibers upward into the cerebral cortex. These output pathways allow the basal ganglia to influence spinal cord as well as cortical motor mechanisms. This massive network of input and output fibers of the basal ganglia apparently serves to facilitate and inhibit a wide variety of movements.

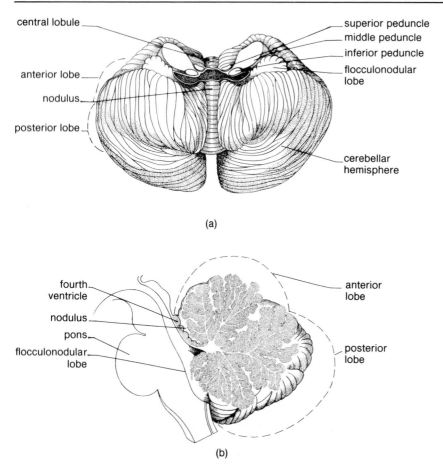

central lobule

superior peduncle

middle peduncle

inferior peduncle

anterior lobe

flocculonodular lobe

nodulus

posterior lobe

cerebellar hemisphere

(a)

fourth ventricle

anterior lobe

nodulus

pons

flocculonodular lobe

posterior lobe

(b)

Figure 12.6   *The cerebellum: (a) a view of the anterior part of the cerebellum. This part is just behind the brainstem. (b) a sagittal view.*

Actually, very little is known about the precise function of most of the various basal ganglia except that they work together as a loosely knit unit to perform controlling functions for coordinated movement. Findings by DeLong and Strick (1974) indicate that the primary motor function is the control of slow movements. This is not to suggest that the basal ganglia function solely in the control of slow movements, but at least a large portion of the basal ganglia is preferentially involved in this manner. Further discussion of the role of the basal ganglia in motor control appears in the next chapter.

The Cerebellum

The cerebellar level is another brain level that is essential to well-coordinated, complex motor function. The **cerebellum** is a large, profusely fissured structure located posterior to the brainstem. It is divided into two hemispheres and a midline connecting portion, the vermis. Each hemisphere is joined to the brainstem by three peduncles—the superior, middle, and inferior—composed of nerve fibers. The superior peduncle connects with the midbrain, the middle with the pons, and the inferior with the medulla. The cerebellum also has indirect connections, by way of the peduncles, with the cerebral cortex and the spinal cord (figure 12.6).

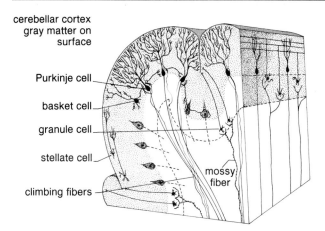

cerebellar cortex
gray matter on
surface

Purkinje cell

basket cell

granule cell

stellate cell

climbing fibers

mossy
fiber

Figure 12.7   *Cross section of interior of cerebellum, showing the network of cells which transmit nerve impulses through it.*

The cerebellum has a cortex of gray matter, similar to the cerebral cortex, and an interior of both white and gray matter. Its cortex is elaborately convoluted to increase its area. In fact, the fissures are much deeper and more closely spaced than those of the cerebral cortex. The interior gray matter consists of four cerebellar nuclei (dentate, emobliform, fastigial, and globose nuclei) that receive collateral axons from the afferent fibers projecting into the cerebellum and efferent connections from the Purkinje cells (described below) of the cerebellar cortex (figure 12.7).

The cerebellum receives input from a variety of sources: the somatosensory, visual, auditory, and motor areas of the cerebral cortex, various nuclei in the brainstem, the reticular formation, and the somatosensory system. Cerebral cortex axons destined for the cerebellum follow a route through the internal capsule to the pons. There they synapse on neurons projecting into the cerebellum. The cerebellum also receives numerous inputs from brainstem nuclei. Sensory signals from the proprioceptors (the receptors in the muscles, tendons, joints, and vestibular apparatus) project into brainstem nuclei, where they synapse on cerebellar afferent neurons whose axons ascend to the cerebellar cortex.

Collectively, these signals transmit space-and modality-specific data to the cerebellum. These data can be used in the control of fine movements of the limbs and in the monitoring of information pertaining to location or stages of movement involving an entire limb. Also, afferents from other sensory modalities give off collaterals to brainstem nuclei that in turn project to the cerebellum.

Within the cerebellum, input is served by two types of afferent fibers, the climbing fiber and the mossy fiber. The principal type of cell in the cerebellar cortex is the **Purkinje cell,** whose axons constitute the only output line of the cerebellum. Climbing fibers begin outside the cerebellum in other regions of the brain and project into the cerebellar nuclei and cortex, synapsing on a one-to-one basis with the Purkinje cells. Climbing fibers have a strong excitatory effect on the Purkinje cells. Whereas each climbing fiber connects with a single Purkinje cell, the mossy fibers do not synapse directly on Purkinje cells. Rather, the mossy fibers synapse on the interneurons of the cerebellum, thus ultimately but indirectly innervating many Purkinje cells. This form of input supplies both excitatory and inhibitory influences to the Purkinje cells (figure 12.7).

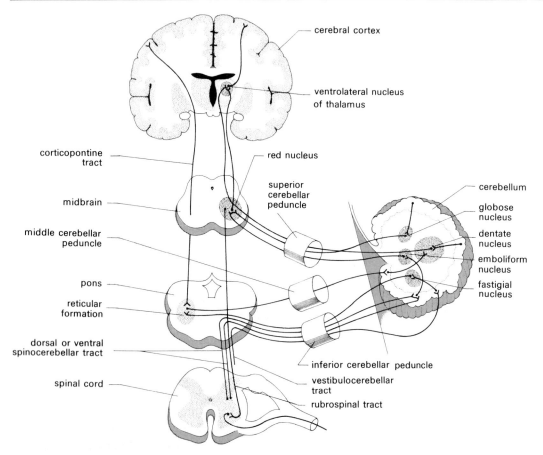

Figure 12.8   *The main cerebellar pathways. The reticulospinal tract is not shown. This tract extends from the reticular formation to the spinal cord, and fibers in this tract terminate on motoneurons.*

Cerebellar output involves two stages. First, Purkinje cell axons project into the cerebellar nuclei and synapse there. The cerebellar nuclei are, then, the principal targets of the output of the cerebellar cortex. Second, the cerebellar nuclei neurons project axons to brainstem nuclei and the thalamus. Purkinje cells are inhibitory, but the cerebellar nuclei neurons are excitatory. The origins of excitatory input to the cerebellar nuclei neurons seem to be the collateral transmissions from the climbing fibers and the mossy fibers (figure 12.8).

Output pathways from the cerebellar nuclei project to various brainstem nuclei where they join the extrapyramidal tract. Thus, there are cerebellar-brainstem feedback loops. Ascending cerebellar fibers enter the ventrolateral thalamic nucleus, which projects to motor areas of the cerebral cortex. It can be seen that signals that leave the cerebral cortex may ultimately return, after further processing, by way of the cerebellum. Thus, the cerebellum is part of a dynamic cerebral-cerebellar feedback loop.

There have been many attempts to correlate cerebellar and body areas to ascertain whether one portion of the cerebellum is concerned with upper-limb function and another part with lower-limb function. Although investigations of this kind have been moderately successful in lower animals, the only localization known with any certainty for humans is that relating a hemisphere of the cerebellum to the same side of the body. Control is not contralateral as it is in the cerebral cortex. It has also been found that upper limbs have greater representation in the cerebellum than do the lower limbs. Investigators are in general agreement that the cerebellum does not contain a precise somatotopic map, such as those found in the somatosensory and motor cortex areas. There seems to be, instead, a large overlap of inputs, and any small region in the cerebellum will receive inputs from a very large number of sources.

Several neuroscientists have proposed models of cerebellar function. With each model there is general agreement that cerebellar output plays a significant role in regulating postural adjustments, locomotion, and many other reflex activities. It also appears to play an important role in the preprogramming and control of rapid, ballistic movements (Llinas 1975; Eccles 1977; Llinas and Wolfe 1977). These functions will be described in more detail in the next chapter.

The Brainstem

The next level for motor integration and control is the **brainstem.** The two major structures of the brainstem, the pons and the medulla, contain numerous nuclei that are concerned with the control of motor activity. Another structure, the reticular formation, extends throughout the brainstem; it also projects ascending and descending signals to influence motor behavior.

Input to the brainstem arrives from many sources. Axons from all of the sensory systems pass through the brainstem and give off many collaterals that then synapse on brainstem nuclei neurons. In addition, the cerebellum, cerebral cortex, and the basal ganglia have projections into the brainstem. This area of the nervous system is, then, an integrative area for combining and coordinating all sensory information with motor information. Information from these various sources is then used to control many of our involuntary movements. Much of our postural, locomotive, cardiovascular, and respiratory activity is mediated by brainstem centers, and a great deal of this activity is carried out in the form of reflexes.

The reticular formation is a critically important brainstem mechanisms for the control of reflex movements and coordination of motor activity. Some reticular formation axons descend into the spinal cord. It is through these descending fibers, called reticulospinal fibers, that the reticular formation exerts many subtle influences in controlling basic patterns of reflex connections to conform with postural needs or specific motor commands from the cortex or related extrapyramidal centers. Reticular formation excitation may cause enough spinal facilitation to produce movements—even complete postural adjustments. Usually, however, the reticular formation functions to facilitate or inhibit motor adjustments and therefore modifies instead of elicits postural and phasic actions.

Ascending reticular formation fibers play a decisive role in activating the cortex and regulating its activity. As noted in a previous chapter, a certain state of arousal is important for effective and efficient cortical function.

The Spinal Cord

The lowest level of the motor system is the gray matter of the spinal cord. In the anterior horns of the cord are two types of spinal motoneurons. The first is called the skeletomotor neuron (also called the alpha motoneuron). Its cell body is located in the spinal cord, and its axons and collaterals pass through spinal nerves to terminate on extrafusal muscle fibers, which are the main skeletal muscles. It is through these neurons that impulses must pass on their way to skeletal muscles. The **gamma motoneuron** (also called the fusimotor motoneuron) is the second type of spinal motoneuron. Its cell body also lies in the cord and its axons and collaterals also pass through the spinal nerves, but the terminals end on the specialized muscle fibers of the muscle spindle, the intrafusal muscle fibers. Impulses from these motoneurons initiate the gamma loop, which will be discussed in the next chapter.

Skeletomotor Neurons

Skeletomotor neurons are the final common pathway for transmission of motor impulses from the brain to the skeletal muscles. They have rather large diameter axons, averaging 8–20 mμ, and they conduct impulses at velocities of around a hundred meters per second. Their axon fibers end at neuromuscular junctions with extrafusal muscle fibers.

Each skeletomotor neuron cell body can have from a hundred to over fifteen thousand synaptic endings on it that converge from many different sources. The activity or inactivity of the neuron depends upon the sum of the excitatory and inhibitory synaptic activity impinging upon it at any moment. If the sum of input is strongly excitatory, the motoneuron fires impulses at a rate reflecting the intensity of the stimulus; if the sum of synaptic input is predominantly inhibitory, the neuron does not fire; if the sum of input is excitatory but not enough to reach a threshold potential, the neuron is said to be facilitated.

Each skeletomotor neuron gives off collateral fibers, and each fiber synapses on an extrafusal muscle fiber at the neuromuscular junction. As you recall, a single skeletomotor neuron and all of the extrafusal muscle fibers innervated by it are called a motor unit (see figure 5.11). A motor unit is the basic building block for control of movement. As such, motor units are designed to match the needs of work required of the muscles. As the total demand for muscle contraction increases, more motor units are recruited, and the strength of contraction is increased by an increase in frequency of discharge of the individual motor units. This will be discussed more fully in chapter 13.

Gamma Motoneurons

Like skeletomotor neurons, gamma motoneuron axons pass through spinal nerves, but their terminals end at junctions on the intrafusal muscle fibers of the muscle spindle. While skeletomotor neuron axons divide to produce upwards of a hundred neuromuscular junctions, gamma motoneuron axons supply only a few different intrafusal muscle fibers, although one gamma motoneuron may innervate several spindles within the same extrafusal muscle. Gamma motoneuron axons are small (2–8 mμ) and conduct impulses at a lower velocity (10–50 meters per second) than the skeletomotor neurons. About 40 percent of the total motoneurons of the spinal cord are the gamma motor type.

Intrafusal muscle fibers that are innervated by the gamma motoneuron fibers do not contribute to contraction of extrafusal muscles. Their contraction, instead, results in stretching their central, noncontractile portions, where the spindle sensory receptors are located, causing these receptors to fire. The consequences of this stimulation of the spindle afferents for kinesthesis were described in a previous chapter; the role of the gamma motoneurons in motor control will be taken up in the next chapter.

Other Spinal Motoneurons

In addition to the skeletomotor and gamma motor spinal motoneurons, many other neurons in the gray matter of the cord are capable of assisting in certain kinds of organized motor activity. You will recall from a previous section in this chapter that most pyramidal system (corticospinal tract) axons terminate on interneurons located in the spinal cord gray matter. Thus, motor impulses are usually transmitted through interneurons before finally reaching the spinal motoneurons that control muscles. Other motor fiber pathways, besides those of the pyramidal tract, terminate on the interneurons as well.

In the anterior horns of the cord there is also an important interneuron, the **Renshaw cell.** One of its main functions when stimulated is the inhibition of the antagonistic muscles of those that are contracting. This activity is called reciprocal inhibition.

Summary

A persisting goal in the study of motor behavior is to infer function from structure. Traditionally, the cerebral cortex has been viewed as the main motor control structure, but recent research has demonstrated that the integration and control of movement is accomplished by a complex set of subcortical as well as cortical structures. A study of motor behavior requires an understanding of various structures that make up the motor system.

Motor transmission is carried over two main systems, the pyramidal system and extrapyramidal system. The first is a rather direct transmission network to muscle fibers, while the latter is more complex and indirect.

The region of the cerebral cortex from which most neurons arise for motor integration and control is called the motor cortex area. This area has a primary area and a secondary area, called the premotor cortex. The motor cortex area is somatotopically organized, with each part controlling specific muscle groups of the body. The most anterior area of the cerebral cortex is called the prefrontal cortex.

One of the most important subcortical levels for coordinated movement is made up of the basal ganglia. Collectively, the basal ganglia coordinate the control of slow movements.

The cerebellum is a profusely fissured structure attached to the posterior of the brainstem. It has a cortex of gray matter similar to the cerebral cortex. This structure has a significant role in regulating postural adjustments, locomotion, and many other reflex activities. It also has an important role in preprogramming and control of rapid, ballistic movements.

The brainstem is made up of the pons and medulla. These structures are primarily integrative centers, combining and coordinating all sensory information with motor information. Information from these various sources is then used to control many of our involuntary movements.

The lowest level of the motor system is the spinal cord. In the anterior horns of the cord are two types of spinal neurons, skeletomotor neurons, which innervate extrafusal muscle fibers, and gamma motoneurons, which innervate intrafusal muscle fibers. The former produce movement, while the latter stimulate the muscle spindle afferents.

13

Motor Integration and Control of Movement

*T*he observer of a smoothly coordinated motor performance usually does not realize that the performance represents a fantastically complex integration of many parts of the nervous system to produce the postures and movement patterns. In a jump shot, a forward pass, or an intricate dance routine, the complete movement patterns consist of reflexes, simple movements, and complex movements with precise spatial and temporal organization, meaning that the appropriate muscles are selected and employed at just the right time.[1]

How the nervous system produces a coordinated motor pattern has long been one of the major mysteries of the neurosciences. What accounts for the graceful performance of the skillful athlete or even the ordinary movements of daily life? For movement to be effective, an appropriate group of muscles must be selected, each muscle fiber must be activated in the proper temporal sequence to the others, and a precise amount of inhibition must be sent to each of the muscle fibers of muscle groups that oppose the intended movement. In addition to producing the contraction of a certain group of muscles, the CNS must monitor the effects of its commands, coordinate the movements of the various segments of the body, and terminate a given phase in a movement pattern and proceed to the next phase.

In this chapter we shall examine the mechanisms of the nervous system that are responsible for the integration and control of human movement patterns. But we must emphasize that much

---

[1] Spatial organization refers to the fact that the appropriate muscles must be selected. Temporal organization refers to the fact that muscle contraction or relaxation must occur at the appropriate time.

is still unknown about this aspect of human behavior. The organization of this chapter is from lower to higher levels because each higher level of organization incorporates into its control functions all the levels below it. As we noted in the preceding chapter, the motor system is hierarchically organized, with the simplest, involuntary responses controlled at the lowest levels of the hierarchy and more complex, finely coordinated, and novel responses controlled at higher levels (Summers 1981).

Muscles and Movement

The first requirement for movement is a muscle, and the second requirement is a system for stimulating the muscle to make it contract in an orderly manner. Therefore, the basic building block for the integration and control of movement is the **motor unit**—one **skeletomotor neuron** and the group of muscle fibers it innervates (see figure 5.11). Motor units differ in two important ways, both of which have important implications for motor control. First, they vary widely in their muscle innervation ratio. Some skeletomotor neurons innervate fewer than five muscle fibers, while others innervate several hundred. For example, the innervation ratio of the eye's muscles averages about 1:3, while the ratio to a limb muscle, such as the biceps, may be 1:150. The consequence of this variability in muscle innervation ratio is that muscles that operate with great speed or that control fine, precise movements have a low innervation ratio; in muscles that move large body masses, such as limbs, and where precision is normally not so important, a high innervation ratio is typical.

A second way in which motor units differ is in the types of muscle fibers they innervate. Some skeletomotor neurons innervate muscle fibers that have great power and speed of contraction but fatigue quickly. Muscle fibers of this type are **fast twitch fibers.** They quickly generate a large peak muscle tension but fatigue rapidly. Fast twitch muscle fibers are controlled by large, fast conducting skeletomotor neurons. Other skeletomotor neurons innervate muscle fibers that lack the

power and speed characteristics of fast twitch muscle fibers, but they are resistant to fatigue and are, therefore, well suited for prolonged contraction. Muscle fibers of this type are called **slow twitch fibers.** These remain active for long periods of time, but they produce relatively little muscle tension. They are controlled by small, slow conducting skeletomotor neurons. Fast and slow twitch muscle fibers represent extremes of a continuum, with many muscle fibers showing mixed characteristics (Edington and Edgerton 1976).

Within a typical muscle, the fibers of fast and slow twitch motor units are intermixed. There are, however, fewer slow twitch muscles. Basically, they are the antigravity extensor muscles—the soleus muscle of the calf is a typical slow twitch muscle. All flexor muscles and most extensor muscles are predominantly fast twitch.

The functional importance of the contrasting types of motor units for the control of movement is related to the way in which the motor units are "recruited" during a movement. Basically, muscle tension is organized in two ways: (1) through control of the number of motor units recruited; and (2) through control of the firing rate of the motor units that have been recruited. With respect to the former, the voluntary contraction of a muscle involves a sequence of motor unit activations within a muscle's spectrum of motor units. The smallest slow twitch motor units, generating relatively little muscle tension but resistant to fatigue, are the first to be activated, since they have the lowest threshold. As more motor units are recruited, there is an alteration of firing among the units, as some discharge and others stop firing in a seemingly random manner. Since these units are small and develop only low contractile tension, the random alteration of motor unit firing does not produce a jerky contraction of the muscle, but rather a finely graded, smooth contraction.

As muscle tension increases, more motor units are recruited, and they tend to be controlled by the larger, high-threshold skeletomotor neurons that innervate the fast twitch muscle fibers. As these larger, fast twitch units are recruited, the amount of muscle tension added with each unit increases. The larger the motor unit, the more the number of muscle fibers and therefore the greater the muscle tension developed by each newly recruited motor unit. Thus, as total muscle tension rises, fewer additional motor units are needed to produce it. But while these larger motor units generate large peak muscle tensions, they are quickly fatigued.

The second way in which muscle tension is organized is by the firing rate of the motor units that have been recruited. The tension produced by a motor unit can be increased greatly by increases in the firing frequency of the skeletomotor neuron, which is caused by more intense stimulation. When a high frequency of nerve impulses is sent to muscle fibers, the muscle tension from one stimulation is unable to relax before the next stimulation causes contraction. The net effect is higher muscle tension produced by the motor unit and greater force generated by a given muscle.

Spinal Motor Control

The spinal cord is a complex structure where much motor behavior is organized and controlled. One of the most important components for sensorimotor integration within the spinal cord is the skeletomotor neuron. Skeletomotor neurons have direct control over the muscles, but are, in turn, under the control of other sources. The

nerve fibers of neurons from throughout the nervous system converge on skeletomotor neurons, which is why they are called the "final common" pathway linking the nervous system to the muscular system.

During the execution of a coordinated movement, the CNS must provide specific patterns of nerve impulses to the skeletomotor neurons to produce appropriate muscle contractions. One of the fundamental questions in the neurosciences is how this is done. To answer this question, investigators have studied movement in **deafferented** animals and in animals whose spinal cord has been surgically severed (the latter are called "spinal animals"). These techniques effectively separate the control of skeletomotor neurons from sensory feedback and from the brain.

The early research of Charles Sherrington (1910) and Graham Brown (1911) established that "spinal animals" could produce coordinate movements. Since that time evidence has become conclusive that there are interneurons in the spinal cord that activate **pattern generators** that serve to produce certain basic movements, such as locomotion (Grillner and Zangger 1974; Pearson 1976). These movements can be produced in the absence of sensory input and without control from higher brain centers. Certain movements can thus be viewed as based on "central programs" originating in the spinal cord.

The role of spinal interneurons in producing an entire movement pattern can be elaborated as follows: A neuron within the spinal cord—called a **command neuron**—activates a pattern generator that is composed of a set of local control centers. The neurons within these centers consist of a network of cells that coordinates the firing of skeletomotor neurons to produce movements. Command neurons have been found for the regulation of posture and locomotion (Bowerman and Larimer 1974; Pearson 1976). It is likely that centrally generated patterns of motor activity underlie all kinds of stereotyped behavior, such as respiration and chewing.

While a command neuron is capable of setting a movement pattern in motion and sustaining it, under normal conditions higher brain centers or sensory feedback cause the stimulation of the command neuron, which triggers the sequence. Moreover, a change in stimulation to the command neuron will lead to a modification in the intensity of response. For example, command neurons that generate the walking sequence can produce, when more intensely stimulated, a fast walking pace and even running (Kupfermann and Weiss 1978).

The existence of command neurons that, through pattern generator centers, can produce coordinated movements without the assistance of sensory feedback does not mean that sensory input is unimportant in these movements. Sensory input can and does influence the central programs so that the movements are adaptive to the particular requirements of the task. Several investigators have found that, in a spinal cat, pattern generators for stepping could be stimulated by afferent inputs from the feet and legs. Once the pattern generators were started, the speed of stepping was controlled by the rate at which the treadmill under the cat's feet moved (Shik and Orlovskii 1976; Smith 1978).

If a rhythmic task, such as locomotion, is being performed, sensory input can alter the amplitude of a movement without affecting the rhythm, or alter the timing without influencing the amplitude of the movement (Stein 1978). A great deal of current research on locomotion is directed toward clarifying the way in which sensory input interacts with central programs. Pearson (1976) has described the role of sensory feedback in locomotion, indicating that the switching of the motor program from swing to stance is triggered by sensory input. This input during locomotion serves two broad functions: to switch the motor programs from one phase to the next, and to alter the motor output within a single phase.

Proprioception and Motor Control

In chapter 11 we examined the function of the proprioceptors in kinesthesis. But the proprioceptors—especially the muscle receptors—also play an important role in motor control.

As noted in chapter 10, lying parallel with the main muscle is the muscle spindle, containing intrafusal muscle fibers with their own motor nerve supply and sense organs, the spindle afferents. Since spindle afferent fibers enter the CNS and synapse on skeletomotor neurons that supply the same extrafusal muscle group of which the spindle is a part, the result of spindle afferent stimulation is a contraction of the extrafusal muscles, opposing increased muscle length.

The second muscle receptor is the Golgi tendon organ, which senses muscle tension rather than length. GTO afferent transmission produces inhibition in the skeletomotor neurons supplying the muscle in which the GTOs lie. Increased muscle tension produces increased GTO discharges that, in turn, reduce muscle tension. Thus, the spindle afferents and GTOs serve as components in a negative feedback system that maintains body segment stability by resisting changes in muscle length and muscle tension (figure 13.1). Evarts (1979) illustrates the operation of this mechanism with the following example:

Imagine a man who is trying, in the absence of any external disturbance, to hold his arm steady while it is extended straight out to the side of his body. Slight unintended fluctuations in position will, of course, take place, particularly as the arm gets tired. For example, occasional involuntary decreases of tension in the muscles opposing the force of gravity will lead to increases in the length of those muscles. Because of the increase in muscle length, the activity of the proprioceptive length receptors will increase, while at the same time (because of the decrease in muscle tension) the activity of the proprioceptive tension receptors will decrease.

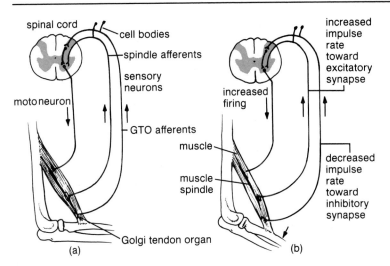

spinal cord
cell bodies
spindle afferents
sensory neurons
motoneuron
GTO afferents
muscle
muscle spindle
Golgi tendon organ
(a)

increased impulse rate toward excitatory synapse
increased firing
decreased impulse rate toward inhibitory synapse
muscle
(b)

Figure 13.1 *Contraction of a flexor muscle in the arm is regulated by two types of receptor. At rest (a) there is some activity in both the spindle and the Golgi tendon organ. A slight stretch of a muscle (b) due to a spontaneous fluctuation in the transmission reaching it leads to increased activity of the muscle spindles (stretch receptors) and decreased activity of the Golgi tendon organs (tension receptors).*

Although these are opposite directions of change, their central effect is not subtractive but additive: the increased firing of the length receptors excites the motor neurons affecting the muscle, and the decreased firing of the force receptors removes the inhibition of the same neurons. This synergistic action of the two kinds of proprioceptive receptors takes effect when muscle-length changes are a consequence of the application or removal of an external force. For example, an increase in muscle length due to an increased external load gives rise to an increase in length-receptor activity associated with an increase, rather than a decrease in the activity of the tension receptors.

Gamma Motor Function in Motor Control

Another spinal mechanism for motor control involves the gamma motoneuron. As described in chapter 10, the activation of extrafusal muscle fibers can occur in two ways: (1) directly, by signals from the skeletomotor neurons; and (2) indirectly, via the gamma motor loop. In the latter case, gamma motor signals cause intrafusal muscle contraction, stimulating spindle afferents,

which, in turn, stimulate skeletomotor neurons, producing extrafusal muscle contraction. This latter way of activating the extrafusal muscle fibers is called the gamma motor loop.

Over the past thirty years there has been considerable controversy in the neurosciences about the role that gamma motoneurons play in motor control. Granit and his colleagues (1955) proposed a follow-up servo theory that suggested that some voluntary movements are actually produced solely by the gamma motor loop system, especially slow movements and postural adjustments. According to follow-up servo theory, the CNS signals the gamma motoneurons rather than the skeletomotor neurons. That is, signals from the motor tracts supply the appropriate impulse code to the gamma motoneurons to bring about, through the gamma motor loop, the appropriate contraction of the extrafusal muscles to produce the intended movement. According to this view, the extrafusal muscle reflexively contracts until it nullifies the stretch of the muscle spindle. The final length of the extrafusal muscle is, therefore, determined by the length of the muscle spindle as set by the gamma motoneuron discharge.

One advantage of driving the skeletal muscles through the gamma motor loop is that the valuable muscle length self-regulating properties of the stretch reflex are maintained at all lengths during the movement. On the other hand, movements initiated indirectly via the gamma loop will suffer delay from transmission time, so for fast starting movements this system will not be very effective.

More recently, a consensus has developed that it is unlikely that any movements are initiated solely by the gamma motor loop. **Coactivation** of the skeletomotor and gamma motoneurons seems to be the more accepted notion with regard to motor control, though each system is perhaps preferential for some types of movements. For example, it has been speculated that for fast starting movements the descending motor tract signals probably converge primarily on the skeletomotor neurons, while gamma motor activation is primarily employed for smooth, continuous, controlled movements. Even here there may be exceptions. Investigators have reported that the extent of movement disorders during gamma motor deprivation is correlated with movement speed (Smith, Roberts, and Atkins 1972; Abbs 1973). Smith and her colleagues (1972) assessed reaction time and dart-throwing performance with gamma motor-deprived elbow extensors. With gamma motors blocked, extension reaction times increased significantly, and the linear velocity contributed to the dart by elbow extension decreased on the average of 1.5 feet per second. The findings suggest that the gamma motor loop normally enhances the rate of acceleration in the initiation of rapid movements.

Another complimentary muscle spindle mechanism can contribute to the initiation of a fast, ballistic movement and so needs to be mentioned here. Frequently, the best mechanical position for the initiation of a rapid movement calls for placing certain body segments in a stretched position, which places the muscle spindles in a favorable position to contribute to excitation of skeletomotor neurons. Taylor and Cody (1974) found that spindle afferent discharge during voluntary movement is often maximal at the stretched position just prior to muscle contraction. Athletes in sports such as basketball have found that stamping one foot hard against the floor, thus stretching muscle spindles in the gastrocnemius (calf) muscle, just before jumping will result in a higher jump than if this is not done. Thus, during jump balls in basketball and spiking in volleyball this foot-stamping technique is employed.

In addition to the role that coactivation may have in the initiation of fast, ballistic movements, there are more fundamental functions for gamma motor coactivation in motor control. The basic notion of coactivation is that signals activating skeletomotor neurons will, at the same time, activate gamma motoneurons. The two efferent systems are activated in parallel. This direct motor discharge of the gamma motoneurons causes intrafusal muscle contraction and enables the spindle to adjust intrafusal fiber length during active contraction of extrafusal muscles. So when the skeletomotor neurons produce extrafusal muscle contraction, which would normally "unload" the spindle afferents and thus produce a "slack" in the spindle, the coactivation of the gamma motor firing compensates for the shortening of the extrafusal fibers due to skeletomotor firing and keeps the spindle "in tune" by resetting intrafusal length. If the gamma motor coactivation did not occur, the shortening of the extrafusal muscle would "unload" the muscle spindle afferents, decreasing their discharges. If the extrafusal muscle shortening continued, eventually all spindle afferent firing would cease.

An important motor control function is served as a consequence of coactivation during a movement. By offsetting the unloading of the spindle afferents, which would otherwise be brought about by the contractions of the extrafusal muscle fibers, coactivation of the gamma motors enables the spindle afferents to take up the slack and thus remain sensitive to minute distortions in movement over the whole range of movement. The net effect of intrafusal muscle shortening over the range of movement to coincide with the shortening of the extrafusal fibers is that if the extrafusal fibers are suddenly stretched, the muscle spindle will be stretched and spindle afferents will discharge, producing increased extrafusal muscle contraction and reflexively reducing the stretch.

The significance of this coactivation function for motor control can be illustrated as follows: Suppose an individual voluntarily bends the elbow to a position and wants to maintain that position. Muscle contractions shorten the extrafusal muscles and, if the intrafusals were not simultaneously shortened, the spindle would become slack. Now suppose some external force suddenly stretches the extrafusal muscle. Since the stretch would not immediately activate the spindle afferents, a great deal of unwanted movement might occur in the arm before enough stretch had occurred to stimulate the spindle afferents to oppose the lengthening of the extrafusal muscles (see figure 10.8). This system, then, permits rapid error corrections. Actually, since coactivation constantly takes up the slack between extrafusal and intrafusal muscles, small perturbations to muscle length can be responded to within 30–80 msecs! (Dewhurst 1967). This is an incredibly fast time, when one considers that visual reaction time is about 200 msec. This fast reaction time, though, helps explain why we can rapidly react to unexpected obstacles to our movements.

In addition to the reflexive adjustment that coactivation provides, there is mounting evidence that coactivation helps to coordinate ongoing movements, especially precise movements. Since muscle spindles are abundantly represented in muscles used for precisely controlled actions, the coactivation enables these movements to be executed as intended.[2] Findings from several investigations suggest voluntary movement commands carry a reference of correctness coded into the signals to the gamma motoneurons that specify the appropriate position for a body segment at any point in time. The gamma motor activity is coordinated with the skeletomotor activity. Gamma motor discharges shorten intrafusal fibers to the "correct" length. Since the gamma motor loop will stimulate skeletomotor neurons and cause extrafusal muscles to contract until the extrafusal muscle length is "matched" by intrafusal length, the gamma motor action can be viewed as "seeking," through the spindle afferents, the appropriate muscle length. Deviations from this length are corrected through the gamma motor loop (Marsden, Merton, and Morton 1972; Schmidt 1976(a); Nashner and Woolacott 1979). In describing this, Granit (1972) commented that spindles "form part of a mechanism for checking the execution of movements in relation to commands."

Spinal Reflexes

A reflex is the simplest functioning unit of nervous activity, and many functions of the nervous system are performed by reflexes. In fact, much human behavior is reflexive. A reflex is a relatively constant pattern of response or behavior that is similar for a given stimulus. Reflex behavior involves glands, (for example, sweating) as well as muscles.

---

[2] Muscles involved with fine motor control have more muscle spindles embedded with them than muscles subserving less precision control. For example, the gastrocnemius and soleus muscles (which together form the calf of the leg) have 5–20 muscle spindles per gram of muscle tissue, while the small muscles of the hand have 120–140 muscle spindles per gram of tissue. The rich sensory innervation probably provides more feedback to the CNS about the length and stretch forces present in the hand muscles, thus providing more accurate correction in producing a precise level of contraction.

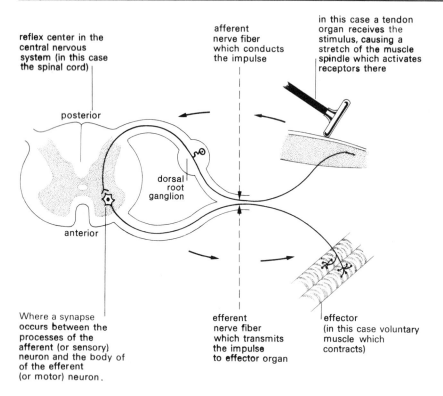

reflex center in the
central nervous
system (in this case
the spinal cord)

posterior

dorsal
root
ganglion

anterior

afferent
nerve fiber
which conducts
the impulse

in this case a tendon
organ receives the
stimulus, causing a
stretch of the muscle
spindle which activates
receptors there

Where a synapse
occurs between the
processes of the
afferent (or sensory)
neuron and the body of
of the efferent
(or motor) neuron.

efferent
nerve fiber
which transmits
the impulse
to effector organ

effector
(in this case voluntary
muscle which
contracts)

Figure 13.2   *Basic nervous unit for reflex behavior.*

The word *reflex* is from the Latin meaning "bending back." This is very appropriate because to bring about a reflex, nerve impulses travel from a sensory receptor along a sensory axon to the CNS. There the impulse "bends back" and moves away from the CNS, along a motoneuron axon to activate a muscle or gland to bring about a response (figure 13.2).

Four basic nerve units are necessary in reflexes.

1. A receptor: all of the sensory receptors in the body are potential receptor organs for reflexes.
2. An afferent neuron: a sensory neuron projecting to the CNS.
3. An efferent neuron: a motoneuron from the CNS to muscles or glands.
4. An effector: all of the muscles and glands are effector organs.

A fifth unit consisting of one or more interneurons is characteristic but not essential. The total pathway is called a **reflex arc,** and it can function independently of higher brain centers. This independence, however, is not typical of reflexes.

The precise role of **spinal reflexes** in coordinated motor behavior is still not fully understood, but increasingly the evidence suggests that normal motor coordination is based, to a large extent, on reflexes. Easton (1972; 1978) claims that they probably underlie all or most volitional movements. Evarts (1979) states that events that underlie voluntary movement "are built up from a variety of reflex processes." He claims, "Some of the most noted scientists in several disciplines accept the notion that 'purposive movements are built in a base of reflex processes.' "

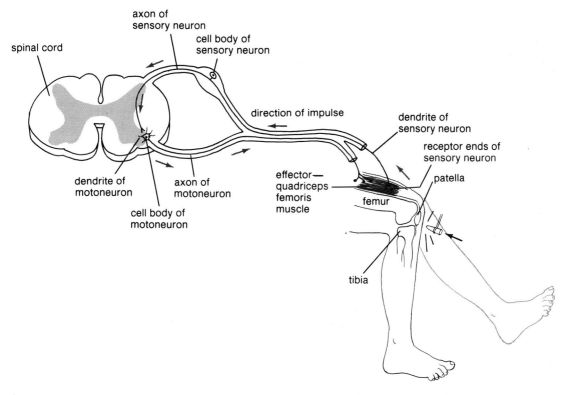

Figure 13.3   *The knee-jerk reflex involves only two neurons: a sensory neuron and a motoneuron.*

Spinal cord reflexes vary from simple two-neuron arcs to complex arcs that involve literally hundreds of neurons. The ones that have been most commonly implicated in serving a facilitating role in coordinated movements are the stretch reflex, flexion reflex, crossed extensor reflex, and extensor thrust reflex.

Stretch Reflex

The **stretch,** or myotatic (muscle-stretching), reflex is the simplest of the spinal sensorimotor reflexes because its basic structure consists of only a single sensory neuron and a single spinal motoneuron. This type of reflex arc is referred to as monosynaptic due to this characteristic.

The knee jerk exemplifies a phasic type of stretch reflex (figure 13.3). To produce the knee jerk, the subject is seated and one leg is crossed over the other at the knee. Then the patellar tendon (located just below the kneecap) of the hanging leg is hit. The tendon stretches the quadriceps (thigh) muscles, which stretch muscle spindles embedded in the quadriceps. The spindle receptors are stimulated and send impulses to the spinal cord, where they synapse on skeletomotor neurons. Efferent signals are transmitted back to the quadriceps. The result is a quick muscular contraction causing the lower leg to jerk forward. While this movement may not have much functional value, it does have clinical significance. If a reflex can be elicited, it demonstrates that both sensory and motor nerve connections are functional.

The primary purpose of the stretch reflex is to oppose changes in muscle length, especially sudden changes. The functional significance of the stretch reflex during voluntary motor activity is not clearly understood, but it is believed that this reflex functions to "damp" movements preventing jerkiness and "overshooting" (hypermetria) during movement. Jerkiness of movement and "overshooting" do result when the stretch reflex is lost from a body segment.

Flexion Reflexes

The arrangement of three or more neurons is the most common reflex arc. In a three-neuron reflex arc, an interneuron mediates between the sensory neurons and motoneurons. Actually, this is an oversimplification, for seldom would we find just a single interneuron in a reflex arc. More often, a number of interneurons connect an afferent and an efferent neuron to form a reflex arc. A whole chain of them may lead up and down the spinal cord from one segment to others. This would be considered a multisynaptic reflex (figure 13.4).

The **flexion reflex** is complex and is considered to be a classic example of a multisynaptic reflex connection. This reflex consists of a contraction of the flexor muscles while reciprocal connections with the antagonistic extensor muscles cause reciprocal inhibition, resulting in relaxation of the extensors. This interaction of muscle groups permits movement of the stimulated limb away from the source of stimulation. In its classic form, the flexor reflex is elicited most frequently by stimulation of receptors through application of a pinprick, heat, or some other painful stimulus. Pain causes withdrawal of any injured portion of the body from the object causing the injury.

The fiber pathways for eliciting the flexor reflex do not project directly from sensory neurons to the skeletomotor neurons. Instead, they pass first into the CNS neuron network. Thus, a three-neuron arc is the shortest possible circuit for eliciting a flexor reflex. Actually, most of the impulses of the reflex travel over many neurons and

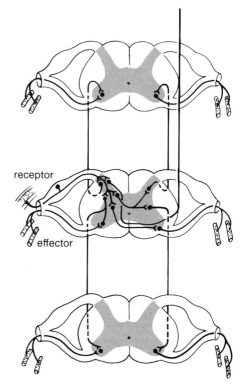

Figure 13.4   Diagram of the connections by which impulses from a receptor reach motoneurons at various levels of both sides of the spinal cord. This accounts for multisegmental, ipsilateral and contralateral responses.

involve diverging circuits to spread the impulses to the necessary muscles for withdrawal and inhibitory circuits to inhibit antagonistic muscles.

Crossed Extensor Reflex

Another type of reflex that often functions in conjunction with the flexor reflex is called the **crossed extensor reflex.** Usually, when a flexor reflex occurs in the limb, impulses pass to the opposite limb, causing it to extend. Extension of the opposite limb, therefore, aids in pushing the entire body away from the object causing the painful stimulus (figure 13.5). A similar reflex appears to play a supportive role in locomotor behavior: A flexion movement in one limb causes a reflex extension of the opposite limb. In the lower limbs, this action assists in supporting the weight of the

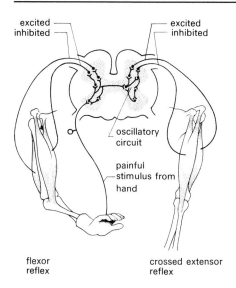

excited
inhibited

excited
inhibited

oscillatory
circuit

painful
stimulus from
hand

flexor
reflex

crossed extensor
reflex

Figure 13.5   *The flexor reflex and the crossed extensor reflex showing their neuronal mechanisms. This also illustrates reciprocal inhibition.*

From *Physiology of the Human Body* 5th Ed. by Arthur C. Guyton, M.D. Copyright © 1979 by W. B. Saunders Company. Reprinted by permission of Holt, Rinehart and Winston, CBS College Publishing.

body and in maintaining the desired posture when the stimulated leg is lifted. So it is at the spinal cord level that postural adjustments are initiated.

Extensor Thrust Reflex

One of the most complex reflexes in the body is the **extensor thrust reflex,** which is another reflex important to postural adjustment. This reflex helps to support the body against gravity. It is initiated by pressure on the footpads. The pressure excites the cutaneous skin receptors in the footpads and reflexively causes contraction of the extensor muscles of the leg. This reaction involves a complex circuit in the interneurons similar to that responsible for the flexor and crossed extensor reflexes.

Pressure on the footpad of a decerebrate animal (brain severed from the brainstem and spinal cord) will cause the foot to extend against the pressure. If the animal is placed on its feet, the footpads will reflexively stiffen and the limbs will

support the weight of the body. Standing posture does not depend upon higher-brain level, but rather is a product of reflexes.

In sum, it can be seen that in the spinal cord are groups of neurons capable of controlling discrete fragments of motor activity resembling parts of coordinated movements. But the role often attributed to the reflexes is that of lending a facilitating influence to volitional effort. The neuron circuits making up the various reflexes are viewed as interacting with command neurons and pattern generators that are employed in structuring such tasks as postural adjustments and locomotion. In this view, reflex patterns can be triggered centrally, and not solely by peripheral stimulation. One source of support for this notion is the demonstration that spinal reflex interneurons are directly affected by various brainstem and cortical activities (Eccles and Lundberg 1959; Lundberg 1966).

Spinal Tuning

A spinal mechanism by which a voluntary movement is translated into appropriate muscle action involves what is called spinal tuning, or preparing spinal motor centers for an anticipated movement. The mechanism is thought to work as follows: The higher-brain levels of the motor system are concerned with only the general parameters of movement execution. The specific details of a movement are left to spinal motor centers. However, the higher centers prepare the spinal centers for the anticipated movement so the movement can be executed as planned. This presetting of spinal motor centers for a particular movement (spinal tuning) can therefore "be regarded as preparation of motor centers to act toward the intentions of the higher center once the trigger for movement is supplied" (Marteniuk and Mackenzie 1980). It appears that motor control centers in the brain adjust the actions of the spinal centers in terms of movement parameters, such as length-tension relationships between agonist and antagonistic muscles for terminal location of movement. (Turvey 1977; Easton 1978).

Brainstem Motor Control

Motor functions of the brainstem are concerned with the control of muscle tone and posture, but this part of the CNS is also important for a number of equilibrium reactions, including the basic spatial orientation or righting reflexes.

Righting Reflexes

Righting reflexes are concerned with maintaining the body in an orientation to gravity. The control center for these actions is in the brainstem. Sensory impulses originating in the vestibular apparatus are sent through the appropriate cranial nerve to the brainstem and synapse on neurons that are used to contract muscles for upright posture and to control muscles of the eyes. Information from the vestibular apparatus is used for two basic purposes: First, to control the muscles that regulate the eyes so that in spite of movements of the head, the eyes remain fixed on the same point; second, for maintaining upright posture.

There are four groups of righting reflexes. They are:

1. the labyrinthine-righting reflexes,
2. the neck-righting reflexes,
3. body-righting reflexes from tactile stimulation, and
4. optic-righting reflexes.

Labyrinthine-righting reflexes can be observed in a blindfolded animal with intact labyrinths. When the animal is held, head down, by the pelvis or hind legs, its head will remain in an upright posture, as far as possible, regardless of how the pelvis is rotated. Such reflex head movements are absent in labyrinthectomized (labyrinths removed) animals. Thus, these reflexes must depend on the functioning of the vestibular apparatus. These reflexes hardly exist in a newborn human, but they develop in the first few months, and as they develop they help the growing child in the various postural tasks of lifting its head, sitting up, and finally standing.

Neck-righting reflexes are concerned with the position of the neck with respect to the head. If the body is tilted, the labyrinthine reflexes restore the head to an upright position. As the head is brought upright, the neck becomes twisted in relation to the head. This triggers the neck-righting reflexes, causing the upper and then lower parts of the body to be brought back in line with the head.

Body-righting reflexes can be induced in a blindfolded labyrinthectomized animal by stimulation of the skin on one side of the body, such as lowering the animal in a side position onto a surface. Even if the head of the animal is held firmly in the lateral position, its body will right itself.

Optic-righting reflexes play a major role in postural orientation in most higher animals because the orientation of the head is controlled mostly by vision. A blindfolded thalamic preparation animal with labyrinths removed will display disorientation of its head until the blindfold is removed and the eyes are allowed to fixate on the environment. At that point, the optic-righting reflexes will cause the animal to attempt to attain an upright head and body position.

In the normal individual, all of these righting reflexes function together to maintain the upright posture. In the disoriented position, a sequence of events, called a chain reflex, occurs. For reorientation, the head leads the way through the mediation of the optic and labyrinthine reflexes, then the upper body is lined up with the head by the functioning of the neck-righting reflexes, and finally the lower body rotates into line with the upper positions.

It is clear that maintenance of upright posture depends on several sensory modalities, in addition to the vestibular receptors. Vision as well as tactile stimulation of the skin plays a critical role.

Much human movement behavior involves the assuming of certain postures, and reflexes play an important role in this behavior. In the adult, postural reflexes as well as other reflexes are incorporated into, and retain their identity within, a hierarchy of complex learned movement patterns (Zelazo 1976). The human infant, however, does not possess a functional cerebral cortex and thus exhibits postural reflexes in a primitive form.

Tonic Reflexes

Another type of postural reflex mediated mainly, but not exclusively, by brainstem centers is called tonic reflexes. **Tonic reflexes** are concerned with the control of the position of one part of the body in relation to other parts, but not in relation to gravity. Tonic reflexes last as long as the head is held in a given position. Two tonic reflexes that are of particular interest in movement behavior are the tonic neck reflex (TNR) and the tonic labyrinthine reflex (TLR). The first results from stimulation of the neck muscle receptors and the second from stimulation of the vestibular apparatus.

Tonic neck reflexes can be noted in human infants during their first six months. During this period the cerebral cortex has not gained control over lower reflex centers. The TNR is evoked by a rotation of the head to one side, causing stimulation of joint receptors in the neck, which results in extension of both limbs on the side to which the face is rotated. At the same time, there is a relaxation of the limbs on the side toward the back of the head (figure 13.6). Lowering of the head (ventriflexion) causes a flexion of the arms and an extension of the legs. Elevation of the head (dorsiflexion) causes an opposite response. This reflex can be seen in the behavior of four-footed animals, such as cats. As the cat lowers its head to eat food on the ground, the forelimbs relax. When the head is elevated, there is usually some relaxation in the hind limbs.

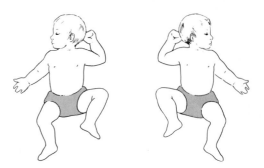

Figure 13.6 *Tonic neck reflex (fencing position) in an infant.*

In humans, TNRs are obscured as motor development continues. They blend into the overall righting reflexes by helping to ensure that the body follows the head in spatial orientation.

In TLRs, isolated from TNRs when the individual is moved into different positions in relation to gravity, the extensor tonus changes in the same way in all four limbs. The tonus is maximal in the supine position and minimal in the prone position. In human infants, the TLR produces stereotyped extension in all the limbs when the child is placed in a supine position. The prone position produces flexion in all the limbs. The TLR is masked by more complex reflexes as the infant matures (figure 13.7).

The TNR and TLR are not easily detected in normal humans after the first few months of life. This does not mean, however, that these reflexes are obliterated in the mature person. It means that they have become subservient to more useful motor control patterns. There is evidence that these reflexes might play important roles in certain motor activities. For example, Fukuda (1961) has shown TNR and TLR postures in archery, baseball, fencing, gymnastics, shot-putting, and other activities. He suggests that in many cases the patterns of these reflexes are the most efficient for performance and that these reflexes provide a facilitating influence to voluntary

Figure 13.7   *Tonic labyrinthine reflexes. (a) all limbs in extension in the supine position; (b) under limbs extended in side position; (c) all limbs in flexion in prone position.*

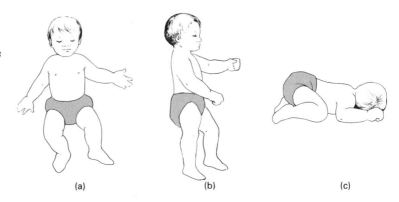

(a)   (b)   (c)

movement. Support for this view has been reported by Hellebrandt and her associates (Hellebrandt and Waterland 1962; Hellebrandt, Schade, and Carns 1962). They have demonstrated the presence of these reflexes in normal adults. Further, they have shown that these reflexes function especially during stressful motor activity to reinforce muscle contraction and extend endurance. More recently, George (1970; 1972) has demonstrated facilitative and inhibitory effects of the TNR upon grip strength of children. When the head was turned away from the hand doing the gripping, there was an increase in force compared to when the head was turned toward the hand. Turning the head presumably actuates the TNR. It appears reasonable to conclude that although these reflexes are not readily apparent, they probably play a role in the coordination of limb and body movements into an organized pattern.

The Reticular Formation

The network of neurons that extends throughout the brainstem and makes up the **reticular formation** plays an important role in motor control. The ascending reticular system plays a decisive role in activating the cerebral cortex and regulating its activity, and it also contributes to the selective attention mechanisms. These functions were described in chapter 7. With regard to motor control, the reticular formation influences the

spinal cord in two seemingly contradictory ways: facilitation and inhibition. The powerful facilitating reticular influence is exerted via descending signals principally to spinal neurons mediating extensor reflexes—facilitating the extensors and inhibiting the flexors. This pronounced extensor facilitation of the extensors makes sense since one of the main functions of the brainstem is postural control, and the extensors are important in the maintenance of posture.

The effects of the inhibitory reticular formation on the spinal reflexes is opposite that of the facilitating influence—flexor facilitation and extensor inhibition. This may sound strange and inefficient, but the action of both of these systems is influenced by higher motor centers in the brain. The facilitating reticular system tends to operate normally at high levels of firing, and this overabundant discharge is harnessed and suppressed by higher brain centers. Conversely, the inhibitory reticular system requires the higher motor centers to stimulate it into action. Without this influence, the inhibitory system is unable to maintain its influence on spinal reflexes. The reciprocal actions of these two systems enables a person to maintain various postures without having to devote much conscious attention to postural control.

The Brain and Control of Movement

The traditional notion about voluntary movement has been that the motor cortex is at the highest level of motor control and subcortical structures are at a lower level. However, recent research suggests that the situation is not that simple. A major purpose of current research on the control of movement by the brain is to develop a better understanding of how inputs from various cortical and subcortical structures integrate their influences to control the final output from the motor cortex to spinal neurons and out to the muscles.

Current interpretations of motor control continue to assign a significant role for the motor cortex. But the outputs of this cortical area are viewed as the result of inputs from other cortical areas, such as the somatosensory and prefrontal cortex areas. In addition, inputs come from subcortical structures such as the basal ganglia and cerebellum, which provide input indirectly by way of still another subcortical structure, the thalamus, are seen as equally important. We shall describe these various inputs to the motor cortex, beginning with subcortical structures, and then return to the issue of the motor cortex's function in motor control.

The Cerebellum

Recent findings (DeLong and Strick 1974; Kornhuber 1974) show that the basal ganglia and cerebellum, as well as the motor cortex, are activated prior to movement. This has changed traditional ideas about the functional relations of these three structures. It now appears that the entire cerebral cortex sends signals to both the basal ganglia and the cerebellum, and these two structures recode this information and then send a new pattern of signals back to the motor cortex via the thalamus.

It has long been known that the **cerebellum** is concerned primarily with the control of complex movements. It is commonly believed that the major role of the cerebellum is the control of movement in response to feedback from the proprioceptors after movement has begun. But recent investigations have shown that changes in cerebellar activity occur well in advance of the initiation of movement (Thach 1970). Several neuroscientists have indicated that the cerebellum actually has a key role in the initiation of fast, ballistic movements through its connection with the motor cortex via the thalamus (DeLong and Strick 1974; Llinas and Wolfe 1977). Kornhuber (1974) has been largely responsible for developing the notion of the cerebellum as the ballistic movement "function generator."

This is not to suggest that it does not have a feedback role in movement control, because the cerebellum does indeed appear to have as one of its functions a kind of feedback loop circuit during motor activity. It receives data from various sensory modalities concerning the position of the body in space. It also receives information from cortical areas concerning the position of the body in space and the direction and amplitude of the intended movement. When the body parts deviate from the intended movement pattern, the cerebellum appears to initiate necessary adjustments via its connections with the cerebral cortex and brainstem motor pathways. This model, then, suggests that one of the cerebellar functions is to compare efferent and afferent signals, adjusting the movement so that the two sets of signals coincide.

Damage or destruction of the cerebellum results in various movement disabilities, depending on the damage. This fact supports the model of this structure as a regulator of motor activity. Disequilibrium, tremor, disturbances in timing and coordination, and overactive reflexes are some of the common effects of cerebellar damage. Cerebellar damage causing coordination deficiencies results in voluntary movements that are slow to start, have inaccurate direction of movement (so the moving part stops too soon or too late), and display wild, jerky movements made in an effort to correct directional errors. Characteristic of cerebellar damage is muscular tremor that is most severe during rapid voluntary movement and least severe when the muscles are at rest. Since voluntary modification of the functions of the cerebellum seems to be impossible—we are never directly conscious of the functioning of the cerebellum—defects resulting from cerebellar damage or disorders cannot be voluntarily controlled or modified in any way.

The Basal Ganglia

Basal ganglia appear to have a complimentary function with the cerebellum. The primary motor function of the basal ganglia is to generate slow movements. DeLong and Strick (1974) recorded activity in both the basal ganglia and cerebellum prior to voluntary movement and found that basal ganglia cell discharge was greatest during slow movements, suggesting a preferential role for the basal ganglia in the control of slow movements.

The victim of a basal ganglia disease, such as Parkinson's disease, can frequently carry out high velocity movements quite normally, but may have great difficulty starting a slow movement with the same muscle group. The condition is just the opposite of cerebellar dysfunction whereby, as noted above, muscular tremor is more severe during rapid voluntary movement and less noticeable while the muscles are at rest.

The Somatosensory Cortex

With respect to the cerebral cortex, it appears that all of its various areas contribute unique input to the motor cortex. It has been suggested that there are four cortical components of cortical control of voluntary movement, each of which originates in a different part of the cortex (Luria 1973;

Granit 1977). The first component emanates from the somatosensory area, which lies just behind the motor cortex and blends into it. Indeed, since many somatosensory fibers terminate in the motor cortex and many pyramidal tract neurons arise in the somatosensory cortex, some neuroscientists refer to these two areas as the sensorimotor area.

Although simple ballistic movements can be performed without feedback from the somatosensory system, humans find it difficult to regulate complex coordinated movement patterns only by way of efferent signals from the brain to the muscles. The **somatosensory cortex** receives inputs from a performer's proprioceptors and cutaneous receptors, and evidently relays signals to the motor cortex. These actions complete a feedback loop (sometimes called transcortical loop) that is undoubtedly quite helpful for movements requiring precise, fine control (Evarts and Fromm 1978). The dependence of convergent inputs to the motor cortex from muscle, cutaneous, and joint receptors to mediate movements has been described by several investigators (Marsden, Merton, and Morton 1972; Wiesendanger 1973). This mediation plays an important role in correcting impulse codes directed to the muscles.[3] If the somatosensory cortex is damaged or destroyed, the individual not only loses certain sensations, but is unable to execute familiar voluntary movements.

Parieto-Occipital Association Cortex

A second component of voluntary movement is that of spatial organization. A voluntary movement must be precisely oriented toward a certain point in space. This spatial analysis depends upon **association areas** of the **parieto-occipital lobes.**

---

[3] It has been found, however, that motor performance, and even learning, can occur in the absence of proprioceptive information. This will be discussed more fully in chapter 14.

Malfunctions in these parts of the cortex result in a disturbance in which the sensory base of the movements is normal, but the individual fails to exhibit precise spatial organization of the movement. Right and left spatial relations can be confused. Inability to make appropriate spatial movements even in a familiar place can result. Even the ability to distinguish east from west on a map or the position of the hands on a watch may be lost.

The Prefrontal Cortex

Another component of voluntary movement involves purposive conduct, or stable intention. An effective movement must be carried on in a goal-directed manner, taking in all of the factors about the present stimuli, previous experiences, and the consequences of just-performed movements. According to Luria (1970), the **prefrontal cortex** functions as an executive control center. Damage to this area disconnects the processes of memory, which integrate current input and translate it into patterns of behavior appropriate to its context (Filskov, Grimm, and Lewis 1981). There is an inability to foresee the consequences of a course of action and to act accordingly, so this area plays a prominent role in such things as judgment and planning for the future. Lesions in this part of the cortex reduce the ability to use good judgment; the individual responds rapidly, impulsively, and with no apparent evaluation of the consequences. In a way, then, the prefrontal area may have somewhat of an inhibitory effect on other brain areas, causing one to hesitate and plan one's response and its possible consequences before responding.

A related role of the prefrontal cortex is concerned with regulatory activity in the form of correct evaluation of external impressions and the purposive direction and selection of movements in accordance with the evaluation. With prefrontal damage, the somatosensory and spatial organization components of movements remain, but goal-directed movements are replaced by inappropriate repetitions of already completed movements or impulsive responses to the stimuli. Luria (1966) reported that humans with a massive lesion of the prefrontal cortex cease to compare their performance with their original plan, and they can no longer ascertain whether the action does in fact correspond to the original plan. Thus "prefrontal" patients are perseverant. They find it difficult to change from one solution of a problem or form of response to a different one. They lose flexibility and the capacity to make adjustments in the face of changes in problems or situations. As an example of this condition, Luria (1970) describes a patient with damage to the prefrontal lobe who wrote a letter to the noted Russian neurosurgeon, Burdenko, that went like this: "Dear Professor, I want to tell you that I want to tell you that I want to tell you. . . ." This was repeated page after page.

Damage or destruction to this part of the brain also produces striking personality changes. There is a loss of drive and ambition, but the most dramatic changes are a lack of self-consciousness and freedom in social relationships, sometimes to an obnoxious or embarrassing degree.

Finally, extensive loss of abstract thinking or reasoning ability accompanies prefrontal area lesions. Simple problems requiring reasoning become extremely difficult to solve (Filskov, Grimm, and Lewis 1981).

The Motor Cortex

We now return to the **motor cortex,** for it is this area of the brain that is the final relay, the summing point, upon which the widely dispersed subcortical and cortical inputs are focused. On the basis of these inputs, the motor cortex formulates the overall plan of action and initiates the motor commands, while subcortical and spinal centers supervise the details of the movement.

Motor cortex activity is involved with both slow and fast movements. The basal ganglia are preferentially active in slow movements, while the cerebellum is preferentially active with fast, ballistic movements. Damage to the motor cortex produces paralysis, whereas damage to the basal ganglia or the cerebellum causes abnormality instead of abolition of movement (Evarts 1973).

Most of the motor cortex output to spinal neurons is indirect and travels via multineural chains. It is also influenced by convergent effects from the basal ganglia, cerebellum, and reticular formation via the extrapyramidal tract. However, the distal segments of the limbs, especially the hands, have more direct cortical regulation, which is important for their precise control.

As noted in chapter 12, lying immediately anterior to the motor cortex is a secondary area called the **premotor cortex,** which functions as a motor association area. It operates in intimate relation with the motor cortex (some neuroscientists do not separate the motor cortex into two zones) and is concerned with the integration and refinement of complex motor actions. A voluntary movement requires temporal organization, or sequential linking. In Luria's (1966) words, "A skilled movement is a kinetic melody of interchangeable links." As one part of a movement is completed, the motor impulses must be shifted to another link, and so on. Only in this way can an organized movement pattern be made. It appears that the premotor cortex is responsible for the organization of the sequential interchange of individual links of a movement pattern. When this part of the cortex is damaged, many skilled movements disintegrate. The individual loses the ability to block, or inhibit, one of the links of a movement and to make a transition from one link to another (Roland et al. 1977).

It should now be clear that the old notion that voluntary motor behavior is formed in the narrow area of the motor cortex is inaccurate. The areas of the brain contributing to the creation of a voluntary movement include a complex of cortical and subcortical structures, each playing a very specific role in the entire functional system. Moreover, a great deal of human movement is under the control of lower motor centers, which regulate reflexes. The reflexes, in turn, are under the influence of brain structures, thus providing the potential for control over the enormous variability in motor behavior.

Much is still unknown about the control of complex movements, and this whole area of study is still in its infancy. The next few years promise to be exciting ones for more precisely specifying the role of the various mechanisms in voluntary motor control.

Summary

We usually do not realize that a coordinated motor performance represents a fantastically complex integration of many parts of the nervous system to produce postures and movements. The way in which the nervous system produces a coordinated movement has long been one of the major mysteries of the neurosciences.

The motor system is hierarchically organized, with the simplest, involuntary responses controlled at the lowest level and more complex responses controlled at higher levels. The basic building block for the integration and control of movement is the motor unit, and motoneurons scattered throughout the spinal cord are the final common pathway for efferent signals from throughout the nervous system. It is, then, at the spinal cord level where much of the neural activity that results in movement occurs. Movement can be produced through the actions of specific command neurons without control from higher brain centers.

Both skeletomotor and gamma motoneurons are coactivated during the execution of a movement, though each system is perhaps preferential for certain types of movements. This mechanism makes it possible to control fine, precise movements and to correct unexpected disturbances in a body segment during movement.

Reflexes underlie much of human behavior. A variety of spinal and brainstem reflexes play supportive roles in voluntary movement. Most of the motor functions of the brainstem involve reflex activity.

The entire brain is involved in the production of voluntary movement. Input to the various sensory projection areas is transmitted to other cortical areas as well as to subcortical structures, where it is recoded and transmitted to the motor cortex. Signals converging on the motor cortex are translated into spatial and temporal codes that are then sent to the appropriate motoneurons for the execution of a movement.

14

Motor Programs and Motor Behavior

The fact that nerve impulses by the motor system can produce muscle contraction and bring about movement of certain body segments does not explain how motor output is organized to produce a coordinated movement pattern. It does not explain how movement patterns can be employed to bring about specifically intended motor acts, such as serving a tennis ball or shooting a basketball. And it does not explain how the movement patterns for carrying out these acts are acquired.

It would be highly desirable to know how the exquisite control and organization that typify the performance of a skilled athlete are structured and carried out. Yet, at present no definitive explanation encompasses all we want to know about this phenomenon. One of the most noted researchers in the field of motor behavior, Richard A. Schmidt, has observed: "Without a doubt, one of the most heated and persistent controversies throughout this century in the field of motor behavior has concerned the competing ideas about the locus of movement control" (Schmidt 1980). In this chapter we shall describe some of the historical as well as current views on motor control and learning.

(a) open loop

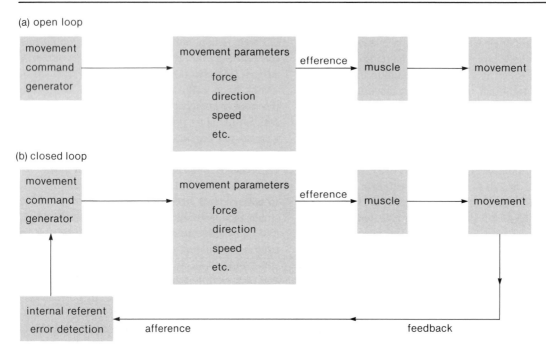

Figure 14.1   *Open- and closed-loop models. Part (a) depicts an open-loop system and part (b) depicts a closed-loop system.*

Closed- and Open-Loop Motor Control Theories

Historically, two major explanations have been proposed for the control of movement. The first emphasizes the role of sensory feedback and has, therefore, been labeled the **closed-loop theory** of motor control. The second proposes that movements are structured centrally within the CNS and executed without feedback; this notion is called the **open-loop theory** of motor control. The processes involved in these two modes of control are very different. Closed-loop control emphasizes the utilization of feedback and the initiating of corrective movements on the basis of feedback to achieve the movement goal. Open-loop control is postulated to involve the generation of a series of movement instructions prior to the movement, and de-emphasizes the role of feedback. The central mechanism for this latter process is commonly called a motor program (figure 14.1).

A **motor program** is viewed as an abstract memory structure that is prepared in advance of a movement. One of the best-known advocates of motor programming, Steven Keele, describes a motor program in the following way:

A motor program is a hierarchical representation of action that proceeds from general goals to specific selection of muscles. Much of the learning is concentrated at higher levels in the hierarchy that specify the general sequence of action. Lower levels are free for alternative specification such as speed of arm. Final details may partly be taken care of by innate reflex patterns (Keele 1982).

Although there have been respected proponents of each of these theories of motor control over the past eighty years—and persuasive arguments have been advanced for each—present evidence does not provide compelling support for either a totally closed-loop or open-loop system of motor behavior. Instead, the control of skilled movement appears to involve the integration of both feedback and motor programming processes (Summers 1981). A recently accelerating trend has been to integrate the two theories into a more comprehensive theory that explains motor control on the basis of the type of movement pattern being employed. As one advocate of integrated control incorporating closed-loop and open-loop systems noted, "Such a . . . control system seems to provide a more adequate description for the organization of rapid sequences of skilled actions and the appropriate modifications and error correction that might occur" (Glencross 1977; also see Brooks 1979; Bizzi 1980). One scientist has even recommended that the dichotomy between central and peripheral control should be removed from psychological theorizing (Reed 1982). Given that the organization and control of movement is probably a result of both closed- and open-loop mechanisms, we shall review the characteristics of each, emphasizing the role of each in various types of movement.

As noted in chapter 11, one of the first closed-loop notions of motor control was the S-R chaining hypothesis that proposed that a movement pattern is performed via a stimulus-response (S-R) process. In one version of this hypothesis, movement is postulated to be based on a "serial chaining"—each component of the movement pattern is assumed to be triggered by feedback from various sensory receptors. This notion, then, proposes that once a movement pattern is initiated, the response of one component of the pattern produces a stimulus (via proprioceptors) that serves as the stimulus for triggering the next response component, and so on.

Adams (1971; 1976a) proposed a recent closed-loop theory of motor behavior in which feedback, error detection, and correction play a major role. According to Adams, a movement pattern is selected and initiated by a **memory trace,** a "modest" motor program developed

through previous experiences. During a movement there is a comparison between a **perceptual trace,** a mechanism for evaluating the correctness of the response generated by the memory trace, and the sensory feedback from the movement in progress. Any resulting error signal serves as a stimulus for triggering corrective action.

The perceptual trace is viewed as a mechanism that develops as the learner receives error information in the form of sensory feedback from task performance. It is assumed that visual, kinesthetic, and auditory feedback contribute sensory information to the building of the perceptual trace. This mechanism, then, develops as a result of experiencing the feedback stimuli with each performance. The learner uses it as the reference to modify the next execution of the movement based on the knowledge of results that is obtained with each execution. Once it has been developed, the perceptual trace functions as a reference mechanism to evaluate the ongoing feedback from movement leading to error detection and correction processes. This closed-loop approach appears to be especially applicable to slow, self-paced movements, since in movements of this type feedback is important in the production of each component of the total movement.

Open-loop ideas of motor control regard the organization and control of a movement as being governed by a central mechanism that, as we have said, is called a motor program after a computer analogy. Woodworth (1899) over eighty years ago suggested that the pattern for simple motor responses is set in advance of their beginning and is uninfluenced during the execution by any feedback, while complex responses can be performed and initiated as a unit. More recently others have provided evidence for motor programs that function without sensory feedback. According to this notion, what one has acquired during the learning of a skill is a motor program that contains the information for commanding a movement pattern. Once the motor program is activated, the movement pattern is executed without recourse to peripheral feedback.

It is obvious that the major difference between these two notions is in the role of feedback. Closed-loop theory specifies the necessity of feedback for movement, while in open-loop control feedback is not essential. The mechanisms capable of supplying feedback during movement are readily apparent, but the argument for the existence of motor programs in humans is much more problematic because at the present time we have only fragmentary evidence for such a mechanism.

Evidence for Motor Programs

In order for motor program control to be a persuasive explanation for motor behavior, it is necessary to demonstrate:

(1) that skilled movements can be performed in the absence of feedback;
(2) for some movements feedback is not used, even though it is present;
(3) movements can be planned in advance of movement rather than as the movement progresses (Schmidt 1981; 1982; Summers 1981).[1]

Movement without Feedback

The earliest support for a closed-loop model of motor control came from research by the esteemed neurophysiologist Charles Sherrington and his colleagues (Mott and Sherrington 1895). They deafferentated the forelimbs of monkeys and observed the postoperative use of the limbs. They reported that though random movements were made after recovery from surgery, the monkeys did not make purposeful use of the limbs. This finding provided strong support for the S-R chaining hypothesis because the deafferentation was presumed to eliminate the feedback and thus eliminate movement capabilities. For many years Sherrington's work stood as the definitive evidence that motor control was a function of a closed-loop, serial chaining mechanism.

About the only serious challenge to the **peripheral hypothesis** in the first half of the twentieth century was a study by Karl Lashley (1917) of a man who had a gunshot wound to the spinal cord, which had deafferented the proprioceptive input to the legs. Lashley reported that the man could produce positioning movements that were about as accurate as "normal" people. He concluded that feedback from the periphery was *not* necessary for movement production. He proposed, therefore, that movement was controlled centrally by some kind of motor program.

But the strongest challenge to closed-loop notions of motor control has come from research over the past twenty-five years. Numerous investigations of lower animals (locusts, birds, mice) whose sensory feedback mechanisms have been severed have demonstrated that normal movement patterns can still be executed in a manner quite similar to the movement that was performed prior to the loss of afferent input (Wilson 1961; Nottebohm 1970; Fentress 1973). More important, the findings of Sherrington on the consequences of deafferentation of the limbs of monkeys have been directly challenged by Taub and his colleagues (Taub and Berman 1968; Taub, Heitmann, and Barro 1977). Using more sophisticated surgical techniques and structuring the postoperative environment to encourage the use of the deafferentated limbs, Taub and his co-workers reported that the animals could use the deafferented limbs to perform a wide variety of motor tasks, and could even learn new tasks. Furthermore, they reported that infant monkeys blinded and deafferented shortly after birth learned to walk (Taub, Perrella, and Barro 1973).

---

[1] The discussion that follows draws heavily on these sources.

Corroborating the findings on lower animals with humans is very difficult since surgical deafferentation is obviously not possible. However, several useful experimental techniques have been employed. Several investigators have used a pressure cuff applied to the upper arm to block sensory input from the arm below the cuff. Under the sensory block conditions, subjects are still able to execute movements, but quality of performance is markedly disrupted (Laszlo 1966; Laszlo, Shamoon, and Sanson-Fisher 1969; Laszlo and Bairstow 1971). The pressure cuff technique has come under severe criticism, however, because it appears that motor impairment accompanies the loss of sensory feedback, suggesting that the disruption in performance during application of the pressure cuff may not be solely attributable to loss of sensory input (Kelso and Stelmach 1974; Glencross and Oldfield 1975).

Another experimental technique for blocking sensory input involves anesthetizing the proprioceptors in a body segment and then testing for motor control in that segment. As with the pressure cuff technique, motor control precision is disrupted, but movements can be made with the affected part (Provins 1958; Smith, Roberts, and Atkins 1972).

Other potential sources of information about the effects of sensory loss in humans comes from people who have had afferent pathways cut to reduce chronic pain and from those who have had prosthetic surgery. These individuals remain capable of performing a wide variety of movements (Cross and McCloskey 1973; Kelso, Holt, and Flatt 1980).

We can conclude from the research on deafferentation that movements can be made in the absence of peripheral feedback. Nevertheless, it is necessary to repeat a point that was made in chapter 11 with regard to movement in the absence of feedback: While motor control of movement is still possible after sensory feedback from

the responding body segments has been eliminated, the elegance and precision of normal movement are usually diminished. Movements are clumsy and lacking in normal, smooth coordination. Thus, while feedback is not essential for the execution of movement, it is likely that it contributes to fine motor control and flexibility in execution.

How can individuals without sensory feedback execute movement patterns, when by classic neurophysiological considerations they should not know where the body segments are, whether they have been moved, and if moved, in what way? Since the movement information cannot be signaled over sensory pathways, it must be conveyed by some central mechanism that does not involve the participation of sensory feedback. The motor program is such a mechanism.

Utilization of Feedback

One of the most persistent criticisms of closed-loop models of motor control has been the charge that sensory feedback is too slow to control rapid and brief movements. In humans, many movements in the limbs are executed with angular velocities of over 100 degrees per second and many are started and completed in less than 100 msec. The basic question with respect to a closed-loop model for movements of this type is how rapid and brief movements can be controlled by feedback when the sensory feedback processing time is longer than the movement time. For example, it appears that processing time for visual information is between 190 and 250 msec (Keele and Posner 1968).

While proprioceptive feedback is often the proposed feedback mechanism for the control of skilled movements—rather than visual feedback—even this mode of feedback appears too slow for controlling rapid, brief movements. Kinesthetic reaction times to stimuli indicating change in force or displacement of a limb have varied from 160 msec (Vance 1948) to 199 msec (Chernikoff and Taylor 1952), and kinesthetic

Figure 14.2 *Oscilloscope tracings for two subjects early and late in practice. The objective was to keep a dot centered on the center line by pressing two keys, one of which made the dot move to the left and one of which made the dot move to the right.*

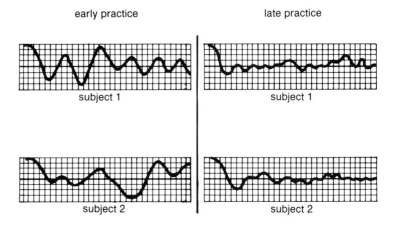

early practice   late practice

subject 1   subject 1

subject 2   subject 2

reactions to amend incorrect responses are characterized by times between 60 and 100 msec (Higgins and Angel 1970; Megaw 1972). Glencross (1977) has suggested that the simple kinesthetic reaction times reported from laboratory studies probably are a poor indication of the time lags that would be typical in a complex skill execution situation. He cites evidence demonstrating that the response to a second kinesthetic stimulus that closely followed a first stimulus is about 300 msec.

Much evidence suggests that sensory feedback is too slow to control brief, rapid movements due to processing time lag, pointing to open-loop control of these types of movements. But there is some evidence that proprioceptive input that is out of the purview of consciousness is capable of producing reflex corrective actions in 40 to 60 msec. This will be discussed more fully later in this chapter.

Assuming a role for feedback in movement patterns that are executed slowly enough to employ sensory feedback, what is the role of feedback as a movement is learned? Here closed- and open-loop models diverge drastically. Closed-loop models typically propose an increased role for feedback as a function of practice (Adams 1976a). Open-loop models propose a diminishing role for feedback with skill acquisition as control becomes vested in a motor program. The classic

work that is usually cited to illustrate the apparent reduced role of feedback during the development of a motor program during skill acquisition is a study conducted by Pew (1966). In Pew's study, subjects were seated before a screen on which a moving dot was displayed. A subject's task was to keep the dot centered on the screen. A button depressed by the right hand accelerated the dot to the right, while the left-hand button, when depressed, accelerated the dot to the left. At first, subjects pressed one button or the other and waited for the dot to move so that they could use visual feedback to see the displacement; then they pressed the other button to correct the error. This strategy produced jerky movements and was largely unsuccessful in maintaining the dot in the center of the screen. As practice continued, the subjects adopted a different strategy. They pressed the buttons quite rapidly in alternation at a rate of about eight per second. The rate of pressing a single button seemed to be altered about every second, depending upon the location of the dot. This suggests that the subjects were emitting a motor program of about eight or so presses, then monitoring the error and correcting it with a new program (figure 14.2). Others have demonstrated a reduction in the use of feedback and an increase in reliance upon some form of motor program control as skill on a task is acquired. (Schmidt and McCabe 1976).

Preprogramming of Movements

Fundamental to motor program theory is the question of how a program is organized into a motor command sequence and whether such organization requires time. Motor program models of motor control expect that the organization of a motor response does take time. Further, the more complex the movements the longer the preprogramming time, since a more comprehensive program must be structured for a complex movement. Beginning with the classic study of Henry and Rogers (1960), who assessed the simple reaction times of subjects who had to perform movements varying in complexity immediately after reacting to a stimulus, numerous studies have found increases in reaction time with increases in movement complexity (see Klapp 1977 for a review of this literature). Christina and his colleagues (Christina, Fischman, Vercruyssen, and Anson 1982) have recently claimed that increases in simple reaction time could have been produced by nonprogramming instead of programming effects.[2] They have called for a more adequate testing of this phenomenon. Until this issue is settled, however, the changes in reaction time as a function of movement complexity will be interpreted as reflecting changes in the time required to organize the appropriate motor program.

Motor Programs and Reflexes

As noted in chapter 13, we now have good evidence that spinal command neurons, when triggered, can produce stereotyped movements that serve as the foundation upon which complex movement patterns can be constructed. Indeed, reflexes can be linked to produce a sequence of movements. Since this topic is discussed at some length in chapter 13, this information will not be repeated here.

Summary of Evidence for Motor Programs

The previous sections describe the various types of evidence supporting motor program models of movement control. It seems clear that at least some movements appear to be controlled by centrally located motor programs. Schmidt (1980) noted that "there is overwhelming evidence that the central nervous system is capable of structuring relatively large segments of movements in advance." Having said this, it seems important to emphasize that while movement patterns can be structured and executed in the absence of feedback, under normal conditions feedback probably plays an important role in motor control and learning. Most contemporary proponents of motor program control emphasize the importance of interaction between feedback and motor program in motor performance and learning (Glencross 1977; Summers 1981).

Functions of Feedback for Motor Program Control

As noted above, even the motor behavior scientists who espouse a motor programming notion of motor control and learning endorse a role for feedback. One of the strongest advocates of motor programming, Steven Keele (1973), has proposed four major functions for feedback that operate before a movement, during a movement, and after a movement. According to Keele, the four functions of feedback are:

1. giving information relevant to starting position;
2. employment as a motor program monitor;
3. making fine adjustments by peripheral feedback loops (motor programs evoke gross motor patterns);
4. acquisition of motor progams.[3]

---

[2] For example, the difference in simple reaction time could have been due to the fact that the amount of inertia to be overcome to release the reaction key was different as the complexity of responses increased. Only the index finger needed to be raised to release the reaction key in the simplest response, while the entire arm had to be moved in the more complex responses.

[3] The discussion that follows draws heavily on Keele (1973).

Feedback Prior to Movement

The first function of feedback is to provide information about the position of the body and its segments as well as the state of the environment just prior to movement. Visual, auditory, and proprioceptive data are integrated in this process of organizing an appropriate motor program to achieve the desired outcome. In the execution of many skills, the body position and the environment may be quite different each time just before executing the skill, so slightly different motor programs must be organized for each execution. In hitting a backhand shot in tennis, one never moves to the ball from exactly the same position; the flight and location where the ball strikes the court are never exactly the same; environmental conditions differ, and feedback is used to signal the current conditions so the correct motor program will be structured.

Feedback for Monitoring the Motor Program

Although motor programming proponents have persuasively shown that movement can be carried out in the absence of feedback, almost all agree that normally feedback can play an important role in movement execution. If a movement pattern is carried out slowly enough and vision is available, visual feedback can be used as a monitor. Likewise, the proprioceptors can serve as movement monitors (Christina, Lambert, and Fischman 1982). If errors are detected, attention can be focused on that feedback mode, and a correction can be initiated by selecting a new motor program.

Another way in which feedback can serve as a program monitor involves the comparison of feedback with what has been called "corollary discharge" by some and "efference copy" by others (Angel 1976). This notion hypothesizes that when a motor program is initiated, the commands to the muscles are accompanied by information that prepares the system for the expected sensory consequences of the movement. This efference copy is then compared with the actual

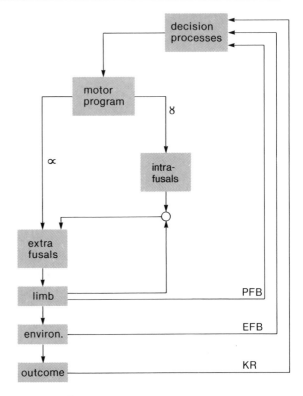

Figure 14.3 *Diagram representing the outside loop for corrections of errors in selection, and the inside loop for corrections for errors in execution. (PFB is proprioceptive feedback, EFB is exteroceptive feedback, and KR is knowledge of results.*

sensory feedback produced by the movement. This comparison process detects errors and may produce corrections at a subconscious level. Thus the corrections are of errors in program execution rather than in program selection. In this instance, when a correct motor program has been selected and something interferes with its execution—such as the limbs not moving to the proper place—signals via the gamma motor loop and the transcortical reflex loop (from proprioceptors to higher-brain centers and back to muscles) produces reflex correction of errors in execution within 40 to 60 msec (Dewhurst 1967; Evarts and Tanji 1974) (figure 14.3). When feedback indicates that an error has been made in program *selection* and that a new program is required for an appropriate response, over 100 msec is required for the corrective movements to occur.

Fine Motor Control and Feedback

The third function of feedback in motor programming described by Keele is closely related to the second and suggests that the muscle receptors are nicely designed for assisting with minute corrections in the motor program, especially through the gamma motor loop. It is suggested that motor program signals activate both skeleto and gamma motoneurons in such a way that they cause the intrafusal muscle fibers to contract to a certain extent while the extrafusal fibers are contracting. If the extrafusal muscle contracts to the same extent as the spindle muscle fibers, this mutual action means that spindle afferents will not be stimulated. However, if there is a discrepancy, the spindle afferents can be stimulated and, through their firing, bring the extrafusal muscle in line. This process may bypass the brain completely or it may occur simultaneously with feedback to the brain. In any case it could result in a compensatory change in the movement to adjust the movement to correspond with the efference copy.[4] This control of skeletal muscle activity via the spindle afferents is discussed in chapters 10 and 13. The important point to note with respect to the use of feedback in correcting errors in motor program selection or errors in program execution is that "feedback is used not to drive the motor pattern but to correct it when the program falls in error. Feedback is the monitor of success or failure" (Keele 1982).

---

[4] Recently an alternative to this view has been advanced, proposing that fine movement control is accomplished by the specification of an equilibrium point between the agonist and the antagonist muscle groups (Polit and Bizzi 1978; 1979; Kelso, Holt, and Flatt 1980).

Acquisition of Motor Programs

Keele's final function of feedback emphasizes that feedback is essential for the complete development of motor programs. Christina and Anson (1981) have provided some empirical support for this position. In outline, the view that a motor program is developed during motor skill acquisition is as follows: First, a template, or image, that corresponds to the task is established. This is based upon the instructions and demonstrations that have been given about the task. Once a template has been established, the learner attempts to select from previously learned motor programs one that produces a movement pattern that most closely resembles the demands of the current task. The learner then performs the task. The feedback from the execution is then compared with the template stored in memory. If there are discrepancies, the motor program is altered and feedback is again compared with the template, and so on, until the "intended" movement and the actual movement correspond and the correct movements are established.

It should be noted that according to this notion, feedback is not conditioned to subsequent movement in a S-R chaining fashion. Instead, feedback is used for making modifications in the motor program. In theory, once the motor program has been established each performance is maintained by an interaction between the motor program and feedback in the manner described for the previous three functions of feedback.

In this interactive view of motor learning, the learner is regarded as an information processor who compares response-produced sensory feedback with a stored representation (template) of what feedback from correct performance should be. Improvement in skill is achieved by the individual through detecting discrepancies between the template and the actual reafference of feedback, then modifying the motor program to reduce or eliminate these discrepancies. Eventually a motor program emerges that brings about the desired performance.

A Generalized Motor Program: The Schema

We now have some evidence for centrally structured plans of action—motor programs—that are structured before a movement is initiated and that control the movement pattern. But there is also considerable evidence that in normal motor responding, response-produced feedback interacts with the motor commands. Schmidt (1981) has described a motor program incorporating these ideas in this way:

A motor program is an abstract representation of action that when activated produces movement without regard to sensory information indicating errors in selection. Once the program has been initiated, the pattern of action is carried out for at least one RT [reaction time] even if the environmental information indicates that an error in selection has been made. Yet, during the program's execution, countless corrections for minor errors can be executed that serve to ensure that the movement is carried out faithfully.

Since no one has ever actually seen a motor program, there has been a great deal of controversy in the motor behavior field over two issues. The first issue is called the "novelty problem" and the second is referred to as the "storage problem" (Schmidt 1976b). The novelty problem is concerned with how a performer can produce novel movements. For example, if one who has never pitched a softball before is asked to make the underhand pitch, usually the movements required to approximate this skill can readily be performed. In another example, a shortstop must field many types of ground balls, and in each case the fielded ball must be thrown to the first baseman. But since each ball is fielded from a different location, a slightly different motor program must be generated to throw the ball to first base. Bartlett (1932) described a similar situation for tennis:

When I make the stroke I do not, as a matter of fact, produce something absolutely new, and I never merely repeat something old. . . . We may fancy that we are repeating a series of movements learned a long time before from a textbook or from a teacher. But motion study shows that in fact we build the stroke afresh on a basis of the immediately preceding balance of postures and the momentary needs of the game. Every time we make it, it has its own characteristics.

Even when the same movements are performed under the same environmental conditions, slightly different movement patterns have been detected through cinematographic analysis (Higgins and Spaeth 1972). These examples raise the same fundamental question: Where do the motor programs come from, if the performers can execute movements that have never been exactly performed before? Early ideas about motor programming did not adequately explain how movements can be performed for the first time or how a movement can be performed with incredible variety and flexibility.

The storage problem concerns how programs are stored in memory. A number of the early motor program advocates implied that for every movement pattern there is a separate and specific motor program that controls it. This raises the question: Given the enormous variety of movements that one can produce—even the variation in speed, force, etc., that one can exhibit in performing one skill, such as the overhand throw—how can the brain store the incredible number of programs that would be required? Even closed-loop models of motor control do not necessarily resolve the storage problem. When movements are hypothesized to be controlled by feedback and error reduction, there is also hypothesized to be some type of reference of correctness with which the movements are compared. This implies that there must be a reference of correctness for each movement with which response-produced feedback can be compared (Adams 1976a). This, also, points to the storage problem.

In an effort to overcome the problems associated with previous notions about motor programs, proposals have been advanced for a **generalized motor program.** The concept most

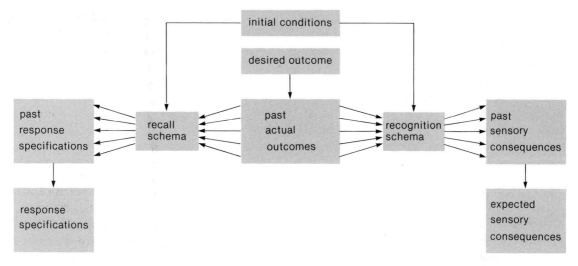

Figure 14.4   *The recall and recognition schema in relation to various sources of information.*

popularly used for this generalized motor program is a "schema" (Pew 1974; Schmidt 1975). Schmidt (1976b) explains that "schema theory evolved from an attempt to take the strong parts of various theoretical positions, adding modifications and extensions so that the new theory would be able to deal with some of the problems" of previous theories, "particularly the storage and novelty problems."

A schema was originally defined as an abstraction of information from a particular class of events that forms a rule governing membership into that particular class (Bartlett 1932). Extending this definition to relate to motor skills, Schmidt (1975) proposed that a motor schema is a "rule" that encompasses the underlying movement principle for a movement response class. More specifically, he proposed that the relationships among four types of information are abstracted from any movement in which an individual engages:

1. The initial conditions that existed when the movement started. Limb and body position as well as environmental conditions are included in this information. Was I standing or running? What was the size and shape of the object I was throwing?

2. The response specifications (parameters[5]) that were employed in the execution of the movement, that is, the motor program and parameters selected to achieve the goal.
3. The actual outcome of the movement, that is, information about the extent to which the response was successful in relation to the desired outcome. Did the jump shot go in? Was the pitch a strike?
4. The sensory consequences of movement, that is, the sensory feedback from making the response. What did the movement feel, sound, and look like?

Given these four sources of information, the theory proposes that two independent schemata are involved in the learning and performance of motor skills—a recall schema and a recognition schema (figure 14.4).

---

[5] As used in this context, a parameter refers to a specification of the motor program for the particular expression of the pattern of movement. Some parameters of movement are speed, force, and movement size. Undoubtedly others exist, but in an empirical sense they have not been adequately defined.

The first mechanism, the **recall schema,** is responsible for movement initiation and execution. In other words, it is the mechanism responsible for structuring the impulses sent to the musculature for producing a movement pattern. When a performer is asked to perform a movement for the first time, such as a tennis serve, a recall schema (or movement pattern) will be selected based on the relationship, built up over past experiences, with similar movements, between the outcomes and the response specifications. When the recall schema has been selected, the next step is the translation of the motor program into a motor command. Various movement parameters are programmed into the command, such as duration of the movement (speed of the movement), the force required, and timing. These produce a particular spatial and temporal organization for the movement. The motor commands activate the muscles, producing a pattern of movement to achieve the intended goal.

The first execution of a new movement will be the best guess of the appropriate movement pattern, based on the relationship between past outcomes and past response specifications for the same class of movements. This is because the recall schema only has a relationship between previous outcome and response specifications from similar tasks on which to draw. But in making a new movement, the performer pairs the response specifications and the actual outcomes on each practice trial for that particular task. After several such trials, there begins to form a relationship between the two variables. This relationship, the recall schema, is updated with each practice trial. After much practice the recall schema becomes well developed. As the strength of the recall schema increases, the predicted specifications more accurately approach the desired outcome.

As a further consequence of the recall schema, an image of the expected sensory consequences of actually producing that movement is also generated. This constitutes the **recognition schema,** which is a mechanism for determining in advance what the movement is going to feel, sound, and look like. Like the recall schema, it is assumed that the recognition schema stores the sensory consequences of past movements along with their actual outcomes. These two sources of information are used to develop the relationship between sensory consequences of a response and actual outcome. Based on the relationship abstracted from these two sources, the recognition schema generates the expected sensory consequences of the correct movement: the best guess about the sensory consquences if this outcome is produced, based on the relationship of past sensory consequences and past desired outcomes. This enables a comparison to be made between the intended movement and the actual movement-produced feedback. An evaluation of the correctness of the movement occurs by having the recognition schema compare the actual with the expected sensory consequence. Such a comparison generates an error signal when a mismatch occurs.

It can be seen that the recognition schema is assumed to be based upon sensory feedback from past movements. The recognition schema evaluates the correctness of a response by comparing feedback from the ongoing response with the expected sensory consequences. In executing a movement, the performer can specify the desired outcome and, through the recognition schema, predict the expected sensory consequences of the movement. A mismatch between feedback and the reference for correctness generates an error signal that tells the recall schema to update the instructions to the muscles, and consequently, produces a more accurate response. This process is assumed to function during the execution of slow, graded movements and upon the completion of the response in fast, ballistic movements.

The roles of the recall and recognition schema depend strictly upon the type of movement being executed, but basically the recall schema is responsible for the generation of motor commands to the musculature that produce the movement (or movement corrections); the recognition schema is responsible for evaluation of response-produced feedback that enables the generation of error information about the movement. To illustrate, if the movement is rapid, with a completion time of less than 200 msec, the movement is carried out under the complete control of the recall schema. The motor program determines all of the details of the movement in advance, and any stimulus that signals the ongoing movement needs to be modified must wait one reaction time (between 120 and 200 msec) before a *new* motor program can be *selected* and initiated. Thus, when a movement is completed in less than one reaction time, the performer completes the programmed movement even though the situation might indicate that the movement selected will be incorrect. For this type of movement, the recognition schema operates after the movement is completed by providing expected sensory consequences against which the movement-produced feedback is compared. Any resulting discrepancies indicate that an error has occurred, and this information can be incorporated into the recall schema the next time the movement is executed.

A slow movement is carried out using both schemata. In this case the performer makes a short programmed movement and then compares the movement-produced feedback against the expected sensory consequences. If there is a mismatch, a modification in the original program is made. The comparison process is repeated until the difference between the expected sensory consequences and the movement-produced feedback is zero. Here the role of the recall schema is to produce short movements only, and the basic determinant of movement accuracy is the comparison of the expected and the actual feedback. So for slow movements there is a dependence on the recognition schema, even though the performer may be modifying the original movement with the recall schema.

Motor learning is viewed as rule learning through the development of the schemata with practice. **Schema theory** predicts that the strength of both schemata, for a particular class of movements, is directly related to the amount and variability of practice. In the case of the recall schema, the relationship is built up with practice between the response specifications and actual outcomes, as modified by initial conditions.[6] The strength of the recall schema is assumed to be a function of the number of practice trials and the variability of prior experiences. It is assumed that increased amount and variability of experiences will lead to the development of an increasingly robust recall schema. As a consequence, a performer confronted with a novel situation that is governed by the schema will be able to generate the appropriate response specifications, given the desired outcome and initial conditions. The extent of success in the initial trial with the novel response will be directly related to the variability of practice that the performer has experienced that is governed by that class of movement prior to the novel response. The theory predicts, therefore, better performance on the initial trials of a novel movement, and an accelerated rate of learning, as a function of increased variability in previous movement experiences of a similar type (see Shapiro and Schmidt 1982 for a review of research on this prediction of schema theory).

---

[6] Recent research has indicated that initial conditions might not be as important for certain kinds of movements as schema theory originally proposed (Polit and Bizzi 1978; Schmidt and McGown 1980). For certain movements apparently the motor program specifies an end point directly, and the body segments move to it regardless of the initial conditions.

Increased variability of practice also enhances the development of the recognition schema because it leads to a stronger relationship between the actual outcome and the sensory consequences. As a result, once the recognition schema has been developed through practice, a performer asked to execute a novel slow movement can move to the correct position by comparing the movement-produced feedback and the expected sensory consequences as generated by the recognition schema. For a novel rapid movement the performer can generate the expected sensory consequences of the movement and can compare the expected sensory consequences and the actual outcome to ascertain the extent of error (if any) on that particular practice trial. We shall have more to say about variability of practice in chapter 17.

Advantages of Schema Theory

Summers (1981) has nicely summarized the advantages of schema theory over other models of motor behavior:

There are many advantages of the schema theory over traditional open- and closed-loop models. There is no necessity for a separate motor program or reference of corrections to be stored for each movement that a person makes. By applying various response specifications to a generalized motor program a large number of movements can be generated from this abstract representation. In this way the tremendous flexibility evident in human skills can be achieved. Furthermore, the model emphasizes the interaction between program and feedback in the control of movement.

It is nonetheless important to note that there is only fragmentary empirical evidence supporting the existence of generalized motor programs. One major limitation of this model is its vagueness regarding how a program is formed in the first place, how one makes the first response before any schema exists, and how the motor schema parameters and sensory consequences are developed. Furthermore, one of the predictions of

schema theory is that the two schemata are separate states and that they should, therefore, develop independently. But the research on this issue is equivocal (Schmidt, Christenson, and Rogers 1975; Zelaznik, Shapiro, and Newell 1978; Wallace and McGhee 1979). No motor behavior model presently provides a complete understanding of motor learning and control, but for the time being schema theory provides a useful framework for attempting to understand this complex subject.

Summary

We have no definitive explanation of the organization of motor control. Historically, two explanations have been proposed for the control of movement, closed-loop theory and open-loop theory. The former emphasizes the utilization of feedback to achieve the movement goal. The latter emphasizes central programming in the initiation and execution of a movement, and the mechanism for this process is commonly called a motor program. The major differences between these two notions is in the role of feedback. Closed-loop theory specifies the necessity of feedback for movement, while in open-loop control feedback is not essential.

Support for motor program control of movement comes from several sources: (1) evidence that skilled movements can be performed in the absence of feedback; (2) evidence that for some movements feedback is not used, even though it is present; (3) evidence that movements can be preprogrammed rather than controlled as the movement progresses. In spite of the evidence that coordinated movements can be made in an open-loop manner, under normal conditions feedback probably plays an important role in motor control and learning.

Feedback has at least four functions in motor behavior: (1) It gives information relevant to starting position; (2) It is employed as a motor program monitor; (3) It is used to make fine adjustments during a movement; (4) It is used in the acquisition of motor programs.

In an effort to overcome the problems associated with older notions about motor programs, especially the novelty and storage problems, Schmidt proposed a generalized motor program theory called schema theory. A motor schema is a "rule" that encompasses the underlying movement principle for a movement response class. This theory proposes the existence of two schemata, a recall schema responsible for the production of movement via open-loop motor programs, and a recognition schema responsible for movement evaluation to determine response correctness. According to schema theory, rapid movements are produced by the recall schema and run off by the motor program. Slow movements, once initiated, come under the control of the recognition schema and are therefore feedback based. While certainly not the final answer in explaining motor control, schema theory provides a useful framework for understanding this phenomenon.

Motor Learning and Conditions Influencing Skill Acquisition

15

Learning and Memory

*P*revious chapters have focused on the role of sensory mechanisms in skillful motor behavior and the neural mechanisms that underlie motor behavior. In the remaining chapters we turn our attention to the processes involved in motor learning and to the effects of certain variables on the learning and performance of motor skills. The use of this information in teaching motor skills will also be described.

Complex motor behavior consists of a variety of movements, and these movement patterns must be learned. Although the individual muscle contractions that allow skilled movement are functional in early infancy, the repertoire of complex motor patterns is very small. The movement patterns that require the selection of certain muscle groups (spatial organization) and the contraction of these muscles in a precise sequential order (temporal organization) must be learned. One way to understand how we acquire motor skills is to study the memory aspects of motor behavior since learning obviously requires memory. In this chapter we focus on the neural processes in learning-memory.

Learning-Memory and the Nervous System

Learning

We have referred to motor programs as plans for action. We now must ask how they are learned. They certainly must have a physical basis—there must be changes in the nervous system when we learn. In chapter 2, learning was defined as a neural change that occurs as a result of experiences with stimuli in the environment. It is the internal process assumed to occur when a change in performance exhibits itself. You may want to return to chapter 2 to review the section on motor learning.

Memory

Closely related to learning is, of course, memory. The ability to learn cannot proceed without it. The word *memory* refers to the retention and subsequent retrieval of information. It is really no more than a label used to indicate that people do retain information. Memory is commonly measured by a recognition or recall test, and evidence of memory retrieval is what we expect of individuals in order to infer that learning-memory has occurred (Adams 1976b). If I practice a tennis stroke today and can perform it tomorrow, it follows that I have retained something that enables me to recall the movement pattern.

Memory is assumed to involve some modification in neuronal structures, and the postulated neural correlate of memory is called a memory trace. Neuroscientist J. Z. Young (1978) has said:

Memories are . . . physical systems in brains, whose organization and activities constitute records or representations of the outside world. . . . The representations are accurate to the extent that they allow the organism to re-present appropriate action to the world.

Learning deals more with the acquisition of new information or skills, and memory deals more with remembering learned information or skills. But in any discussion of learning it is difficult to put memory into one category and learning into another. Learning and memory are inextricably related. It is artificial to speak of the learning process as isolated from memory. We therefore use the term **learning-memory** frequently in this chapter.

Retention and Forgetting

As noted, memory refers to the retention and retrieval of information. We make a distinction between the acquisition and the retention phases of learning. The acquisition phase is the time or trials needed to attain a certain level of proficiency. **Retention** is the savings of proficiency on a skill following periods without practice. What is retained is said to be learned. What is not retained, or at least not retrievable, is said to be forgotten.

Most motor skills, such as sports and industrial skills, are learned with the intention of performing them at a later time. Athletic contests and assembly line performance are examples of occasions that demand the retention of skills learned during prior practice. Instructors of motor skills, as well as learners, must be concerned with retention and forgetting, as well as acquisition, during motor learning.

One might ask why there is any forgetting at all. Why should not skills be retained at a certain level regardless of how much time intervenes between performances? There are two basic theories of **forgetting**: trace decay theory and interference theory. **Trace decay theory** assumes that passage of time causes a weakening of memory traces. If you do not practice basketball shooting, you will forget how just from lack of practice. According to this idea, whatever modifications occurred in the nervous system during learning can decay when practice is not continued to maintain them.

Does forgetting consist of an actual loss of stored information, or does it result from a loss of access to information, which, once stored in memory, remains forever? The issue has been controversial for many years. Some researchers contend that once information is registered in long-term memory it is never lost from the system, although it may be inaccessible (Tulving 1974). Others propose that certain circumstances may cause stored information to be destroyed (Loftus and Loftus 1980). At present we have no satisfactory solution to this issue.

The most powerful opposition to trace decay theory has come from interference theory, which has been and remains the most influential theory of forgetting. **Interference theory** advocates argue that forgetting is the result of competing responses learned either before or after having learned a task. In this view, learning some things tends to interfere with stored memories of previously learned information. For example, learning tennis skills might interfere with the movement patterns built up for basketball shooting skills.

Most research on interference is carried out through experiments on transfer of learning. Transfer is the effect of learning one task upon the learning of a second. Interference theory suggests that forgetting occurs as a result of interference from learning other things. The interfering activity can occur before the main task is learned, in which case it is called proactive interference; or it can occur between learning the original task and the retention test, in which case it is called retroactive interference.

Present Knowledge About Learning-Memory

The physical processes that underlie the functional changes we call learning-memory have provided a fascinating challenge to many scientists. Biological sciences such as neuroanatomy, neurophysiology, and biochemistry, in addition to psychology, have made important contributions to this work. The basic question is exactly what happens when an organism is in the process of learning and remembering. The past fifty years of intense research has produced much information about neural mechanisms in learning-memory, but present knowledge concerning the nervous system's function in learning-memory is far from complete. Nevertheless, students of human motor behavior need to have some understanding of the accumulated knowledge on this subject.

Learning-Memory Functions

A learning-memory mechanism must perform at least four fundamental, interrelated functions. First, external and internal stimuli impinging on the individual, which constitute experience, must be detected, selected, and coded into neural impulses; this might be called a registration function. Second, the coded data about that set of stimuli must be stored; this would constitute a storage function. Third, access to that coded information must be available to retrieve the specific experiences from storage; this would be a retrieval function. Fourth, the retrieved information must again be recoded into neural activity that in some manner recreates the sensations and qualities of the original experience or initiates responses; this might be considered a read-out function (figure 15.1). Failure of any of these functions will lead to faulty memory.

Figure 15.1   *Functions of a learning-memory mechanism.*

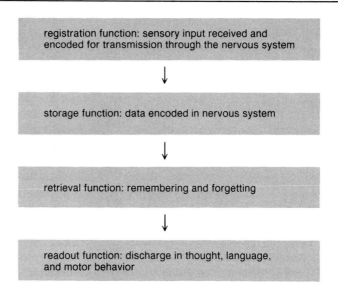

registration function: sensory input received and encoded for transmission through the nervous system

↓

storage function: data encoded in nervous system

↓

retrieval function: remembering and forgetting

↓

readout function: discharge in thought, language, and motor behavior

Previous chapters that dealt with sensory integration and motor integration and control are related to the first and fourth of the functions above. This chapter focuses on the second and third functions of learning-memory. However, since research has been overwhelmingly concerned with memory storage rather than retrieval, we shall have to limit our attention more to this function in examining the neural basis for learning-memory.

Learning-Memory Theories

Theories about learning-memory prior to the twentieth century were mostly based upon myth, superstition, religious teaching, and primitive physiology. Aristotle taught that the heart was the seat of memory and the brain was a structure that cooled the blood. An eighteenth-century scholar, Descartes, in one of the earliest attempts to explain memory in terms of the action of the brain, said:

When the mind wills to recall something, this volition causes the little (pineal) gland, by inclining successively to different sides, to impel the animal spirits toward different parts of the brain, until they come upon that part where the traces are left of the thing which it wishes to remember; for these traces are nothing else than the circumstances that the pores of the brain through which the spirits have already taken their course on presentation of the object, have thereby acquired a greater facility than the rest to be open again the same way by the spirits which come to them; so that these spirits coming upon the pores enter therein more readily than into the others (cited in Lashley 1950).

An even more bizarre approach to describing learning-memory, **phrenology,** was advanced by a group of pseudoscientists of the eighteenth and nineteenth centuries. The phrenologists taught that memory was stored in different compartments of the brain, each of which controlled a separate behavior, or "faculty" (see figure 6.3).

No theory of learning-memory had a scientific basis until the late nineteenth century, when studies of the functions of the nervous system began in earnest. Over the past eighty years an enormous effort has gone into the search for an understanding of the learning-memory process. The learning-memory theory currently favored by neuroscientists proposes that there are several stages to this process; this has been labeled consolidation theory. Recently a rival to this theory

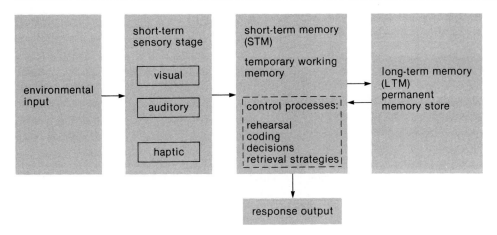

Figure 15.2   *The Atkinson and Shiffrin model of stages of memory consolidation.*

has been gaining support. The new theory is called the levels-of-processing theory. We shall describe both in order. More attention will be given to the former because we have a larger body of empirical support for it.

Consolidation Theory

The original **consolidation theory** was advanced by Muller and Pilzecher (1900). They hypothesized that information is initially stored in some form of dynamic electrical activity and is gradually converted into structural changes in the brain. More recently Atkinson and Shiffrin (1971) and Eccles (1977), to name only some of the more influential scientists in this field, have supported and extended the consolidation theory. Although the details of the theory vary, common basic concepts and hypotheses are easily discernible, and they are sufficiently similar to provide a composite model of learning-memory. Briefly, **consolidation theory** suggests that following a learning experience a continuing process involving several stages takes place until a memory trace is firmly consolidated or stored in the form of some structural or chemical change (figure 15.2).

In line with the notion that several interrelated processes exist in learning-memory, proponents of consolidation theory have identified at least three stages. These stages are called short-term sensory stage (STSS), short-term memory (STM), and long-term memory (LTM). Each is different in storage capacity, the form in which the information is presumed to be stored, and the rate of loss of information.

Short-Term Sensory Stage (STSS)

According to consolidation theory, the **short-term sensory stage** occurs immediately after the experience and can be viewed as an image of a stimulus that is maintained briefly after the physical stimulus ends. As information is received it is transduced at the receptors into a physiological representation that is very briefly stored in a sensory storage system. There is considerable evidence that information persists in a sensory store for two to three seconds for vision and perhaps up to fifteen seconds in other sensory modalities (see Crowder 1978 for a review of STSS). It seems that this representation is transformed into a new code and retained temporarily in another storage system that is also of relatively short duration. This system is STM.

The STSS is capable of processing large amounts of information, but it loses information very rapidly (Sperling 1960). Moreover, STSS handles information in terms of the way it entered the system, in a literal way: The coded information has a strong similarity with the actual stimulus input, in a manner similar to the way camera film records what enters through the lens.

Short-Term Memory (STM)

Short-term memory is a fairly brief period during which the relatively fragile and labile trace of an experience is maintained by a transient reverberative process. This phase decays within a few seconds or minutes, but before doing so the short-term electrochemical process causes a series of actions in the brain that leads to a long-lasting phase, representing a long-term memory (LTM). During this phase the memory trace is consolidated in the form of a structural modification of the nervous system, presumably a specific biochemical or morphological alteration in the neurons (Deutsch and Deutsch 1975).

STM is viewed as having a limited capacity and a relatively short duration (Atkinson and Shiffrin 1971). The initial evidence that humans have the capacity to hold only a limited amount of information in STM was provided by Miller (1956) in the mid-1950s. According to him, STM has a capacity of only about seven (plus or minus two) items. Exactly what constitutes an "item" is not clear, but it has been proposed that separate items, such as letters in a word, might be "chunked" into larger collections. Thus, the word *cat* might originally be three items in STM, but with learning, the entire word may be chunked as one item in STM. Recent research has shown rather convincingly that learning techniques for "chunking" information are successful in increasing the capacity of items in STM (Ericsson, Chase, and Faloon 1980).

Probably several STM systems enable one to process input from different sensory modalities in STM at the same time. In this view STM processing of verbal information can be carried out while STM processing of nonverbal information is occurring (Roediger, Knight, and Kantowitz 1977). The idea of several STM systems is congruent with evidence of special-purpose processors, each with its own attentional capacity (Allport, Antonis, and Reynolds 1972).

STM may also have a role in movement responding in addition to its role in processing incoming information. Klapp (1976) has proposed that STM is where movement programs from long-term memory are readied and held briefly before they are run off.

One thing clearly implied by consolidation theory is that if the electrical events in STM are interrupted, the final stage, or LTM, will not be triggered, and memory of the experience will be lost. This prediction has been supported by numerous studies that have shown that if the brain is disturbed soon after a learning event, memory storage is disrupted.

Evidence for STM

Perhaps the most compelling clinical support for STM comes from head injury in humans. After a severe head injury, a person usually experiences a period of unconsciousness. When consciousness is regained, there is frequently a loss of memory of events just before the accident. Common exclamations are: "What happened?" "Where am I?" "How did I get here?" This condition is known as retrograde amnesia (RA). With RA, memory loss occurs from the second before the accident and becomes less pronounced for events occurring some time before. In other words, there is typically no impairment of memory other than for very recent events. Russell (1959) reported that of over a thousand cases of head injury that he studied, in only about 13 percent was there no report of RA. Amnesia was reported for events occurring from a few seconds to thirty minutes before the injury in about 67 percent of the cases. In the other cases there was RA for periods longer than thirty minutes. It appears that the injury to the head causes electrical disruption of events in STM and thus prevents STM from triggering the LTM stage. There is no memory deficit for events occurring some time before the accident, presumably because they were already in LTM and therefore not affected by momentary electrical disruption caused by the accident.

Experimental work with **electroconvulsive shock** (ECS) also supports an STM stage. In ECS a rather substantial electric charge is passed through the brain. These experiments involve periods of learning separated by the administration of ECS and then testing for retention of the learned material. With humans and with animals, ECS, if given shortly after a learning experience, produces a retention deficit. As the interval between the learning and the application of the ECS increases, the learning deficit decreases; recently learned information is more adversely affected than previously learned information.

It would not be feasible to review all of the pertinent research in which ECS has been used, but one example will help to elucidate the findings from experiments in which this technique was employed. Halstead and Rucker (1968) used ECS to interfere with STM in mice. A mouse was placed on a platform under an intensely bright light. To escape the light, the mouse quickly stepped into a nearby hole. Once in the hole, it received a foot shock. The next day under the same conditions, the mouse would not step into the hole, presumably because it remembered being shocked when it stepped in the hole. However, if an electrical current was passed through its brain immediately after the foot shock, the next day the mouse would not hesitate to run into the hole to escape the light. Apparently, the electrical current disrupted the STM process. But if the current was not passed through the mouse's brain for some time after it received the foot shock, the effect on the mouse's memory was much less. This suggests the information had reached LTM (and therefore was not bothered by electric shock) before the electric current was applied.

Clinical work in which ECS therapy has been used with human patients in an effort to correct certain mental dysfunctions has shown that the patients are not only disoriented immediately after the ECS treatment, but they are also confused about events immediately before the ECS. In other words, the ECS treatment frequently produces a genuine retrograde amnesia (McGaugh and Herz 1972).

Experiments in which anesthetic and convulsant drugs, such as ether, sodium pentobarbital, and pentylenetetrazol, were administered to animals soon after learning trials to interfere with STM have generally yielded results comparable with ECS experiments. On the other hand, when stimulant drugs have been injected into animals shortly after completion of learning periods and the animals tested for learning retention after the drugs had worn off, drug-treated animals demonstrated superior performance over the control animals (those who learned the same task but did not receive an injection of stimulant drugs). Investigators have concluded that the results with the stimulant drugs could best be interpreted as showing that these drugs improve memory consolidation by facilitating the short-term memory process (see McGaugh and Herz 1972 for a review of this work).

Evidence for some sort of short-term memory process that gradually produces a long-term memory trace is rather convincing. However, the exact way in which this short-term mechanism functions has not been ascertained. The most generally accepted hypothesis at this time is that the neurons in the brain record a sensory input by means of a pattern of neural activity. A reverberating circuit is established in a set of neurons, and the nerve impulses circulate many times in a closed, self-exciting circuit until some type of permanent process develops to "stamp in," or consolidate, the data and cause LTM. This process—a reverberating circuit for STM and a permanent storage mechanism—seems to be confirmed in the experiments mentioned above.

Long-Term Memory (LTM)

Long-term memory refers to the stage of memory storage that spans hours, days, and even years. It is manifested in the ability to recognize or recall something after a long delay without rehearsal. As noted above, one of the main functions of STM is to consolidate information into LTM. The transfer process requires time—minutes, hours, perhaps days—but it proceeds much faster when the material is meaningful.

Whereas STM has limited capacity, it seems that LTM has virtually unlimited capacity. Moreover, although information in STM can be lost completely and leave no permanent record, it is possible that no complete loss of memory occurs among materials that have reached LTM. Whether one can retrieve, or remember, certain information may be dependent upon such factors as the precise way the information is stored and the cues available to the individual for locating the information. Loss of information from LTM may involve its being misplaced in the complex associative structure of memory, rather than actually being eliminated. The loss in this case is like losing a golf ball. The ball still exists, out there in the rough, but the owner cannot locate it. On the other hand, there may actually be a loss of information over time or the information may be blocked by previously learned or subsequently learned information.

Two major issues have concerned neuroscientists with regard to LTM. The first issue is where memory is located. The second centers on the structural basis for LTM. Remarkable advances in understanding these issues have been made, but at present we still have much to learn before definitive conclusions can be drawn about both the location and structural basis of LTM. We shall briefly review current knowledge about these issues.

Localization of LTM

During the early years of this century the dominant belief about LTM was that memories are localized in a single region of the brain. This notion was probably a carry-over from phrenological theory. More significant were the findings from electrical stimulation[1] experiments during the latter decades of the nineteenth century. These "brain stimulation" experiments had mapped out the somatosensory and motor areas of the cerebral cortex and had shown that sensations and movements could be evoked in certain regions of the brain, depending on where the stimulation was made. This line of work suggested that a similar localization of function for memories might be present in the brain.

The idea that memories are localized in the brain led to the conclusion that if the site of memories is removed, the memories will be obliterated. Thus, numerous lesion (meaning to destroy tissue) and ablation (meaning to remove tissue) experiments were performed in an effort to find the site of memory. These studies failed to locate the site or the connection of any pathways responsible for memory. Of course, certain behaviors, especially those based upon complex sensorimotor integration, can be severely disturbed by localized brain destruction, but it is difficult to show unequivocally that memory for some specific event is localized in a particular restricted point in the brain.

As we noted in chapter 6, Karl S. Lashley studied the question of brain localization in great detail. His work offered no support for the notion that specific areas of the brain act as repositories for memory. However, particular brain regions may play a critical part in the consolidation of

---

[1] Electrical stimulation of the brain is done by exposing the brain, touching different parts of it with an electrically active probe, and observing the results. With humans this is only done as a concomitant to surgery to correct some dysfunction.

memories about certain specific classes of events in humans (see chapter 6 for details on this subject).

Although there is evidence that certain brain areas may have memory functions, investigators have been moving away from viewing the brain as having centers and regions with specific memory functions. A promising substitute has recently been proposed by John (1972; John et al. 1973), that learning-memory may be reflected in unique spatiotemporal patterns of electrical activity that encompass most of the brain. According to John (1976), "Many brain functions are distributed throughout most brain regions, but . . . some regions contribute more than others to any given function."

Evidence for this idea comes from research examining the electrophysiological correlates of learning, that is, looking for changes in brain electrical activity during learning (Olds 1977). The electrical activity of large populations of cells and single neurons has been monitored in experiments of this type. Although there are many technical and interpretive problems in analyzing vast amounts of electrophysiological data, this work suggests that when we learn something, neurons in many parts of the brain develop a new rhythm of firing that corresponds to the learning. The memory of what is learned is found in its unique cell-firing rhythm, not in any specific region. John (1976) states: "No part of the brain, by itself, holds a particular memory or list of knowledge. The average activity of cells throughout the brain causes us to see, move a finger, or remember our first bicycle ride."

While this work is promising, many unanswered questions remain, and it does not provide a completely satisfactory explanation for the issue of where memories are stored. This approach is incomplete because memory does not depend entirely upon an active mechanism, or purely dynamic process. This, of course, does not preclude the possibility that the initial dependence of memory necessitates reverberating circuits, for the initial experience does trigger the passage of impulses in the nervous system. As we have noted, evidence from studies in which electrical activity in the brain is disrupted shortly after the learning experience has shown an impairment of memory.

Structural Basis for LTM

How memories are consolidated and stored for LTM has challenged the efforts of numerous scientists. Although there is little agreement on the neural basis of LTM, current theories can be grouped into two major categories: chemical theories and morphological theories. These theories are certainly not mutually exclusive, because a change in structural relationships (morphological change) is possible through a modification in molecules (chemical change). Indeed, this is exactly what Sir John Eccles, the Nobel laureate in neurophysiology, has recently proposed (1977). We shall discuss this theory later.

A growing body of research on the subject of LTM points very clearly to chemical processes. The biochemical bases of memory are the subject of widespread current investigations. One of the most important factors stimulating biochemical studies on memory has been the remarkable advances in the field of molecular biology in the past two decades.

Current chemical work on memory is focusing on the possibility that the neural change is in a modification of the chemical structure of the neurons of the brain. Basically, it has been proposed that slight changes occur in the molecular structure of brain cells as a result of learning, and these molecular changes "store" the information in coded form.

Scientists interested in the chemical correlates of memory have performed experiments in which they taught various things to animals and then analyzed the chemical composition of the animals' brains. They have theorized that the brain from an untrained animal should be chemically different from that of a trained animal, and their research has tended to support this belief. These experiments have generally confirmed the view that an organism's brain chemistry is subtly altered by the organism's experiences (see Dunn 1980 for a review of this research).

The nucleic acids and nucleoproteins have been studied extensively over the past fifteen years. At the present time, the more promising substances appear to be the nucleic acids. Ribonucleic acid (RNA), an essential intracellular chemical found in every neuron in the nervous system, is believed by a number of scientists to be the substance that is modified in LTM and, therefore, to be responsible for storing information. An RNA molecule is a large complex unit, consisting of thousands of subunits. The potential number of different arrangements of subunits within the RNA molecule is enormous, and each arrangement creates a distinct RNA molecule capable of causing the synthesis of distinct protein molecules.

The amount and structure of RNA seem to be altered by neural activity; this altered state could result in modified protein synthesis and, therefore, modified functions of the cell. For these reasons RNA has been proposed by some scientists as the structural component for the memory process, or the "memory molecule." Considerable recent evidence has accumulated that suggests that RNA must play a vital role in memory consolidation (for reviews of this research see Rainbow 1979; Rose and Longstaff 1979; Dunn 1980). Studies have demonstrated that—

- RNA synthesis is increased in nerve stimulation.
- There is an increase of RNA synthesis in learning situations.
- Base ratios of RNA change during learning.
- A decrease in RNA adversely affects learning and performance.

- Chemical stimulators of RNA synthesis accelerate the rate at which consolidation is achieved and sometimes increase learning.
- An increase in RNA facilitates the storage of information and its retrieval.
- RNA can be transferred from one animal to a second animal, and the conditioned responses of the first animal will be transferred to the second.

Even though we have a variety of evidence that RNA is implicated in memory consolidation, some studies suggest that perhaps RNA is not the primary agent for data storage, but instead is an agent for the transfer of information to protein. These investigations suggest that the synthesis of new brain proteins is crucial for the establishment of the LTM process. According to this view, if new proteins are prevented from forming in the brain, the LTM process never becomes established, even though the STM process is not interfered with (see Quartermain 1976 for a review of this research).

While the evidence seems convincing that biochemical changes accompany learning-memory, correlation of neurochemicals and retention does not establish the physiological basis for memory, but merely suggests the possibility. Much remains to be done to specify the biochemical basis of learning-memory.

Morphological theories of memory have been popular among neuroscientists for over seventy years. These theories suggest that changes in the relationship between neurons occur during the formation of a memory trace. Since it is known that nerve impulses pass from one neuron to another via the synapses, the synapse has long fascinated learning theorists. This juncture has seemed to be a likely candidate for involvement in learning-memory because of its key role in the transmission of impulses.

It has been suggested that new synaptic relationships are established or that existing synapses become more efficient when new information is transmitted to the brain. These modifications of synaptic relationships might take the form of enlarging or shrinking of synapses or increasing or decreasing the actual number of synapses as the result of use or disuse. They might also take the form of increasing or decreasing secretion of transmitter substance (Deutsch 1973).

Several investigators over the past thirty years have reported that dendritic branching is considerably greater in the cerebral cortex of animals raised in groups in a complex environment than in litter mates raised individually in laboratory cages. The increased branching in neurons presumably provides increased surface for synaptic contacts. The increased branching and the reported alterations in the size of individual synapses together might conceivably underlie some forms of information storage in the brain.

An interdisciplinary group of scientists at the University of California has also reported more dendrite spines[2] in animals exposed to an "enriched" environment than in litter mates from an "impoverished" environment. In addition, they found that the synaptic junctions of the animals from the enriched environment averaged about 50 percent larger in cross section than similar junctions in litter mates from impoverished environments (Rosenzweig, Bennett, and Diamond 1972). Research on the effects of experience on the morphology of the brain has been extended by other researchers with essentially the same results—experiences do affect the morphology of the brain (Greenough, Juraska, Volkmar 1979).

The eminent neuroscientist Sir John Eccles has proposed that *both* chemical and morphological changes occur in the consolidation of memory. He suggests that in the process of learning, the experience leads first to specific RNA modification, and this in turn to specific protein synthesis, and "finally to synaptic growth and the coding of the memory" (Eccles 1977).

---

[2] Dendrite spines are tiny "thorns," or projections, from the dendrites of a nerve cell that serve as receivers in many of the synaptic contacts between neurons.

Present Status of Consolidation Theory

It should be evident from the discussion above that we have no definitive answer as to exactly what changes in the nervous system correlate with the behavioral modifications that we call learning-memory. Although some changes must occur, our present stage of understanding about the nature of the changes and where they occur is largely based on suggestive and correlational evidence. It admittedly is very general and imprecise. The consolidation theory seems to provide the best approximation of the learning-memory process at the present. The evidence for consolidation memory theory suggests that it is at least useful to divide memory into STSS, STM, and LTM stages. A theory can be useful "for describing and explaining events without being an exact literal account" (Klatzky 1975).

Levels of Processing and Learning-Memory

An alternative to the conceptions of the consolidation theory of stages of memory is the **levels-of-processing** notion proposed by Craik and Lockhart (1972; also see Craik 1977; Cermak and Craik 1979). They suggest that memory of an event is a function of the *depth* to which the event is processed. The greater the depth, the more elaborate, longer lasting, and stronger the memory.

The "shallow" levels of processing (or "Type I processing," as Craik and Lockhart call it) are concerned with the analysis of physical or sensory features of input. "Deeper" levels ("Type II processing") involve matching the input against a stored abstraction from past learning. According to this formulation of a "hierarchy of processing levels," memory "is a function of the depth, and various factors, such as the amount of attention devoted to a stimulus, its compatibility with the analyzing structures, and the processing time available, will determine the depth to which it is processed" (Craik and Lockhart 1972).

Memory is viewed as a continuum ranging from simple sensory analysis to abstract associative operations. Memory is tied to levels of processing. It is a positive function of the depth to which stimuli have been analyzed, rather than the amount of processing, that leads to a more persistent memory trace.

The levels-of-processing view has been criticized by several psychologists on both theoretical and empirical grounds (Nelson 1977; Baddeley 1978; Eysenck 1978). One of the strongest criticisms of this approach is that it is not *really* a rival of the consolidation theory. According to one critic: "In fact what we see is a single approach with the label 'stages' heavily used in one and that label 'processing' heavily used in the other" (Glanzer and Koppenaal 1977). Craik and Lockhart (1972) themselves acknowledge that their "approach does not constitute a theory of memory. Rather, it provides a conceptual framework—a set of orienting attitudes. . . ."

Perhaps it would be more appropriate to view the levels-of-processing formulation as extending, rather than replacing, consolidation theory. It is possible that a synthesis, stressing both consolidation and levels of processing, will emerge. At present consolidation theory is generally favored because of the vast research tradition behind it. Nevertheless, since several studies in motor behavior have employed a "levels" perspective with some promising results, it is important for a student of motor behavior to be familiar with this memory framework.

Motor Learning-Memory

We now turn our attention to focus directly on motor learning-memory. The majority of theoretical and empirical effort on learning-memory has been concerned with verbal behavior. Investigators interested in motor learning-memory have employed, either explicitly or implicitly, the

same theoretical approaches. Consolidation theory and levels-of-processing frameworks form the basis of most work on motor learning-memory. Although there has been speculation that memory processes for motor memory are different from those underlying other forms of memory, there is no compelling evidence at this time for this position. Therefore, in general, what has been said about learning-memory theories in previous sections of this chapter appears to apply to the motor domain. This is one reason for the extended discussion of these theories and research.

The history of interest in motor memory can be traced to Woodworth's (1899) work at the end of the nineteenth century. But sustained research on this topic did not begin until the late 1960s, following the emergence of extensive research on the neural correlates of learning-memory and work on verbal STM. Early motor memory research was concerned with establishing similarities between verbal and motor behavior, especially short-term verbal memory. As Laabs and Simmons (1981) say, "The question was raised as to whether or not motor short-term retention would obey the same laws as verbal short-term retention." Over the past fifteen years an enormous amount of research literature has accumulated on the topic of **motor short-term memory (MSTM)**.

Motor Short-Term Memory

MSTM research has been basically the study of processing and storing sensory information for simple positioning movements, primarily over short durations. In most experiments, blindfolded subjects have pushed a slide along a linear track to a stop (perhaps a distance of 40 cm) that was preset by the experimenter (see figure 2.10 for an example). Either immediately, or after rest intervals from 1 to 120 seconds, the subjects attempted to reproduce the extent of movement originally performed. There have been a number of variations on this procedure, of course.

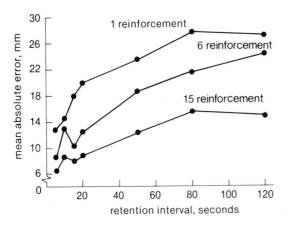

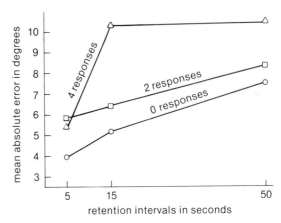

Figure 15.3 *Performance curves for the three reinforcement conditions as a function of retention interval.*

Figure 15.4 *Mean absolute error of target reproduction plotted as a function of retention interval for the 0-, 2-, and 4-prior-response conditions.*

The pioneering study in MSTM, and the one that served as the experimental model for many subsequent studies in MSTM, was conducted by Adams and Dijkstra (1966). They used a linear positioning task in which blindfolded subjects moved to an experimenter-preselected stop that defined the target position. Subjects then returned to the starting position for a retention interval that was varied from 5 to 120 seconds. After the retention interval, they attempted to reproduce the length of the movement that had been made originally (now with the stop removed). Subjects were not given any information about the accuracy of their movements, but they were given varying "reinforcements," whereby the target position was presented one, six, or fifteen times before the retention interval.

Figure 15.3 displays the major findings of this study. As the length of the retention interval increased, the absolute error also increased, with the increase in error almost complete by the eighty-second retention interval. Forgetting appears to be retarded by practice because error scores were systematically smaller with the increase in number of practice trials before the retention interval. Thus, the results are similar to the findings for verbal STM in that accuracy of MSTM was a decreasing function of time and was

a positive function of number of practice repetitions. Adams and Dijkstra interpreted the forgetting as a decay of the motor trace. Others have reported similar findings (Posner and Konick 1966; Posner 1967).

As with verbal STM, investigators have been interested in the effects of various interfering events on MSTM. One line of research has been concerned with proactive interference—meaning the effects of prior movements—on the recall memory for a particular position presented later. While early investigators (Adams and Dijkstra 1966; Posner and Konick 1966) reported no proactive interference, subsequent researchers have demonstrated substantial proactive interference (Ascoli and Schmidt 1969; Stelmach 1969a). Stelmach had subjects move to zero, two, and four positions before moving to the position to be recalled. Retention intervals of five, fifteen, or fifty seconds followed before the subjects were asked to move to the position to be recalled. Results of this study are displayed in figure 15.4. Significant proactive interference effects can be seen with the four prior-position group, especially with a retention interval of at least fifteen seconds. The results of the zero prior-position group further support those of Adams and Dijkstra; accuracy of MSTM was a decreasing function of time since, for this group, there were no movements prior to the criterion position.

Substantial evidence had accumulated by the late 1960s from clinical neurology, experimental neurophysiology, and from verbal behavior research that STM is adversely affected via retroactive interference (as predicted by consolidation memory theory) by various stimuli that are introduced shortly after the learning experience. By the early 1970s investigators began to wonder whether the same applied to MSTM, and a number of studies were conducted on this issue during the decade of the seventies. The typical design of these studies was similar to other MSTM studies, except that shortly after the learning experience—presumably while the learned information is in MSTM—subjects were required to perform an interpolated task.[3]

Some investigators found that just as with STM for verbal responses, the pattern of retention of movements declined significantly when subjects had to perform interpolated motor tasks. In other words, movement recall is subject to retroactive interference when the interpolated task involves certain types of attention-demanding movement tasks. This is consistent with verbal STM results. Others did not find adverse effects on MSTM due to the interpolated task. This latter finding, of course, is not in agreement with verbal STM work and suggested that there may be separate STM processes for verbal and motor information (for a review of this research, see Stelmach 1974).

Although the findings have been contradictory with regard to the effects of an interpolated task on MSTM, it appears that the more similar the interpolated activity is to the movement that the individual is trying to remember, the more the interference. In other words, interpolated motor

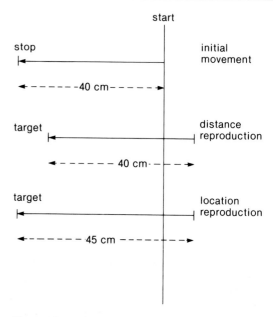

Figure 15.5   *The method for the separation of location and distance cues with linear positioning tasks.*

activities that are similar to the criterion task tend to degrade MSTM more than unrelated motor tasks or verbal tasks (Patrick 1971; Jones 1974). In summary, task-related interference is a powerfully adverse force in MSTM. Conversely, "unrelated" tasks that subjects perform as interpolated tasks have not produced consistent interfering effects.

Distance and Location and MSTM

Distance and end location are two of the more salient cues available to a performer for the reproduction of a movement. In the laboratory, these cues can be separated by using different starting points for the standard position and the reproduction position, making one cue unreliable at recall (Laabs and Simmons 1981) (figure 15.5). Several investigators have found that recall of movement location (specifically the end point of a response) is more accurate than recall of movement distance (Martiniuk and Roy 1972; Laabs 1973; Diewert 1975). Even when subjects are permitted to select the movement distance to be recalled, end location recall results in less error

---

[3] An interpolated task is a task of some kind that is inserted between trials in an experiment. The subject must perform the interpolated task during a retention interval.

than recall of distance (Kelso 1977a; b). It appears that people have a hard time remembering movement distance cues and that positioning movements seem to be based on memory of location. More probably, however, movement-accuracy memory is a complex combination of these two cue sources. "Neither terminal location nor distance are coded independently, and memory for movement is based on interaction between these cues" (Walsh et al. 1979; also see Ashby, Shea, and Tolson 1982). While these findings suggest that some movement cues are differentially stored and employed in the memory of movement information, the neurological substrate for memory of location and distance is uncertain.

Preselected Movements and MSTM

In the early MSTM studies, the target position was chosen by the experimenter, and the subject moved until a stop terminated the movement. This became the target for reproduction accuracy after the retention interval and after the stop was removed. A question arose about the possible differences in MSTM if subjects were allowed to choose their own movement target position, and therefore a preselection method has been employed by several investigators. With this method, the subject is instructed to move to a position of choice, then return to the starting position. After a retention interval, the subject attempts to reproduce this position. In general, MSTM is much better with the preselection technique because recall of the target position is more accurate than in the experimenter-defined method (Kelso 1977b; Roy 1978; Toole, Christina, and Anson 1982).

The reason for the superior reproduction accuracy of preselected movements over experimenter-selected is not clear. Some researchers have suggested that cognitive mechanisms that produce more task-relevant attention and allow subjects more adequately to formulate encoding strategies are responsible. One variation of this

view postulates that when one preselects a movement, an "image" is formed, generating anticipatory signals that prepare the individual to accept certain kinds of feedback that make the memory of the movement more robust and resistant to forgetting (Kelso and Wallace 1978). Another view suggests that preselected movements employ efference copy to a greater extent than experimenter-defined movements, and the movement and its feedback produce greater memory consolidation.

Levels of Processing and MSTM

We have very little research from a levels-of-processing framework for explaining retention of information in MSTM. As noted in an earlier section, this approach implies that recall memory can be attributed to the depth of the processing level attained during learning. If the learner processes newly acquired information by relating it to information already stored in memory, it will be retained much better than if only the physical features of the new information are stored.

The originators of the levels-of-processing framework predicted that when attention is diverted from an item, information will be lost at a rate appropriate to its level of processing—lower rates for deeper levels (Craik and Lockhart 1972). Ho and Shea (1978) inferred from that idea that if verbal labels for position cues result in a deeper level of processing, as was indeed found by Shea (1977), then the addition of an interpolated attention-demanding task should result in less forgetting for subjects using verbal labels than for subjects not using verbal labels. To test this notion, using a curvilinear positioning task, Ho and Shea provided one group of subjects with a verbal label describing the position they were to learn. Subjects were instructed that the use of the label would help in remembering the position. Subjects in a second group were allowed to make up their own labels for the position to be remembered to help them in recalling the position. Two groups of subjects were not given labels and did not receive instructions concerning labels. The "verbal label" groups had greater accuracy at recall for retention intervals of zero seconds and thirty seconds with no interpolated activity, as well as for a thirty-second retention interval filled with an interpolated task. The investigators interpreted the data as suggesting that verbal labels allowed subjects to process the criterion positions to a deeper level of analysis and that the labels facilitated the retrieval of information. The findings are not surprising. It has long been known that associating new information with stored information produces a resistance to forgetting.

Current Status of MSTM

Investigations so far provide only a few tentative conclusions about MSTM. The evidence is still in conflict about whether memory for movements over short periods is similar to that for verbal materials. Research prior to 1975 suggested that there may be separate short-term memories for motor and verbal information. But, while some differences in memory characteristics have been reported for verbal and motor STM, many similarities have also been demonstrated. So at present there is no definitive reason to propose entirely different processes. According to Laabs and Simmons (1981), "Studies of motor short-term memory that are being reported currently indicate that the research is once again trying to establish a correspondence between verbal and motor memory."

A persistent complaint leveled at MSTM research is that the only types of responses used have been slow, self-paced, single-limb, positioning responses. These types of responses represent a very narrow range of possible human movements. Some critics believe that these responses are not representative of the human movement repertoire and that little can be learned about how MSTM *really* works from these responses. Despite these criticisms, the work in MSTM has the potential to aid greatly our understanding of motor learning-memory.

Long-Term Motor Memory

Long-term motor memory (LTMM) is usually studied by motor behavior researchers within the context of retention. Studies of LTMM typically involve considerable practice of a motor skill until some proficiency has been attained, then a period of no practice (the retention interval) that might be several days, months, or even years, and finally a retention test requiring performance on the previously learned task. LTMM is primarily concerned with well-learned tasks that presumably have become consolidated into modifications in the nervous system. The substantial body of literature about LTMM is framed almost exclusively in behavioral terms, and is not concerned with morphological or biochemical changes that occur in the nervous system (although many of the LTM studies with lower animals have used motor responses).

Numerous writers have noted that motor skills, once learned, are remarkably resistant to being forgotten. Once a person has learned to swim, ride a bicycle, or throw a ball, these skills can be performed again even after years without practice. Furthermore, although long intervals without practice may produce some decrement in performance, this can often be overcome with a few practice trials. It is commonly thought that motor skills are retained better than verbal tasks, but an exact comparison cannot be made between the two because it is virtually impossible to equate them for difficulty. Moreover, it is impossible to ascertain how much learning on one task corresponds to a certain level of learning on the other task. Thus, it is difficult to conclude that motor skills are remembered best, although the few studies that have attempted to ascertain this relationship found that memory for the motor tasks was better than for verbal or procedural tasks (Mengelkoch, Adams, and Gainer 1971).

Continuous Motor Tasks

Motor skill retention with continuous motor tasks has been the subject of numerous investigations over the years. Most of these studies report little or no forgetting, even over extended intervals of no practice. The small decreases in performance that do occur are regained rapidly when practice is resumed. Although the motor skills used in many of these studies have been fine motor skills, the sparse research with gross motor tasks corroborates the findings with the other tasks. Several examples of these studies will give the reader a feel for this work.

Jahnke and Duncan (1956) investigated retention, using a rotary-pursuit task, for intervals ranging from ten minutes to four weeks. They found no evidence whatever of forgetting. Indeed, with some retention intervals there was improvement in performance. Fleishman and Parker (1962) studied retention on a complex tracking task for intervals from nine to twenty-four months. They reported "virtually no loss in skill regardless of the retention interval." Meyers (1967), using the Bachman ladder-climbing task, found no significant loss in retention for layoff periods varying from ten minutes to thirteen weeks. Ryan (1962) found that retention was high for both rotary-pursuit and stabilometer tasks up to twenty days, although the pattern of retention was not the same for both skills. In a subsequent experiment, Ryan (1965) tested for retention on a stabilometer task after three months, six months, and twelve months. He found significant loss on the first trial of the retest by all three groups, with the twelve-month group suffering the most loss of proficiency. Relearning was rapid, however, with the twelve-month group requiring more trials to regain their initial proficiency. Melnick (1971) reported that each of four groups that had originally practiced to a criterion level of proficiency on the stabilometer saved over 50 percent of the trials they spent in attaining the learning criterion on retention trials one month after the original learning. A group that had considerably overlearned the task had a savings score of 97.5 percent.

Discrete and Serial Tasks

While there is an abundance of evidence that continuous motor skills are retained quite well even after prolonged periods of no practice, it appears that retention characteristics for discrete and serial motor skills are different because substantial losses in proficiency have been found by several investigators (Adams and Hufford 1962; Lersten 1969). Schmidt (1975) has noted that "tasks that show the greatest retention are continuous tracking tasks and those that show the poorest retention are serial manipulative tasks; discrete tasks appear to be approximately intermediate in retention."

Several reasons have been advanced to explain why continuous tasks are retained better than serial or discrete: Continuous tasks are more highly overlearned than the other types because of the repetition involved in practicing these types of tasks; discrete and serial tasks are similar to verbal tasks because they have a heavy cognitive component, and verbal-cognitive components are more quickly forgotten, or more easily interfered with, than motor components; memory traces for continuous tasks are typically more meaningful, allowing the learner to utilize principles and relationships from prior learnings.

Effects of Certain Variables on Motor Skill Retention

The amount of retention and its persistence are dependent on a variety of factors. Some of the most prominent are degree of proficiency attained during original learning, meaningfulness of the task, interval between original learning and retention measurement, nature of the task, and practice schedule under which original learning occurred.

Original Proficiency and Retention

Several investigators have indicated that the most important factor in the retention of a motor skill is the level of proficiency achieved during the original learning phase. Fleishman and Parker (1962) found a near linear relationship between the degree of proficiency attained during original learning of a simulated piloting task and the amount of proficiency retention following intervals of nine to twenty-four months of no practice. Purdy and Lockhart (1962) reported that the higher the original level of skill on several gross motor skills (a foot volley, lacrosse throw and catch, and balancing on a teeter board), the greater the retention. They found that after one year of no practice, as much as 94 percent of original proficiency was retained. As noted above, Melnick (1971) found some relationship between amount of overlearning and retention on the stabilometer.

From the perspective of both consolidation and levels-of-processing theories, the fact that higher original proficiency yields stronger memory effects makes sense. In the former, practice constitutes rehearsal of the information, thus renewing the information in STM so that is not lost. STM transfers the data about the rehearsed information to LTM, which in turn builds up the strength of LTM. For levels of processing, the repetition of practice enables the information to be coded in deeper levels, thus making retention and retrieval more robust.

For verbal tasks, forgetting is most rapid immediately after the cessation of practice and then is less pronounced with time. While motor skill retention does not follow exactly the same pattern, the general pattern of rapid retention loss is similar to verbal retention (Adams and Dijkstra 1966). Retention loss can be retarded by increased practice before the retention interval.

Meaningfulness and Retention

Memory storage depends to a large extent on meaning or relating new information to stored information. Several studies have shown that meaningful tasks are remembered better than meaningless tasks. Naylor and Briggs (1961) found that motor tasks arranged in an organized sequence were remembered better than arbitrarily arranged tasks. Similarly, retention is enhanced by perceptual organization of the information into a close, meaningful relationship (Gentile and Nacson 1976; Diewert and Stelmach 1978; Dunham 1978). In other words, grouping, categorizing, imposing meaning, and associating new information with stored information during the learning phase will improve retention (for a good review, see Puff 1979).

Interference with LTMM

The effects of interference seem to differ between verbal LTM and LTMM. While interference seems to influence strongly verbal retention, it does not affect motor skill retention as dramatically. However, in the motor domain very few new responses are learned that would potentially interfere with the original skill. To use bicycling skill as an example, after bicyclists stop regular riding, they learn many things, but few that would directly interfere with the pedaling, balancing, and steering necessary to ride a bicycle. Subsequent motor experiences, then, typically do not interfere with a previously learned motor skill.

Serial Position and Retention

A serial position effect on retention has been consistently found for verbal materials. When subjects learn a list of items in their serial order, typically the first few and the last few items are retained best, with the items in the middle retained least. This is referred to as the serial position (or **primacy-recency effect**), and it is clearly seen in the results of a study by Craik (1970)

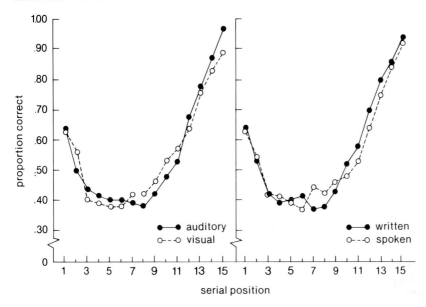

Figure 15.6   *Serial position curves for different input and response modes.*

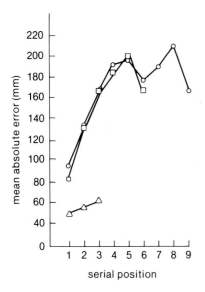

Figure 15.7   *The serial position curves for the recall of a series of three, six, or nine movements on a linear positioning task. The triangles equal the three movement series, the squares equal the six movement series, and the circles equal the nine movement series.*

shown in figure 15.6. Recent studies have demonstrated that when the length of a movement series is greater than five movements, the **primacy-recency** effect occurs for movements too (Magill and Dowell 1977; Wilberg and Girard 1977). In these studies, blindfolded subjects were initially provided with several positions on a positioning task. They were to remember the positions for later recall. This movement series consisted of between three and nine movements (figure 15.7). During the recall phase subjects either recalled the movements in the same order in which they had been originally presented, or they were allowed to recall freely the movements.

Although the few studies of the serial position effect in motor behavior have used simple positioning tasks, many motor skills require a sequential ordering of movements. If one wishes to make inferences about teaching methodology from the research, students of serial tasks will have the most retention difficulty with the middle portions of the task, so certain techniques may have to be employed to enhance retention of this part of the routine. One technique might be to divide the sequence into several smaller segments with individual practice on these segments; another might be to emphasize continually the middle parts of such serial routines as gymnastics and dance. These techniques allow concentrated practice on the middle part and thus improve retention.

Several theoretical accounts of the primacy-recency effect have been given, with Atkinson and Shiffrin's (1971) being perhaps the best known. This account draws on consolidation theory and proposes that the incoming information enters STM, which has only a limited-capacity chamber for storing information. But while it is in STM, it is "rehearsed" as preparation for transfer to LTM. At the beginning of learning, the STM chamber is empty. Successive information enters until the STM store is filled. Thereafter, as each new piece of information enters the STM rehearsal chamber, it replaces some of the information already there. The transfer of information from STM to LTM is believed to depend on the length of time a piece of information remains in the STM rehearsal chamber: the longer the time, the more rehearsal the information receives and thus the more transfer of information to LTM. Since information presented first in a series enters an empty or partly empty STM rehearsal chamber, it remains longer than later information and consequently receives considerable rehearsal. This extra rehearsal produces more transfer of information to LTM for the first information, producing the primacy effect. Information still being rehearsed when the final information is presented is immediately recalled by the learner, giving rise to the recency effect.

Using levels-of-processing concepts, Craik and Lockhart (1972) provide a description of primacy-recency effects by proposing that since learners know they must stop attending to initial information in order to deal with subsequent information, the initial information is subjected to deep processing. This accounts for the primacy effect. Final information survives on physical or sensory encoding, which gives rise to good immediate recall. This accounts for the recency effect. Because once attention to information is diverted and the memory trace is lost at a rate appropriate to its deepest analyzed level, information presented in the middle of a series is given only brief attention. Preceding and succeeding information imposes on it. This accounts for the poor retention of information in the middle.

Reminiscence

The passage of time does not always lead to a diminution of performance when practice is resumed. It may result in a higher level of performance than existed at the end of the last practice. This phenomenon of an increase in performance after a period of no practice is called **reminiscence.** Hilgard (1957) defined reminiscence as . . . "a psychological term for the occasional rise in the curve of retention before it falls; that is, when under some circumstances more may be retained after an interval than immediately upon completion of learning."

Reminiscence has been found on a wide variety of verbal and motor tasks, using rest intervals from a few minutes up to a year after the last practice trial. In addition to the basic finding, these studies rather consistently show that reminiscence is inversely related to the degree of original learning. They also show that motor skills seem to yield greater reminiscence over longer intervals than verbal materials.

The majority of investigations on reminiscence in motor learning have used the rotary-pursuit apparatus. Only a few studies of reminiscence have been done in which the learning of sports skill was involved. Fox and Young (1962) studied reminiscence in two badminton skills (a wall volley and short-serve task) using nonpractice periods of six weeks and twelve weeks. Reminiscence did occur on one of the skills but did not occur on the other. Fox and Lamb (1962) tested for reminiscence of softball skills after five weeks of no practice (first retest) and seventeen weeks after the first retest. There was no significant reminiscence for the first nonpractice interval. Reminiscence did occur during the longer interval without practice.

Theories of Reminiscence

Reminiscence has been frequently interpreted in terms of Clark Hull's (1943) inhibition theory, which postulates that in every learning situation there develops an inhibition (reactive inhibition) caused by a reluctance to repeat a response—an inhibition to further activity of the sort demanded by a specific task. The greater the work demanded by a task, or the more often the task is continually repeated, the greater the inhibition. For Hull, reactive inhibition restricts performance. Rest allows recovery from inhibition and so allows improved performance. Strong support for Hull's concept of reactive inhibition has been demonstrated by Hsu and Payne (1979).

In an attempt to explain certain criticisms of inhibition theory as an explanation of reminiscence, Eysenck and Frith (1977) have proposed a theory of reminiscence, the main feature of which is the employment of consolidation memory theory. With regard to the consolidation theory, they propose that performance sets up cortical events which, in order to become available to the performer as learned behavior, require a rest period during which they consolidate. Improved performance after a rest period results from a consolidation of learning that occurs during rest.

This is another topic in learning-memory in which the processes underlying the performance have not been resolved. How a rest period after practice enables a performer to begin the next practice session at a higher level of proficiency than existed just prior to the rest is uncertain.

Limits of Motor Learning

What are the limits in learning a motor task? Does learning continue with practice? For how long? There are definite limits to the level of proficiency that one can achieve in any particular movement task. But this limit is never known, and proficiency approaches these limits so slowly that it is difficult to ascertain when individuals have reached their optimum proficiency for that task.

Usually, several conditions affect the upper limits that one achieves on a motor skill. Frequent and intense practice is usually required in order to continue to improve performance levels. When practices are infrequent or short, performances remain static. Nor are high levels of skill achieved by repetitious, halfhearted practice. Motivation is one of the most important factors limiting level of motor performance; when motivation wanes, performance is affected accordingly. Champion athletes improve their skill because of their interest in their performance, whether for financial or personal reasons. Certainly, other factors might be identified, such as aging and lack of feedback or standards of mastery. But prolonged practice and motivation are certainly two of the most critical factors affecting ultimate skill level.

Evidence for Prolonged Periods of Skill Improvement

Several studies have shown that proficiency can be improved almost indefinitely. A study by Crossman (1959) has become the classic example of this phenomenon. He found continued improvement of performance from subjects whose practice on a fine motor skill extended over several years. The subjects were operators of hand-operated cigar-making machines. The speed of performance on this task improved for up to four years and only leveled off because the cycle time of the machine set a limit on the rate of work that was possible (figure 15.8). Crossman concluded that skill in performance in simple motor tasks

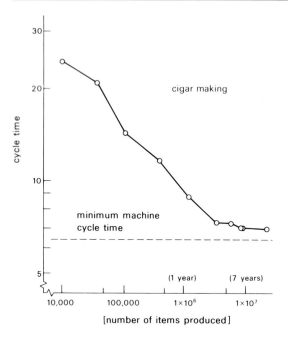

Figure 15.8 *Performance on a fine motor task over a prolonged period of time.*

increases gradually and continually for many practice trials, provided that motivation for improvement is maintained.

Further evidence for the continued improvement of performance in motor skills comes from case histories of championship performers in various sports. In order to reach performance levels to compete successfully in national or international sports events, many years of intensive practice are usually necessary. The typical Olympic figure skater, skier, or fencer has intensively practiced the sport for at least ten years. Professional golfers or bowlers have many years of amateur competition behind them before they can survive as professionals. The successful modern dancer or ballerina usually has been in constant practice since early childhood. When performance does level off, it seems to be due to loss of motivation, or in some cases the effects of aging, rather than the reaching of a true limit in capacity for further improvement.

Summary

Complex motor behavior must be learned. One way to understand how we acquire motor skills is to study the memory aspects of motor behavior. Learning is a neural change that occurs as a result of experiences with stimuli in the environment. The ability to learn requires memory. Memory is assumed to involve some modification in neural structures, and the postulated neural correlate of memory is the memory trace.

The learning-memory theory currently favored by neuroscientists is consolidation theory. This theory suggests that learning-memory occurs through several processing stages. First, stimuli that impinge upon the sensory organs are transduced and coded in the form of nerve impulses and transmitted to the brain. This process probably initiates neural activity that momentarily outlasts the stimulus. Second, this activity then becomes recoded, possibly in the form of reverberating circuits. This phase, so-called short-term memory, has a capacity of about seven to eight items or stimuli. The "hold time" for items in STM seems to vary from a few seconds up to an hour or more. Gradually, the neural representation of the stimulus event is transformed into a structural change in the brain, representing a third stage. This transformation from a dynamic activity to a consolidated memory is the so-called long-term memory. If the STM process is disrupted, the long-term process cannot take place and the stimulus event cannot be recalled. Present knowledge does not permit a definitive explanation of LTM, but recent studies of the biochemical correlates of learning-memory suggest that molecular changes occur in the neurons whenever an individual learns something. The molecules most frequently identified as being involved in LTM are RNA and protein. There is also evidence that morphological changes in the form of changes in the relationship of synapses may also be involved in LTM.

An alternative to consolidation theory is the so-called levels-of-processing notion, which suggests that memory of an event is a function of the depth to which an event is processed.

Motor learning-memory research has employed the same theoretical approaches and research designs as those used in verbal learning-memory. The general findings are that the memory processes for motor memory are not much different from those underlying other forms of learning-memory.

Much motor learning research has focused on short-term memory. Several studies have found evidence to support a trace decay interpretation of forgetting. Studies that have examined the effects of prior learning on skill acquisition have produced no conclusive evidence about proactive interference. Results of retroactive interference on motor short-term memory have been quite variable, but interpolated tasks similar to the criterion movement produce learning decrement. Interference is reduced by increasing the number of practice trials. Using verbal labels to identify various movements reduces forgetting. Motor short-term memory is better when learners are permitted to preselect their movements instead of performing experimenter-defined movements. Recall of movement location is more accurate than recall of movement distance.

It is commonly believed that long-term memory for movements is superior to long-term memory for verbal materials, but there is no way to test this notion adequately. Continuous motor tasks are retained better than serial or discrete tasks. Higher original proficiency yields stronger memory effects. Meaningful tasks are remembered better than meaningless tasks. Subsequent motor experiences typically do not interfere with a previously learned motor skill. A serial position effect on retention has been found for motor skill learning.

Reminiscence has been found in a wide variety of motor skills, but its effect is generally very temporary.

Improvement in proficiency in motor tasks can continue for years. Indeed, in many sports skills it takes years of practice to become a top-level athlete.

16

Motor Abilities and Motor Behavior

Key Terms and Concepts
Ability
Correlation
Factor analysis
General motor ability
Intelligence quotient
Motor ability
Motor educability
Skill

*W*e indicated in the previous chapter that we would be focusing on some of the most important factors that affect motor learning and peformance in the remaining chapters of this book. One of the most important of these factors is perceptual-motor[1] ability. The nature and development of human abilities have been of interest to psychologists for many years. Some have devoted their entire careers to devising and perfecting ability measurement instruments—the intelligence tests would be the most obvious example. Others have studied the relationship of certain kinds of ability to behavior. To use intelligence tests again as an example, many investigators have studied the relationship between intelligence, as measured by intelligence tests, and such things as scholastic achievement, occupational achievement, and so on.

Paralleling the interest in intellectual abilities, a few psychologists and many physical educators have been concerned with motor ability, its nature and development. There is a substantial body of knowledge on this topic. In this chapter we shall examine the issues and problems that have been evident through the years and suggest some implications in light of the current state of the art.

---

[1] Although the term *motor ability* will be used throughout the remainder of this chapter, the use of the term *perceptual-motor* here is deliberate. It is used to emphasize that motor skill acquisition and performance are dependent upon *both* perceptual *and* motor systems. Motor learning is as often the result of improved perceptual functioning as it is improved motor functioning. Or more accurately, motor learning is a process of integrated improvement in perceptual *and* motor functioning.

Definition of Motor Ability

In chapter 2 **motor ability** was defined as a general trait or capacity of an individual that is related to performance on a variety of skills and that is rather enduring and permanent after childhood. Abilities serve as the foundation stones for the acquisition of **skills,** which are specific responses for the accomplishment of a task. A skill is learned through practice and depends on the presence of underlying abilities. Balance, speed of reaction, and flexibility are examples of abilities that are important for the execution of a variety of skills, such as the tennis serve, the breaststroke, and the forward roll.

Neural Mechanisms and Ability

Biological forces are presumed to be primarily responsible for an individual's basic **ability.** Although the bodily structures and functions are similar for each individual, no two people have *exactly* the same structural makeup, and bodily processes function a little differently for each person. There are differences in sensitivity of the sensory systems, making for individual differences in ability to detect and discriminate among stimuli; there are differences in actual number of muscle fibers, neuromuscular connections, and differences in relative muscle fiber composition.[2] There are differences in the chemical, anatomical, and functional makeup of each person's brain, producing variations in cognitive function. We could go on detailing the various structural and functional differences among individuals, but the point is that these differences play an essential part in determining basic abilities.

---

[2] Slow twitch muscle fibers are able to contract repeatedly when stimulated without much fatigue, while fast twitch fibers develop tension rather fast but fatigue easily. On the average, the relative muscle fiber composition is 40–50 percent slow twitch and 50–60 percent fast twitch, but some people have over 80 percent slow twitch fibers, while others have over 80 percent fast twitch fibers. Differences in composition of fast and slow twitch fibers have been found to be related to performances in short, speed events and long, endurance events.

Of course, within biological limits environment plays a significant role in the development of basic abilities. Research on the young of various species, including humans, indicates that early environment is critical for development of the basic abilities, especially motor abilities. Studies have shown rather conclusively that both lower animals and human infants raised in environments that restrict sensory experiences or motor activity have a narrower range of perceptual and motor abilities throughout their lives (Solomon et al. 1961; Gregory and Wallace 1963; Held and Bauer 1967). It is, then, generally believed that the greater the variety of sensory and motor experiences individuals have during their early years, the fuller will be their motor ability repertoire, within the limits set by their genetic heritage.

General Motor Ability

One of the most persistent bits of folklore of physical education and coaching is the notion of a **general motor ability** (GMA)—a singular, unifying motor ability that enables certain individuals to perform well or to acquire quickly a high proficiency on any motor task. Phrases such as "a natural athlete" or "an all-around athlete" characterize this so-called ability. At the same time industrial psychologists have employed motor aptitude tests for selecting employees in the belief that these tests are predictive of performance levels on the job. *Aptitude* refers to the potential of people to perform a specific kind of activity, and an aptitude test is designed to detect underlying abilities within people and to predict how well they will perform after they have had practice on a task.

A wealth of information has accumulated over the past twenty-five years that suggests that the notion of general motor ability is a myth and that selecting personnel through the use of a motor aptitude test battery is, at best, ineffective and may even be counterproductive. The evidence for this statement is presented later in the chapter.

Statistical Techniques Used in Motor Ability Assessment

A brief description of correlation and factor analysis statistical techniques will help the reader understand how various motor ability studies have been done and how their findings are used to advance our understanding of motor abilities. **Correlation** is one of the most frequently used measures of relations. A correlation coefficient is a statistic that describes to what extent and in what way two variables are related to one another. It is ascertained from scores from at least two tests, and is expressed as some number between +1.00 and −1.00. Numbers between 0 and +1.00 indicate a positive relationship, meaning high scorers on one test tend to be high scorers on the second test. Numbers between 0 and −1.00 indicate a negative relationship. High scorers on one test tend to be low scorers on the second test (figure 16.1).

The magnitude, or strength, of the relationship between the test scores is indicated by the size of the correlation. Correlation coefficients that are near zero (0 to +0.20 or 0 to −0.20) indicate little or no relationship between the tests; in the latter, the relationship is said to be inverse; +1.00 or −1.00 correlations indicate a perfect association. Correlations between +0.80 and +0.20 or −0.80 and −0.20 show moderate relationships, the strength of relationship depending upon how close to 0 or 1.0 they actually are. Finally, correlations between +0.80 and +0.99 or −0.80 and −0.99 are considered strong relationships.

Frequently, correlation techniques are used to determine whether or not two tests are measuring the same ability. If two motor tests are administered to a set of subjects and the correlation coefficient is found to be +0.95, it can be inferred that both tests are assessing the same motor ability. But if there is a +0.08 correlation coefficient, it can be inferred that the two tests are not measuring the same ability or that the ability contributing to the performance on one is not the same as that on the other.

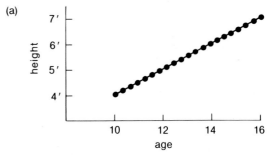

(a)

A positive correlation. The hypothetical heights and age of a sample of people show that the older people are, the taller they are.
(correlation coefficient = +1.00)

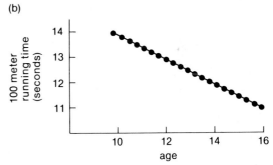

(b)

A negative correlation. The hypothetical time to run 100 meters for a sample of people, showing that the older the age, the less time to run the 100 meters.
(correlation coefficient = −1.00)

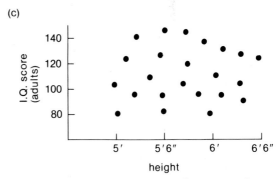

(c)

A zero correlation. The hypothetical I.Q. scores and height of a sample of adults show no relationship between the two.
(correlation coefficient = 0.00)

Figure 16.1 *Graphic example of hypothetical correlations (actual scores would not be this way). Each dot represents a person's score on each of the two variables. The line drawn in a and b merely illustrates the direction of scores.*

Coefficients of correlation are themselves subject to extensive and elaborate forms of analyses, one of which is factor analysis. **Factor analysis** is a statistical technique for identifying, on the basis of scores from a number of test items given to a large group of subjects, a relatively small number of common qualities. It tells us, in effect, which test items belong together—which ones measure virtually the same thing, in other words, and to what degree they do so. It reduces the number of variables, or test items, with which one must cope. It also helps to locate and identify unities of fundamental properties underlying tests and measures. For example, if twenty test items were administered to a group of individuals and the results showed that three of these test items intercorrelate highly, then one factor is identified. Additionally, if three of the other test items correlate highly but do not correlate with the first three, a second factor has been identified. Once the various factors emerge from the analysis, the experimenter subjectively names each factor by some descriptive statement.

The use that researchers have made of correlational and factor analytical techniques will be described throughout the remaining sections of this chapter. It is important to understand that these techniques have served as the basic tools for advancing our knowledge of motor abilities.

Development of Motor Ability Tests

Although it is always hazardous to speculate about the origin of one idea, the notion that there is such a thing as general motor ability was probably triggered by the work done by psychologists in identifying a so-called **intelligence quotient.** In the early part of this century, psychologists who developed intelligence tests contended that the tests measured a general ability to utilize abstract concepts effectively, implying reasoning, imagination, insight, and adaptability as the mental processes involved in intelligent behavior.

The claim was that general intelligence was being measured and intellectual ability was believed to be represented by this term. The primary purpose of these tests was to determine scholastic aptitude, and they did predict to some extent academic achievement (Cronbach 1960).

There is no question about the popularity of intelligence tests. During the 1920s, '30s, and '40s, schools used intelligence test scores to group, counsel, and even to screen students for college admission. The popularity of intelligence tests may have been the primary stimulus for those who were working with motor activities—physical educators, coaches, industrial psychologists—to seek a similar assessment instrument for motor ability.

In any case, between 1920 and 1940 several physical educators devised instruments for the measurement of general motor ability. In 1927, David K. Brace (1927) published a test battery (made up of many motor task items) designed to measure "inherent motor skill." At the University of Iowa, Charles McCloy (1937), one of the most esteemed physical educators of the 1920–1940 era, revised the Brace test and attempted to produce a test that would measure **motor educability,** meaning the "ease with which an individual learns new motor skills." Other test batteries were developed by Granville Johnson (1932), whose battery of tests was designed to measure "native neuromuscular skill capacity," and by Frederick Cozens (1929), who developed a test that purported to measure "general athletic ability."

The basic idea behind the notion of a general motor ability is that there is an underlying ability that enables certain individuals to be able to perform well in any motor task and that they will learn new motor skills to a high level of proficiency quickly. In essence, the suggestion is that there is a motor equivalent of general intelligence.

The various general motor ability tests caused quite a stir throughout the field of physical education for about a decade. Physical education classes were grouped on the basis of the scores, and prospective athletes were selected for teams from the scores. But then evidence began to accumulate that indicated that, in fact, motor ability tests did not do what it was first claimed they could do. One of the first attacks on these general motor ability tests came from a developer of one of them, David K. Brace. In 1941, in a study designed to ascertain the efficacy of several tests of general motor ability and motor educability, Brace (1941) reported that none of the tests, including his own, was predictive of ability to learn motor skills. He wrote: "Conclusions from the data would appear to indicate that either the so-called learning tests do not measure ability to learn or that the other measures obtained have little relationship to the ability to learn motor skills."

More damning evidence came a year later. Gire and Espenschade (1942) correlated the scores on the Brace, Iowa revision of the Brace, and the Johnson test with students' ability to learn basketball, volleyball, and baseball skills. Their findings pretty much destroyed the creditability of these instruments. They said, "Thus, it may be concluded that no test of 'motor educability' studied measured accurately the ease with which the subjects in this study learned new skills or relearned old ones in basketball, volleyball, and baseball. . . ."

More recently, the most persistent and consistent opponent of the general motor ability notion has been Franklin Henry. His own research and the research of his graduate students have shown rather convincingly that there is no such thing as GMA. Two basic strategies have been used by Henry and his students in dismantling this concept. First, they tested groups of athletes and nonathletes on a variety of motor skills (but not sports skills) and found that the athletes performed no better on these tasks than the nonathletes. A second strategy was to administer two or more different motor tasks to the same subjects and assess the relationship between performance on the various tasks by correlational analysis. If the notion of GMA is valid, the performers who score well on one task should score high on other tasks—the correlation between any two motor tasks should be rather high. Several studies designed to assess this relationship found that the correlation coefficients between the performance and learning motor tasks were very low. For example, Bachman (1961) had over three hundred subjects perform on the stabilometer and a freestanding ladder task that he designed and built (thus the name Bachman ladder climb). Correlations between both performance and learning the tasks were mostly below 0.20 for age groups from six to twenty-six. Bachman concluded that the "results show little more than zero correlation between performance of the two tasks . . . [and] motor learning is remarkably task specific. No correlation was found that was significantly different from zero. . . ." A number of other similarly designed investigations have reported low correlations for an individual's performance across even the most similar of tasks, suggesting that skill is a specific and not a general ability (see Marteniuk 1974 for a review). Although the evidence is rather clear that the notion of GMA is unfounded because of the low correlations between motor tasks, there are some abilities common to certain motor tasks. Eckert (1964) reported moderate correlations between speed of limb movement and strength, and Nelson and Fahrney (1965) found moderate to high relationships between tests of strength and movement speed. Nevertheless, these findings do little to support a GMA position.

Classifying Motor Abilities

The work of Edwin Fleishman and his colleagues over the past twenty-five years provides a clarification of the two extreme positions (general motor ability and specificity of motor ability) concerning the abilities underlying performance on a motor task. Fleishman has employed factor analysis to extract factors from a large group of motor tasks. Each factor is believed to represent a basic underlying motor ability, and each motor ability has been named according to the tasks that make up a factor. (For reviews of this work see Fleishman 1972 or Fleishman 1978).

Using over two hundred different tasks and administering them to thousands of subjects, Fleishman has been able to account for performance on this wide variety of tasks by a relatively small number of abilities. He has classified these motor abilities into two broad categories, one of which he calls "psychomotor abilities" and the second "physical proficiency." The first set of abilities was derived from studies of manipulative and limb coordination tasks, while the second came from gross motor tasks.

The psychomotor abilities and their characteristics are:

1. **Control precision.** This ability requires fine, highly controlled muscular adjustments, primarily in situations in which large muscle groups are involved. This ability extends to arm-hand as well as to leg movements.
2. **Multilimb coordination.** This is the ability to coordinate a number of limb movements simultaneously.
3. **Response orientation.** This ability is general to visual discrimination reaction tasks involving rapid directional discrimination and orientation of movement patterns.

4. **Reaction time.** This ability is simply the speed with which a person is able to respond to a stimulus when it appears.
5. **Speed of arm movement.** This is the speed with which a person can make gross, discrete arm movements in which accuracy is not the requirement.
6. **Rate control.** This ability involves making continual anticipatory motor adjustments relative to changes in speed and direction of a continually moving target or object.
7. **Manual dexterity.** This ability is demonstrated by skillful, well-directed arm-hand movements in manipulating fairly large objects under speeded conditions.
8. **Finger dexterity.** This involves making still-controlled manipulations of tiny objects involving, primarily, the fingers.
9. **Arm-hand steadiness.** This is the ability to make precise arm-hand positioning movements where strength and speed are minimized.
10. **Wrist-finger speed.** This ability is best measured by printed tests requiring rapid tapping of the pencil in relatively large areas.
11. **Aiming.** This ability is best measured by printed tests requiring the rapid placement of dots in very small circles under highly speeded conditions.

The abilities identified as physical proficiency abilities are:

1. **Extent flexibility.** This is the ability to flex or stretch the trunk and back muscles as far as possible in either a forward, lateral, or backward direction.
2. **Dynamic flexibility.** The ability to make repeated, rapid, flexing movements in which the resiliency of the muscles in recovery from stretch or distortion is critical.

3. **Explosive strength.** The ability to expend a maximum of energy in one or a series of explosive acts.

4. **Static strength.** The maximum force that a person can exert for a brief period.

5. **Dynamic strength.** The ability to exert muscular force repeatedly or continuously over time.

6. **Trunk strength.** A dynamic strength factor, specific to the abdominal muscles.

7. **Gross body coordination.** This is the ability to coordinate the simultaneous actions of different parts of the body while making gross body movements.

8. **Gross body equilibrium.** This ability involves individuals maintaining their equilibrium, despite forces pulling them off balance, while they are blindfolded.

9. **Stamina.** This is the ability to continue maximum effort, requiring prolonged exertion over time.

The essence to the compilation of this list of motor abilities is not a single, general ability, but can best be described in terms of a number of broad, relatively independent abilities. People typically are high on some abilities and low on others. The individual who is high, or low, on all of these motor abilities is extremely rare.

Fleishman (1967) warns that the list of motor abilities that he has extracted is not to be considered a final, complete list. He says, "We do not present these factors as any kind of final list of perceptual motor categories." Limitations such as the number and types of tasks that were used as well as the subjective nature of some steps in factor analysis necessitate that the work on this subject be continued. Indeed, recent investigations have demonstrated the existence of additional perceptual-motor abilities (Keele and Hawkins 1982).

Changing Role of Motor Abilities during Skill Acquisition

Fleishman's work has helped to clarify the issue of generality versus specificity of motor skill performance and learning. Another of his most interesting findings is that as the learning of a motor skill proceeds, changes occur in the *particular combinations* of abilities contributing to performance. As noted above, several studies have found low correlations for motor learning when the same subjects had to learn two or more motor tasks. Fleishman and his colleagues (Fleishman and Hempel 1954) have demonstrated that the particular combinations of abilities contributing to performance on motor tasks changes as practice on these tasks continues. This finding, combined with their extraction of a number of relatively independent motor abilities, provides a partial explanation for the findings of motor learning specificity: The rate of learning and ultimate proficiency level depend upon the unique ability structure of each person. This suggests, then, the presence of certain potentials for learning a skill.

The pioneer experiment that demonstrated the changing structure of abilities contributing to performance as learning proceeds involved a piloting-type task, requiring the subjects to manipulate a stick and rudder in response to visual patterns. Scores were obtained at eight different points during the practice and were correlated with performance on a battery of tests of hypothesized abilities. The results were then subjected to factor analysis. The analysis showed: (1) the particular combination of abilities contributing to performance on the task changed as practice on the task continued; (2) the changes were progressive and systematic and eventually became stabilized; (3) a factor specific to performance on the task itself increased with practice;

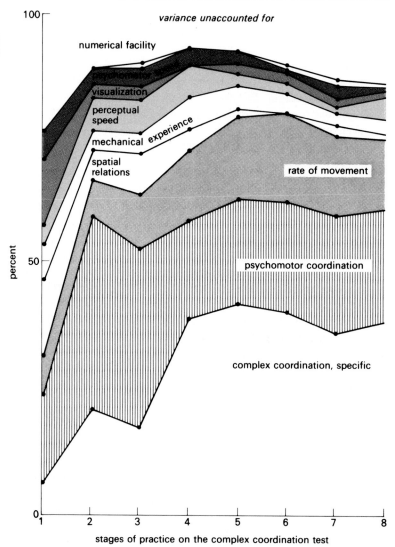

Figure 16.2 *Changes in factor structure as a function of practice. Percentage of variance (shaded area) represented by each factor at various stages of practice.*

indeed, it became the major component of the skill in the late stages of learning (figure 16.2) (Fleishman and Hempel 1954). Using a discrimination reaction time task, a later study also demonstrated a shift in the nature of abilities contributing to performance for early-to-late learning (Fleishman and Hempel 1955).

The finding that different abilities contribute to performance at different stages in learning suggests that people who possess those abilities

that contribute to performance in the initial stages of learning will begin at a relatively high level, and those who possess abilities that contribute to performance at later stages of learning will achieve high proficiency levels later in learning. To test this possibility, Fleishman and Rich (1963) gave a visual-spatial test and a kinesthetic sensitivity test to a large group of subjects. They then divided the subjects into groups high and low on visual spatial ability and into groups high and low

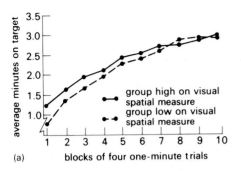

(a)

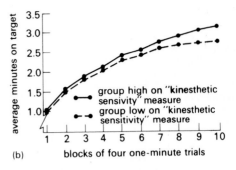

(b)

Figure 16.3 In (a) the superior visual group (high spatial measure) clearly has an early advantage but, as training progresses, the poorer visual group catches up. In (b) the two kinesthetic groups begin at the same level but, in the later stages as kinesthesis becomes more important, the kinesthetically more sensitive group surpasses the less sensitive group.

on kinesthetic sensitivity. Then the subjects learned a two-hand coordination task. The superior visual-spatial ability group exhibited early advantage, but as practice continued the poorer visual group caught up. Conversely, the superior kinesthetic sensitivity group began at about the same initial level as the poorer group, but as practice continued the former pulled away and performed much better than the poorer group in the later stages of learning (figure 16.3).

These findings seem to indicate that if visual cues are predominant in early control of the task, individuals who have superior visual spatial ability do better in the early learning stages of the task. On the other hand, if kinesthetic cues are dominant late in the learning of a task, people with superior kinesthetic perception will outdo others in late stages of learning.

One salient conclusion in these studies by Fleishman is that visual-spatial ability tends to be a major factor contributing to proficiency in the early phase of learning a variety of motor tasks. In the piloting coordination task (Fleishman and Hempel 1954), visual spatial relations were significant only in the first stages of practice; in the discrimination reaction time task (Fleishman and Hempel 1955), they were the main factor at the beginning of practice, but decreased in contribution to performance in the final

phase; and in the two-hand coordination task the group with superior spatial orientation showed initial performance supremacy (Fleishman and Rich 1963). Subsequently, Stallings (1968) confirmed the earlier findings. In her study the group scoring high on spatial orientation maintained superiority of performance in the early learning stage, but spatial orientation became progressively less important as practice continued. Recent research has further corroborated these findings (Beltel 1980).

Relationship of Initial Proficiency to Ultimate Proficiency

Another salient conclusion that has some interesting implications for motor skills instructors is that individual differences in initial proficiency have relatively little relation to ultimate proficiency. There are slow learners and fast learners for particular tasks, and early performance is not predictive of final proficiency. Many motor skill instructors assume that initial performance is related to ultimate proficiency and the rate at which it will be attained. Some athletic coaches, for example, select their teams on the basis of player performance on a few practice trials because they believe that the best performers at that point have

Figure 16.4 *The effects of instruction on learning a tracking task. The task required subjects to keep a dot in the center of an oscillograph display while at the same time trying to keep a pointer centered on an instrument dial. Group 1 received no formal guidance at all. Group II received "commonsense" or traditional instruction. Group III received the same instruction as Group II but also received special guidance on the visual-spatial aspects of the task in the early stages and kinesthetic-coordination aspects of the task were emphasized later in the learning; knowledge of task components was emphasized near the end.*

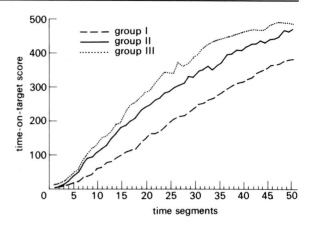

the best potential for further improvement. Findings consistently show that the abilities that underlie early superiority are not necessarily the abilities that underlie later proficiency. This should make coaches pause before they quickly dismiss the poorly skilled.

In two studies done in Canada, Percival (1971) divided performers into two groups, an "initial high performer" group and an "initial low performer" group. One study employed a baseball throw for accuracy and another involved shooting a hockey puck at a target. In both studies, after twelve practice sessions the "initial low performer" group attained the same level of proficiency, or better, than the "initial high performer" group.

In his book *The Search for Ability,* Goslin (1963) nicely sums up the problem of predicting future performance on the basis of ability scores. He says:

Attempting to predict future performance on the basis of [ability] test scores is much like trying to guess the ultimate size and shape of an oak tree by measuring a sapling in pitch darkness with a rubber band as a ruler, and without taking into account the condition of the soil [or] the amount of rainfall. . . . The amazing thing is that sometimes we get the right answer.

Although it is little more than a hunch at this time, shifts in abilities underlying performance suggest that instructors might carefully analyze the task they are teaching for the specific abilities needed to perform it. Then they should either use teaching methods that emphasize those abilities at each level or that emphasize the abilities needed to perform at the high proficiency level. A study by Parker and Fleishman (1961), in which three groups learned a motor task under different instructional conditions, demonstrated that the group receiving guidance with emphasis on the ability components of the task, as they changed over the course of learning, learned faster and reached a higher level of performance than the other groups (figure 16.4).

Despite the enthusiasm of teachers for ability grouping, there is little research support for this method when measures of physical performance are the standard for judgment. In a comprehensive review of the literature, Nixon and Locke (1973) state, "In general, homogeneous grouping appears to be no better than ordinary methods of assignment to class." When the literature on the specificity of motor skill learning is considered, it is quite understandable why homogeneous grouping is ineffectual: Motor skills classes are typically grouped by scores obtained on some general motor ability test.

Intelligence and Motor Behavior

Ever since the Greeks coined the saying, "A sound mind in a sound body," the notion has existed that there is a positive relationship between intelligence and motor ability. At the same time there have been those who have believed that there is an inverse relationship between the two—perhaps the term "dumb jock" characterizes this belief. Actually, we have very little evidence to support either of these two extreme positions.

In one of the first texts on motor behavior, Clarence Ragsdale (1930) reviewed the studies that had been done up to that time and concluded that there was no consistent finding that intelligence and motor behavior are related. Overall, the large body of research on this topic since that time has yielded essentially the same results. The results of the studies can best be summarized with this statement: There is a low, but positive, relationship between intelligence and motor ability (see Rarick 1980 for a review).

This conclusion could probably be expected, given the variety of motor ability test batteries used and given that correlational and factor analytic studies have demonstrated that intelligence is not a single, unitary ability. It should be noted, though, that Ismail and his colleagues (Ismail and Gruber 1967) at Purdue University have found significant positive relationships between a few motor task items, especially coordination and balance items, and intelligence. Factor analysis was used in this work (Ismail, Kane, and Kirkendall 1969).

The statements above apply to people with so-called normal intelligence. Research with retarded people has demonstrated a consistent finding that retardates perform most motor tasks less effectively than those with normal intelligence and are slower at acquiring motor skills. There is an active controversy in the motor behavior literature over the reasons for these differences.

Summary

The nature and development of human abilities has been a central topic in psychology. *Ability* refers to a general capacity of the individual in relation to performance on a variety of human tasks, while *skill* refers to proficiency on a specific task.

Biological forces are presumed to be primarily responsible for an individual's basic ability, but environment also plays a significant role in the development of abilities. The view that there is a general motor ability is not supported by the research.

Research on the relationships between motor ability and performance and acquisition of motor tasks is typically done using correlational and factor analytical statistical techniques.

During the 1930s and 40s several motor ability tests were developed with a view of being able to predict future performance and ease of motor skill learning on the basis of the test scores. The validity of these tests was found to be quite poor. Beginning in the 1950s, Henry and his students demonstrated that skill is a specific and not a general ability.

Over the past twenty-five years Edwin Fleishman has helped to clarify the relationship between motor abilities and motor behavior. He has used factor analysis to extract factors from a large group of motor tasks. Fleishman has been able to account for performance on a wide variety of tasks by a relatively small number of abilities.

In addition to identifying motor abilities, Fleishman has demonstrated that as the learning of a motor skill progresses, changes occur in the particular combinations of abilities contributing to performance. This finding suggests that people who possess those abilities that contribute to performance in the initial stages of learning will begin at a relatively high level and those who possess abilities that contribute to performance at later stages of learning will achieve high proficiency levels later in learning. Moreover, individual differences in initial proficiency have relatively little relation to ultimate proficiency.

The research on the changing nature of abilities in motor learning rather consistently shows that visual abilities tend to be a major factor contributing to proficiency in the early phase of learning a variety of motor tasks.

While there is a popular notion that a positive relationship exists between intelligence and motor ability, the empirical evidence does not support such a view. There is, instead, only a low, positive relationship between these two variables.

17

Practice and Motor Behavior

*M*otor skill acquisition is dependent upon a variety of conditions, and practice is one of the most important of these. Complex motor skills required for riding a bicycle, driving an automobile, shooting a basket, or hitting a baseball must be practiced many times before they can be done effectively and efficiently. As noted in previous chapters, motor learning involves the establishment of appropriate motor programs that correspond to proper movement execution. Motor programs are developed through practice.

Practice may take various forms. In this chapter we examine several of the more important practice considerations. Other conditions (such as feedback, transfer of learning, and motivation) that are normally present during practice will be treated in separate chapters. But although these factors are treated separately, in real teaching-learning situations they are, of course, interrelated with practice.

The General Effects of Practice

The four most obvious effects of practice on the learning of motor skills are:

1. increased speed of performance;
2. increased accuracy, or reduction of errors;
3. increased adaptability to meet the demands of the task;
4. decreasing attentional demands in executing the task movements.

Most improvement in skilled performance is dependent upon increasing the speed and accuracy of movements. As was noted in chapter 11, many motor tasks can be performed the first time if done slowly enough for various sensory mechanisms to guide the performance. However, the difference between the skilled and unskilled performer is that the skilled performer can perform with very little sensory guidance. This has the effect of increasing speed of performance. Accuracy of performance also normally increases with proper practice—basketball players become better shooters and baseball hitters make contact with the ball more frequently. One of the characteristics of a highly skilled performer is adaptability—the ability to perform a task in a variety of different ways according to variations in the immediate situation. An example is the tennis player who can hit the backhand cross court or down the line, depending on the position of the opponent. Finally, with practice, longer motor programs, producing longer sequences of action, are developed. Once a motor program has been selected and initiated, attention can be turned over to other things for a period of time.

There are more subtle effects of practice on the acquisition of a motor skill. Those listed above are only the most easily discerned as one observes a learner become more proficient.

Instruction before Practice

The time given over to instruction to learners of motor skills can be viewed as part of the practice period. Instructions are commonly thought to be an important factor in the learning experience. Other than some general guidelines, there are few specific prescriptions for instructional techniques that have proven to be equally effective for enhancing learning rate across many motor tasks.

Fundamental to all motor learning is the ability to produce an appropriate sequence of motor commands—the generation of a motor program. In order to do this, before practice on a task the learner needs to know what to do, how to do it, the goal of the movement, and the means by which the goal can be accomplished. Only then can an overall image, an internalized picture, of the skill be established prior to actually performing the task. The formulation of this image or internalized representation provides the basis for forming a plan, a schema, that will guide the movement.

All our skilled movements are guided by images of what is to be done. (Schema theory considers this the schema.) The establishment of an appropriate image not only serves as the basis for the motor commands, but also generates a model, or template, of how feedback should appear or feel if the movement is performed correctly. Motor learning is then accomplished by the process of matching the feedback from movement with the model for the movement. If there are discrepancies, the motor program can be altered and feedback again can be compared with the model, and so on, until the appropriate movement pattern is established (Summers 1981).

The notion that the learner must develop an image of the task suggests that an important first job of the instructor is to instill in the learner's memory a perfect image. This can be done in several ways, but the two most commonly used techniques are verbal instruction and demonstration.

Verbal Instruction

Verbal instruction and advice can no doubt assist the learner in developing a motor template, and some verbal instruction is almost a necessity. But verbal descriptions of movements are relatively crude and imprecise. Moreover, verbalization about the execution of a movement tends to be very time consuming. Finally, excessive verbalization often results in diminished attention, thus reducing the effectiveness of the instruction.

Demonstration

Much human behavior is learned by observation of **demonstration.** From observing others one forms an idea of how certain behaviors are performed. We have a rather substantial literature demonstrating the effectiveness of observational learning (Bandura 1977). Having learners observe a skilled performer demonstrate a task before they actually practice would seem to have promise. Observational learning studies have demonstrated marked learning facilitation for a variety of motor tasks following observation of a model's demonstration (Landers and Landers 1973; Landers 1975; Martens, Burwitz, and Zuckerman 1976; Thomas, Pierce, and Ridsdale 1977).

Televised or symbolized models are sometimes as effective as live models (Feltz and Landers 1977). The results of one study (Landers 1975) are shown in figure 17.1. The two groups that received demonstrations before practice began ("before" and "interspaced") performed better on the initial trials than did the group receiving demonstrations only midway through the session ("middle"). Moreover, performance of the group that received another demonstration midway through the practice session ("interspaced") surpassed the group that had only received a demonstration prior to practice. This suggests that demonstrations can enhance learning rate when given before practice begins as well as later in the learning sequence.

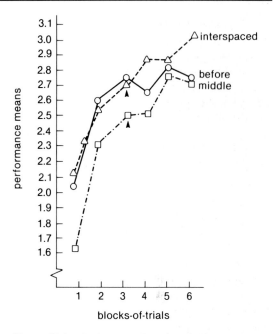

Figure 17.1 *Performance (in rungs climbed) for the three model spacing conditions as a function of trials.*

The method of providing demonstration and requiring learners to observe models has some drawbacks to which an instructor must be sensitive. When models are observed, the learner may not perceive critical aspects of the movement pattern or the tactics employed in execution. Another problem is that some learners can see others perform, but cannot translate this information into a usable model for their own performance. Finally, the research on observational learning of motor skills suggests that the effectiveness of demonstrations varies for males and females, for learners of different ages, and for different motor tasks (Feltz 1982). Demonstration is not an equally effective method for all learners in every situation (see Gould and Roberts 1981 for a review).

A prepractice technique that is related to observation of a model, but requires somewhat more active participation on the part of the learner, is called **verbal pretraining.** Learners are required to learn certain aspects of a task, such as the sequence of events, in the hope that they will transfer this learning when they actually begin to practice. An example of verbal pretraining was employed by Adams and Creamer (1962). They asked subjects, who were to learn to follow an alternating wave form by moving a hand control, simply to watch the wave before trying to track it and respond to the changes in direction with vocal responses. Subjects who received the verbal pretraining subsequently performed the tracking task more accurately than did subjects who did not have the pretraining. Similar findings have been reported by other investigators (Trumbo, Ulrich, and Noble 1965). Shea (1977) has demonstrated that when learners give verbal cues to themselves to make learning a positioning task more meaningful, positioning accuracy (in terms of recall scores) is enhanced. It appears, then, that some type of active experience related to the task demands, before learners actually practice a task, may facilitate performance on the initial practice trials; verbally cueing oneself about movement demands may enhance motor memory.

Another form of instruction often employed during the introduction of a motor task is verbally describing the mechanical principles that underlie the correct execution of the movements. Since this topic is discussed in some detail in chapter 19, it will not be dealt with here.

Practice Intentions

Practice is essential for acquiring complex motor skills. No one ever learned to shoot a jump shot or serve a tennis ball by merely watching someone else or by just thinking about these skills. It is only through repetition of the desired movement pattern that skillful response sequences are developed. Practice will not, however, necessarily result in proficiency. Skill improvement will occur and proficiency is maintained only if conscientious attempts to improve are made. The learner must view the task as desirable to learn and approach practice with the intention of improving.

The fallacy of the old adage "practice makes perfect" can be seen by observing the typical adult's handwriting. Although the task (handwriting) is practiced daily, most individuals' handwriting does not improve and, in fact, gets worse in many cases. Practice may actually perpetuate errors. Our everyday experience with recreational athletics also illustrates this point. Recreational golfers, tennis players, and swimmers typically do not improve, despite playing the sport for years, because they do not try to improve.

The value of positive **practice intentions** is nicely illustrated in a study by Dickinson (1978). He had subjects produce and recall a series of four arm-positioning movements. One group of subjects was given instructions that would give them no particular reason for wanting to learn the positions. The other group was given instructions designed to promote intentional learning on the part of the subjects. After ten practice trials the groups were administered a recall test after 0, 30, 60, and 600 seconds. There was a greater retention of skill for the group that practiced with the intention to learn, and their superiority of recall increased the longer the retention interval. The results are shown in figure 17.2.

Explanations for Intention-Learning Relationship

Several possible explanations exist for the fact that there is little improvement in proficiency unless there is intent to improve. One explanation is based on the assumption that motor learning occurs to some extent as a result of the pairing of

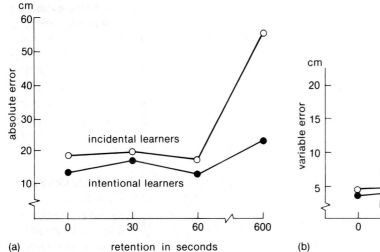
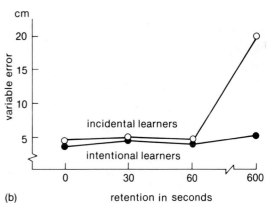

Figure 17.2   *(a) Mean total absolute error for four movements in retention for intentional and incidental learners; (b) mean modified variable error in retention for intentional and incidental learners.*

feedback resulting from the execution of a movement pattern. If the movement pattern is successful (the basketball goes into the basket), an emotionally satisfying state results for the individual who is intent upon becoming proficient. When executing the movement again, the learner will attempt to perform correctly so as to receive the satisfaction again. If one performs and does not experience the emotionally satisfying set of stimuli because correct performance is not important, the feedback does not become paired with a satisfaction. There is no particular effort to perform correctly in subsequent practice (Dickinson 1977).

Another explanation might go like this: We assume that learners incorporate the feedback from a performance into a verbal-cognitive process of some sort, and that this process facilitates forming hypotheses and strategies for making modifications in subsequent performances. A learner who has no particular interest in improving will probably not employ this process to any extent. The result will be little improvement in performance.

A third explanation for no or little improvement without intent to improve makes use of consolidation memory theory. As you recall, unless the short-term memory stage is allowed to persist, there will be little long-term memory. Information that has entered STM can be enhanced by cognitive rehearsal; maintenance of information in STM seems to facilitate transfer to LTM. People who are intent upon improving probably do more thinking about the task and their movements between actual practices. They cognitively rehearse, thus strengthening the process that leads to LTM. A study by Tulving (1966) illustrates that unless there is intention to remember, mere repetition is not sufficient for storage into LTM.

Amount of Practice

Assuming intention to improve, the more one practices, the higher the level of proficiency and the more one retains proficiency when practice is terminated or interrupted. In other words, active rehearsal serves to prevent forgetting and to increase the resistance of stored information to subsequent interferring events.

Active practice is a form of repeating the process that results in memory. The transfer of information to long-term memory seems to require repetition through rehearsal. The more often a task is repeated, the more likely it is to be embedded in long-term memory. In addition, active rehearsal acts to organize material in memory, and such organization facilitates memory (Keele 1973).

In terms of **schema** motor program **theory,** both schemata are developed through practice. In the case of the recall schema, since it is the relationship, built up over practice trials, between response specifications and actual outcomes, the strength of the recall schema is a positive function of the number of practice trials. Similarly, the recognition schema is developed by practice, enabling the learner to generate more accurate expected sensory consequences of the movements involved in performing the skill. Thus, during execution of the movement the learner can compare the actual and expected sensory consequences and make accurate error determinations.

The obvious implication for instructors of motor skills is that the number of practice trials should be maximized. Of course, physical ability limits the ultimate proficiency attainable, but there is no current method for assessing what the ultimate limit may be. In many cases improvement in performance occurs over many years. (See chapter 16 for a fuller discussion of this topic.)

Practice Schedules

In education, industry, and the military, where motor skills are taught, the issue of the most efficient practice-rest ratio has been of special interest because there is typically a limited amount of time available for practice and numerous skills to be taught.

The major questions with regard to **practice schedules** are: Should learners continually practice on a skill with only a few brief rest periods, or should they practice for short periods of time with more frequent and prolonged intervals of rest? Which practice schedule is best for speed of skill acquisition? highest levels of skill? retention?

The two basic variables with which practice-schedule studies have been concerned are the time of continual practice and the interval between practice trials. A practice schedule that requires continual practice with short and/or infrequent rest intervals between trials is called **massed** (or "unspaced") **practice.** When rest intervals are longer and/or more frequent between trials or between a set of trials, this is called **distributed** (or "spaced") **practice.** This description of the two types of practice schedules may strike the reader as imprecise. But the characterization of "massed" and "distributed" has varied from experiment to experiment, so research on distribution of practice in motor tasks has been beset by inadequate and inconsistent definitions.

Regardless of the definitional problems associated with research on this topic, advocates of massed practice suggest that performance and learning are most efficient and effective by practicing continually over an extended period with few and short rest periods. Conversely, supporters of distributed practice have argued that performance and learning are best accomplished when practice trials are separated by frequent rest intervals, with the rest between practice being at least as long as the time of practice itself.

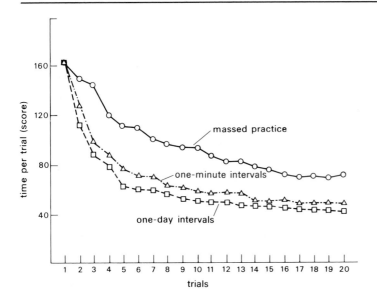

Figure 17.3 *Performance curves under three different schedules of practice on a mirror-tracing task. One-minute rest intervals between trials and one-day intervals were nearly equal, and both were better than massed practice. The lower the score, the better the performance.*

Most investigations designed to test these two contentions have used rather simple motor tasks, such as the rotary-pursuit, mirror tracer, and other fine motor skill tasks. These tasks make it possible to control many variables, but some questions arise as to the feasibility of generalizing from the findings to motor tasks such as those found in sports, industry, and dance. However, several studies using gross motor skills have corroborated the basic findings obtained in studies using fine motor tasks.

Massed and Distributed Schedules and Motor Skills

For most fine motor tasks that have been studied, the results show that performance tends to be superior for the distributed group, especially after the first few trials. On the other hand, the results for learning are not so clear-cut; it appears that there is actually little difference in the two schedules when learning is assessed. Since most of the early investigations did not differentiate between performance and learning, only the performance data were reported. Hence the superiority of distributed practice for performance was commonly incorrectly applied to learning, too.

The results of two studies illustrate how the use of only performance scores leads to the conclusion that distributed practice is superior to massed practice. In what has become one of the classic studies, Lorge (1930), using mirror drawing, mirror writing, and a code substitution task, found that subjects who had practiced with a rest period of one minute or one day between trials produced better performances after twenty trials than did a continual-practice group (figure 17.3). In an often cited study of rotary-pursuit learning, Digman (1959) reported that performance under the massed condition was poorer than under the distributed condition. In some sessions performance actually deteriorated under the massed condition. However, the performance of the massed group was better at the beginning of each new session than it had been at the end of the previous session, and over the course of the experiment the level of performance approached that under the distributed condition (figure 17.4).

Figure 17.4 *Mean performance for distributed and massed practice groups on the rotary-pursuit apparatus.*

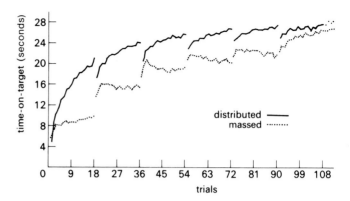

In 1960 Dorothy Mohr reported that a review of the motor behavior literature turned up forty-five studies related to massed and distributed practice. Of these studies, forty reported results favoring distributed practice, three favored massed practice, and two found no significant differences. These findings were of performance results, and they show the clear superiority of distributed practice for performance.

While the results of studies of practice schedules have rather consistently shown that performance tends to be better for the distributed group, several related findings suggest that what is true for performance is not true for learning. First, performance scores after both groups have had a substantial rest interval (five minutes or more) regularly show that the actual proficiency of the massed group is very similar to the distributed group; after the rest their performance scores at the beginning of the new practice period nearly match those of the distributed group. Digman's results illustrate this nicely. Second, when massed-practice learners are shifted to a distributed schedule, they perform like the distributed learners, implying that the learning of a motor task is not necessarily much affected by practice schedules. Finally, when learning formulae have

been employed to assess the effectiveness of practice schedules, few learning differences have been found. Overall, then, massing appears to be detrimental to performance but not to learning fine motor skills (Whitley 1970).

Massed and Distributed Schedules and Gross Motor Skills

Studies of the distribution of practice for gross motor skills have generally corroborated the findings of studies using fine motor tasks for performance, but the findings for learning have been less clear-cut. Two major factors, other than the type of skills involved, may be responsible for the differences in findings for learning. First, the practice and rest periods tend to be quite different. Studies with fine motor tasks often use practice and rest periods of from a few seconds to a few minutes, whereas investigations with gross motor tasks often employ practices of several minutes to several hours and rest periods from several minutes to several hours. A second reason for the differences is that the fine motor tasks used in the studies have typically been continual tasks (like the rotary-pursuit), while the gross motor skills have usually been discrete or serial in nature. Given these differences, evidence is growing that massing is not detrimental for most gross motor skill learning.

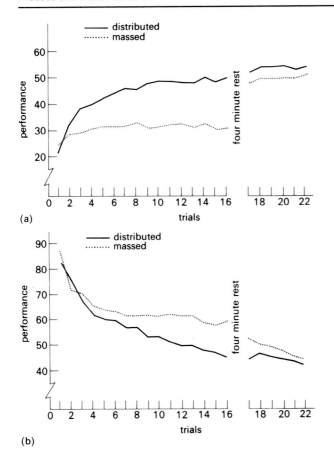

(a)

(b)

Figure 17.5 In (a) the performance curves for the distributed and massed groups on the Bachman ladder; scores were determined by the total number of rungs climbed in a thirty-second period. In (b) the performance curves for the distributed and massed groups on the stabilometer; scores represented total amount of board movement as measured by a work adder during a thirty-second interval, with one movement unit equivalent to 12 degrees of board movement (thus the lower the score the better the performance).

Two studies will be summarized to illustrate the research on practice schedules with gross motor tasks. Stelmach (1969b) designed a study with four groups of subjects. Each subject in a group performed on one of two motor tasks (the stabilometer and the Bachman ladder) under one of two conditions. Distributed practice consisted of alternating thirty-second trials of practice and rest; massed practice was continual for eight minutes. Performance during the last minute of practice prior to the rest interval was significantly poorer for the massed groups. After a four-minute rest period, both groups performed on a distributed schedule. No difference was found in the amount of learning (figure 17.5). Dunham (1976) assigned subjects to massed and distributed groups while practicing on the Bachman ladder. After eight minutes of practice, all subjects were given a four-minute rest. Following the rest, four groups were created, with half of the subjects who had practiced under distributed schedule transferred to massed practice and half who had practiced under massed practice transferred to distributed practice. The results are shown in figure 17.6. Distributed practice produced superior performance, and massing of practice led to a decrement of performance but not of learning.

Figure 17.6   *Performance curves for distributed and massed practice on the Bachman ladder.*

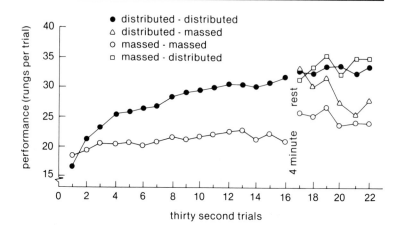

Explanation for Superior Performance with Distributed Practice

Why is performance under distributed schedules superior to that under massed schedules? The most commonly proposed interpretation is that massed practice produces physical fatigue in the performers. This explanation can be dismissed because many of the tasks are quite brief and not very physically demanding. Another proposal suggests that massed practice produces some kind of an inhibitory effect on performance, with little effect on learning. Diminution in the inhibitory effects during rest periods is proposed to account for both reminiscence and for the fact that performance under the two conditions approaches the same level after a rest interval.

The classic statement of inhibitory effects is that of the esteemed behavioral psychologist Clark Hull (1943), who postulated an inhibitory process he called **reactive inhibition** (I_R). With regard to I_R, Hull said, "Whenever any reaction is evoked in an organism, there is left a condition or state which acts as a primary, negative motivation in that it has an innate capacity to produce a cessation of the activity which has produced the state." According to this notion, as a consequence of making any response, there is an increase in a tendency not to repeat it. In addition, the longer the individual practice session, the more I_R builds

up—and the greater is the drive not to respond as the practice continues. The reaction decrements that Hull attributed to I_R bear a resemblance to the decrements commonly attributed to fatigue, but I_R denotes a decrement in action evocation potentiality, not an exhaustion of the energy available to the performer.

Applying reactive inhibition to practice schedules, in distributed practice conditions where the ratio of work to rest is at least somewhat equal, I_R accrues and dissipates in equal amounts; performance is not adversely affected. But in massed practice conditions, I_R builds up as the performer continues to practice, thus depressing performance. Extended rest intervals allow inhibition to dissipate and, when practice resumes, performance levels are initially much better than just before the rest period. As noted in chapter 15, support for Hull's concept of I_R has been recently demonstrated (Hsu and Payne 1979).

Hullian theory is formulated in behavioral, rather than in neurophysiological, terms. Neurophysiological explanations for differences in performance under massed and distributed schedules make use of information about variations in brain activity to stimuli, especially repetitive stimuli.

As noted in chapter 2, it is possible to record the electrical activity of the brain with an electroencephalograph (EEG). When a person is in an alert but resting state, the EEG commonly shows the alpha wave pattern. This consists of relatively high-amplitude, synchronous waves of 8–13 Hz. The neurological response to a novel or unexpected stimulus involves the appearance of low-amplitude, fast, desynchronized wave patterns. Normally, these replace the alpha waves, producing what is known as alpha block. **Alpha block** is associated with behavioral arousal, orienting movements, and widespread autonomic changes (such as increased heart rate and dilation of the eyes). It is assumed that this arousal response results in an increased ability to detect, classify, and respond appropriately to incoming stimulus information. In short, the individual is able to perform well in this state. A continuing repetition of stimuli, however, leads to a habituation of the arousal response. Habituation of the arousal response includes changes that decrease the sensitivity to a stimulus as well as the readiness to respond (Mackworth 1969).

With regard to practice schedules, the neural response to the initiation of practice is undoubtedly an alpha block and the arousal response. Under distributed practice, the frequent rest periods followed by a new practice period are likely to provide enough novelty and changed conditions to maintain the alpha block and, therefore, high performance. On the other hand, the prolonged repetition under massed conditions is likely to result in habituation, and, therefore, a decrement in performance as practice continues.

The notion that the decremental effects of massed practice are due to inhibition, habituation, and decreased arousal addresses the issue of performance (Catalano 1967; Catalano and Whalen 1967; McIntyre et al. 1972), but it is not clear why these processes are not detrimental to learning during massed practice. It has been suggested that the processes responsible for long-term memory are not affected by massed practice conditions (only the processes responsible for immediate memory are temporarily rendered inaccessible to recall, resulting in performance decrement) and, given a rest period, the actual learning that has occurred can more readily be exhibited (see Eysenck and Frith 1977 for a review of this idea).

Changing Practice Schedules

No consensus exists in the research literature concerning the effectiveness of changing practice schedules (for example, from distributed to massed) as learners acquire proficiency. Since there seems to be no consistent superiority of one practice schedule with respect to learning, the decision to switch from one practice schedule to another at some point appears to depend on the task to be learned and the practice time available.

Practice Schedules and Total Practice Time

In most studies of practice schedules, the total time is allowed to vary as shown in table 17.1. Thus, in 105 sec the massed group has had 90 sec of practice, while it has taken the distributed group 180 sec to get the same amount of practice. Given, for example, thirty minutes for a practice session, the massed group would have about twenty-five minutes of "actual" practice, while the distributed group would have fifteen minutes of practice. Clearly, then, the massed group would get more "actual" practice. Intuitively one might conclude that massed practice is more efficient, when total time is considered. While this may be true in many cases, it appears that the issue is more complex than it seems.

Table 17.1 *Types of practice schedules*

Massed schedule		Distributed schedule	
Practice	*Rest*	*Practice*	*Rest*
30	5	30	30
30	5	30	30
30	5	30	30
90	+ 15 = 105	90	+ 90 = 180

Note: Schedules measured in seconds.

In one of the few studies of total practice time and time spent in actual practice, Graw (1968) had learners spend varying amounts of time practicing either the Bachman ladder or the stabilometer in a total practice session of thirty minutes. The results demonstrated that practice-rest ratios are not equally effective across tasks. The most effective practice distribution for the Bachman ladder task was from 30–57 percent of total time spent in practice; for the stabilometer the most effective distribution was 57–77 percent of total time spent in practice. Results of the first task suggest distributing the practice-rest ratio is most effective, but a relatively massed practice schedule is more effective for the second task.

Retention and Practice Schedules

The effects of practice distribution on retention have not been studied to any extent, and the few studies of this topic have produced equivocal results.

General Guidelines for Practice Schedules

It is obvious that the research findings on the distribution of practice do not justify the formulation of any hard and fast "laws." However, drawing on the results of the various investigations reported above and many others that could not be included several guidelines can be proposed.

1. Distributed practice produces superior performance.
2. There is very little difference in learning between distributed and massed schedules, but distributed schedules have a slight advantage.
3. Distributed practice is preferable when the energy demands of the task are high, the task is complex, the length of the task performance is great, the task is not meaningful, and motivation of the learner is low.
4. Massed practice is preferable when the skill level of the learner is high and when peak performance on a well-learned skill is needed.
5. In situations that require that learners acquire proficiency in as short a time as possible, the instructor need not be overly concerned about whether a massed schedule will adversely affect learning, although its effects on immediate performance may be detrimental.

Practice under Fatigued Conditions

Practicing motor skills is often physically fatiguing, hence the question of how practicing in a fatigued state affects performance and learning. The literature on the effects of fatigue on motor behavior is both vast and depressing: vast because the topic of fatigue has been of interest to motor behavior researchers as well as applied scientists in industry, the military, and sports; depressing because this topic has been beset by conceptual and methodological problems that have rendered much of the findings confusing and contradictory.

The conceptual inadequacies of fatigue research stem in large part from the word *fatigue* itself. The word suggests a unitary phenomenon, yet it is obvious that there are a number of separate and diverse dimensions of the word. There is first the subjective awareness of tiredness, and second the objective measure of tiredness. It is clear that reports performers make about their feelings of tiredness bear little relation to objective measures of performance; there may even be a negative correlation. At the same time, objective measures of fatigue are not easily made, and the relationships between the various measures are not altogether satisfactory.

Two of the most evident methodological problems of research on this topic have to do with the time of task performance in relation to the induced fatigue and the amount and extent of induced fatigue. Most investigations have had subjects perform the motor task to be learned immediately after inducing a fatigue state, but several recent investigations have had the subjects perform the motor task while they were simultaneously performing a "fatiguing task." With regard to the amount and extent of induced fatigue, there has been no uniformity. Investigators have used treadmills, bicycle ergometers, and bench step-ups, and fatigue has been indexed by various work loads performed by the subjects, various heart rates, and even subjective feelings expressed by the subjects.

Effects of Fatigue on Performance

A rather substantial body of literature shows that fatigue induced before performance or interpolated between trials to maintain the fatigue condition throughout practice hinders performance on a variety of tasks (Schmidt 1969; Pack, Cotten, and Biasiotto 1974; Williams and Singer 1975). But performance on some tasks seems to be enhanced by previously induced fatigue (Phillips 1963), while performance on others is unaffected by induced fatigue (Gutin 1970). Although these findings appear contradictory, most evidence indicates that physical fatigue is detrimental to performance; how detrimental depends upon such factors as condition of the subjects, the demands of the task, and the actual extent of the fatigue.

Effects of Fatigue on Learning

Research regarding the effect of fatigue on learning is contradictory. Several investigations have found that learning was unaffected by fatigue (Carron 1969; Schmidt 1969; Cotton et al. 1972). However, most of these earlier studies induced fatigue only before performance of the task to be learned, so recovery from fatigue during practice was likely. But studies in which fatigue was severe and was maintained throughout the practice period have produced conflicting findings as well. For example, Godwin and Schmidt (1971) had subjects perform a rapid arm movement task, with one group performing under fatigued conditions and another group performing in a nonfatigued state. The nonfatigued group performed significantly better than the fatigued group on the first day. However, the two groups were very similar in performance on the second day, when both groups performed under nonfatigued conditions (figure 17.7). This shows that the groups learned about the same amount.

A study by Pack and his colleagues (1974) produced quite different results. Their study assessed the effect of fatigue on learning the Bachman ladder climb. Fatigue was manipulated by having subjects perform on a treadmill until they reached an assigned heart rate. Then they practiced the Bachman ladder, returning to the treadmill after each practice trial. The learning score data indicated that subjects whose assigned heart rate fatigue level was 150 to 180 beats per minute showed a decremental effect on learning of the task. It appears, then, that practicing this motor task under conditions of severe fatigue impaired the learning process.

Figure 17.7 *Mean movement times for fatigue group (F) and nonfatigued group (NF) over two days of practice.*

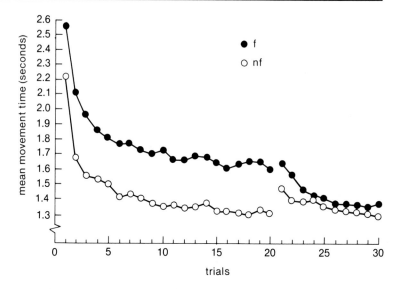

Most research on the effects of fatigue on motor learning has employed the fatiguing conditions before or during the practice—they have been concerned with the proactive effects of fatigue. Common experience and consolidation-memory theory would suggest that fatigue induced immediately after a learning experience might disrupt memory consolidation and thus inhibit learning. Hutton and his colleagues (1972) reported findings from two animal experiments in which fatiguing exercises were introduced after the learning trials. Results suggested partial support for the hypothesis that fatigue introduced after practice on a task depressed learning. More research is needed on this topic before firm conclusions can be made.

Explanation for Findings about Fatigue and Motor Behavior

The nervous system is the primary limiting factor for all kinds of work. A wealth of neurophysiological data indicates that exhaustive exercise tends to depress neural mechanisms associated with alert, attentive behavior. Afferent and efferent neurons lose sensitivity and reactivity with long-repeated, rapid stimulation and thus show a fatigue effect: receptors fail to respond to stimuli

and motoneurons either fail to transmit impulses or eject an inadequate supply of transmitter substance at the neuromuscular junction to fire the muscle fiber. In the CNS, fatigue produces an increase in the resting EEG wave pattern, suggesting that the person is less attentive to stimuli. There is also a reduced effect of stimulants on arousal responses of cortical and subcortical structures (Pineda and Adkisson 1961). All of these physiological responses to fatigue will tend to depress performance. But they apparently do not affect the processes that transfer information from STM to LTM because fatigue seems to have less adverse effects on learning.

Mental Practice

It is possible to facilitate the learning of a motor skill by mentally practicing the skill between practice trials. Although numerous studies have confirmed this fact, little systematic application of it has occurred. The general belief that "physical" learning is different from "mental" learning and the knowledge that actual practice of the movements of a task is necessary for skill acquisition have probably perpetuated the notion that the only way to learn motor tasks is actually to perform them.

The rehearsal of a motor task without overt movement is called **mental practice** or **cognitive rehearsal.**[1] The word *mental* means that a person is thinking about a particular task and imagines performing it. When tennis players imagine themselves going through the movements of serving a tennis ball, they are involved in mental practice. Basketball players who think through their jump shots while not actually performing are mentally practicing.

Since the classic implication of the word *mental* carries with it the notion of a nonphysical phenomenon, perhaps the term *mental practice* is unfortunate. The activity of the nervous system during mental practice is certainly "physical" in that nerve cells are functioning and electric current is being passed along these cells, producing a pattern of neural impulses in the brain. Although several terms have been used to describe this form of practice, the term *mental practice* is most commonly used, so we will use it in this book.

Mental practice investigations date back more than forty years, yet there is a sustaining interest in this topic. Over fifty studies have been explicitly concerned with the effectiveness of this technique for motor skill learning in the past fifteen years.

Mental Practice and Motor Learning

Typically, experiments on mental practice contain three groups: (1) a physical practice group; (2) a mental practice group; and (3) a group that uses a combination of physical and mental practice. Sometimes a group that does not use any form of practice is used. The literature is too extensive to describe all of the studies on mental practice, but we shall cite a couple of these studies to illustrate the work on this topic involving motor tasks.

Vandell et al. (1943) reported the pioneer study on mental practice and motor skill learning. They used junior high, senior high, and college students as subjects and had them practice free throw shooting and dart throwing. These investigations found that the physical- and mental-practice groups improved, while the nonpractice groups did not improve. They concluded that mental practice is almost as effective as actual practice, for the conditions of their experiment. The value of this investigation, however, is limited because there was no statistical analysis and only twelve subjects were used.

In a recent study, McBride and Rothstein (1979) had subjects practice hitting a whiffle ball with a paddle at a target. Subjects were divided into mental, physical, or physical-mental groups. The first group mentally practiced the task, the physical-practice group actually hit the balls, and the combined physical-mental practice group alternated between actually hitting balls and mentally hitting balls. The combined practice group showed the most improvement, supporting the effectiveness of mental practice when combined with physical practice for facilitating motor skill acquisition.

Many other studies showing the effects of mental practice on motor learning could be identified. Instead, Weinberg's (1981) conclusions, made after an extensive review of mental practice studies, will suffice to place this topic in perspective. He says:

Although some studies did not find significant effects for MP [mental practice], the majority of the studies have provided evidence that MP can facilitate performance. MP should not be used as a substitute for PP [physical practice], however, but rather in conjunction with PP. . . . If MP is employed under the proper conditions, . . . it can definitely aid in enhancing motor learning and performance.

---

[1] One psychologist, Richard Suinn (1980), calls a cognitive rehearsal technique he teaches visual motor behavior rehearsal (VMBR).

When to Mentally Practice

At what time during the interval between physical practices is mental practice most effective—immediately after a practice trial, at a point midway between practice trials, or just before a practice trial? Unfortunately, this question has not been studied to any extent. In the studies that have been done, investigators have employed mental practice at different times during the interval between practice sessions with rather consistent positive findings, regardless of when the mental practice was done. So it appears that this form of rehearsal can be effective at any time between practices (Suinn 1980; Weinberg 1981).

Skill Level and Mental Practice

A great deal of controversy exists as to whether mental practice is more effective for novices or for the highly proficient. Overall, most of the research on mental practice has been done with beginners, and learning rate has rather consistently been found to be facilitated. Several investigators have argued on theoretical grounds that mental practice should be most effective with beginners, since at this stage the cognitive aspects of a task are salient as the learner attempts to construct an image of the goal of the task and how to accomplish it. Indeed, when the cognitive and motor aspects of a task have been studied, mental practice seems to enhance the learning of the cognitive components more than the motor components. Minas (1978; 1980) had subjects learn to throw balls into target bins in a particular sequence under different mental- and physical-practice conditions. Mental practice facilitated learning the sequence (the cognitive component), but enhanced very little the learning of the throwing movements (the motor component). Ryan and Simons (1981) corroborated this finding with two other tasks.

Although not as numerous, there are several investigators who have reported that mental practice can be effective with highly skilled performers (Suinn 1976; 1980). Moreover, many top athletes report incorporating mental practice into their performance routines. Jack Nicklaus (Nicklaus and Bowden 1974) says that his good shots are 10 percent swing, 40 percent setup and stance, and 50 percent mental picture. He describes his mental practice process:

I never hit a shot, not even in practice, without having a very sharp, in-focus picture of it in my head. It's like a color movie. First I "see" the ball where I want it to finish, nice and white and sitting up high on the bright green grass. Then the scene quickly changes and I "see" the ball going there: its path, trajectory, and shape, even its behavior on landing. Then there is sort of a fadeout and the next scene shows me making the kind of swing that will turn the previous images into reality.

Rather than an emphasis on skill acquisition with the highly skilled, mental practice emphasis appears to have good potential for correcting errors in execution, increasing concentration, and strategy rehearsal.

Mental Practice Time

Apparently it is not necessary to devote a great deal of time to mental practice; indeed, it seems that learners can fully concentrate on mental rehearsal for only a few minutes at a time. The few studies that have attempted to examine this variable suggest that three to five minutes of mental practice at one time produce the best results (Shick 1970).

Retention and Mental Practice

The effects of mental practice on skill retention have not been studied to any extent. At present there is no evidence that mental practice produces better or worse retention, when the proficiency level is controlled before the retention interval.

Techniques of Mental Practice

Mental practice can be used immediately preceding, following, or during a performance. Two general strategies can be employed in the rehearsal. First, learners might focus on the task and visualize themselves executing the correct movement pattern. This could be likened to a closed-loop filmstrip, with learners performing over and over in their minds. A second technique, which is especially appropriate for games and sports, involves rehearsing game tactics between contests or even during lulls in a contest. In this technique, performers think through what they should do if the ball suddenly comes to them, or if their opponent or teammate makes a certain maneuver. One of the oldest coaching dictates in baseball makes use of this technique: "Before each pitch, think of what you should do if the ball is hit to you."

Explanation for the Effects of Mental Practice

Why does mental practice facilitate motor learning and performance? As with many other questions in motor behavior, there is presently no satisfactory answer. But several theories have been advanced to account for this phenomenon.

It has been hypothesized that motivation is partly responsible for the effectiveness of mental practice. In this view, mental practice groups become more motivated than nonmental practice groups because the former groups become "ego-involved" when asked to mentally rehearse a task. The result is an enhanced learning rate.

Another interpretation might be called the cognitive-perceptual hypothesis. According to this idea, mental practice allows the learner to gain cognitive-perceptual "insights" into the movement pattern. These new insights result in reduced errors and improved performance. There is some support for this notion in what is called the "general factors" theory of transfer of learning. This will be discussed more fully in chapter 19.

The functioning of memory mechanisms can be employed to explain how mental practice enhances learning. Memory for anything requires rehearsal to achieve ultimately long-term storage. This rehearsal can take the form of overt movements or, apparently, of covert rehearsal. In other words, mental rehearsal may have some of the same characteristics of activating and maintaining short-term memory processes as overt practice, and in so functioning will bring about a more robust long-term memory. Mental practice can be viewed, then, as a process of reperception to maintain material in STM, the effect of which is to enhance the consolidation of the materal into LTM. The evidence is substantial that differences in proficiency on various tasks is due in large part to differences in rehearsal strategies and that rehearsal is an effective method to move information between STM and LTM (Chi 1976; Ornstein and Naus 1978).

Another dimension of this issue is that mental practice activates many of the neural components in the brain that are responsible for actually directing movement. The component that is not, of course, fully activated in mental practice is the motor component. Nevertheless, although all of the motor units that are activated when a movement is actually executed are not mobilized during mental practice, there is convincing evidence that *some* of the motor units that are normally activated during movement execution are activated when a person mentally practices the movement. Many years ago Jacobson (1930; 1932) and others discovered, by placing electrodes on muscle groups and recording the electrical activity of subjects while they imagined themselves performing a task, that muscular activity during the mental practice was localized to the muscle groups that would be involved in the actual performance of the imagined activity. Jacobson noted, "When the subject imagines that he is steadily bending one of his arms, electrical phenomena simultaneously occur in the biceps

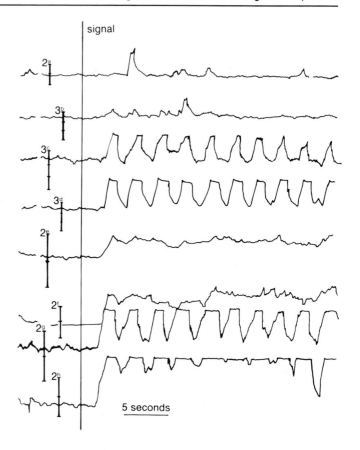

Figure 17.8   *EMG leads: a, biceps-brachial muscle group; b, right extensor muscle group; c, right hand flexors; d, right hand extensor; e through h, same muscle groups on the left side. Instruction: "Upon first signal, imagine that you are rowing a boat." Strikingly positive rhythmical results are notable chiefly in tracings c, d, g, and h, namely from extensors and flexors of both hands.*

region of the arm." Figure 17.8 is from a publication by Jacobson (1973) and vividly illustrates his point.

The picture that emerges is that as a learner mentally rehearses a sequence of movements, there will be an activation of some of the relevant motor units. This being the case, the cognitive activity employed to produce a recall schema to activate the motor units and the recognition schema that accompanies this appear to be capable of facilitating subsequent performance. According to some motor behavior scientists, the value of mental practice is quite congruent with schema theory. One might hypothesize that the more accurately a learner can imagine a particular movement pattern, the more effectively the learner can mentally practice and smooth out the errors in the movements (White, Ashton, and Lewis 1979).

Variability of Practice

As noted in chapter 14, a person never executes a movement in exactly the same way each time. A performer must produce a response that is actually different from any other response the person has ever before produced. In tennis the forehand stroke is one of the basic ground strokes of the sport. In any given match a player will have to use the forehand hundreds of times, but it will never be executed in exactly the same way. It will be used to hit a ball that is always in a different location on the court, traveling at a different speed and height; and the player will have approached the ball from a different angle each time. Finally, the ball will be hit to a different location on the opposite side of the court each time. In basketball a player will use the jump shot many times during a game, but due to the distance from the basket, location of opponents, and other environmental conditions, the shot will never be made in exactly the same way. Even with closed tasks, such as a gymnastic stunt or a springboard dive, there will be variations in execution each time the skill is performed.

Variability raises the question of the most efficient and effective way to practice. As you recall, schema theory assumes that a movement is carried out by a generalized program that can be run off in a variety of ways depending upon differences in initial conditions and variations in the way the movement is to be executed, that is, fast or slow, strong or weak force. A fundamental prediction of the schema theory is that **variable practice** on a given class of movements, such as a forehand stroke or a jump shot, will result in better performance on any unique variation of that same movement class.[2] As Schmidt (1975) says:

Increased amount and variability [of practice] will lead to the development of an increasingly strong recall schema, so that when the subject is transferred to a novel situation governed by the schema, he will be able to determine more effectively the appropriate response specifications, given the desired outcome and the initial conditions. In addition to improved performance on the first trials of the novel movement, the theory predicts increased rate of learning for the new task as a function of increased variability in previous movement experiences.

---

[2] This notion runs somewhat counter to the "specificity of learning" view described in chapter 16. This merely illustrates the need for more research to clarify the apparent differences.

To illustrate: Given that one basketball player practices only a ten-foot jump shot from directly in front of the basket (which would be a 90-degree angle from the basket), another practices only a fifteen-foot jump shot from a 45-degree angle from the basket, and a third practices jump shots from various distances between ten and fifteen feet and from various angles between 90 degrees and 45 degrees. If all three are tested on a twelve-foot jump shot from a 60-degree angle from the basket, schema prediction suggests the variable-practice player will produce the best performance at this novel distance and angle because the same class of movements is involved. The acquisition of a diversified schema seems to be particularly relevant in learning open skills that are executed under constantly changing conditions.

Research has provided moderate support for variability of practice when male adults have been the subjects, while stronger support for variable practice has been generated when children and females have been the subjects (see Shapiro and Schmidt 1982 for a review). Figure 17.9 summarizes the results of one of the most often cited studies of variability and practice (McCracken and Stelmach 1977). The investigators used a task in which subjects moved their hand from its starting position over a specified distance to break an electrical contact on a barrier at the end of the movement. The goal of the movement was to time the movement through the specified distance so as to break the contact in exactly 200 msec. The task could be altered to modify the distance the subject had to move. A constant practice group (low variability) was divided into four subgroups, each of which practiced 300 trials on one of the following distances: 15, 35, 60, and 65 cm. The variable-practice group (high variability) was given the same number of trials, but the trials were variable in that all four distances were practiced, with 75 trials for each distance.

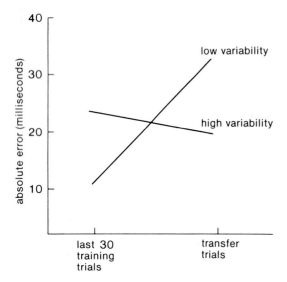

Figure 17.9 *Absolute error on the 50-cm task for high- and low-variability groups under the training and transfer conditions.*

At the end of the practice period, the two groups were given a series of trials at a novel distance (50 cm)—a distance that had never been practiced by either group. In figure 17.9 the results for the last 30 trials of training show that the average timing error was considerably larger for the variable-practice group compared to the constant-practice group. This is as one would expect, since the latter subjects were being scored on their performance on a single distance, while the former had been practicing several distances and therefore had not had as much practice on any one distance. The critical test, with regard to schema theory, is the performance of the groups when they were switched to a novel distance. Here the higher performing group was the variable-practice group, suggesting that variable practice is more effective than constant practice for producing a novel movement of the same movement class.

Although findings up to now have been supportive of the variability-of-practice notion, the topic is relatively new. More research is needed to clarify such things as the kinds of tasks and characteristics of learners for which this form of practice is most beneficial. Also, the issue of retention of learning under variable-practice conditions needs further study because the findings up to now are equivocal (Carson and Wiegand 1979).

Explanation for the Effects of Variable Practice

Schema theory specifically predicts that variability of practice will result in enhanced performance of a novel version of the same movement class. Since schema theory has been described in detail in chapter 14, and since the variability of practice and prediction was discussed in the previous section, this will not be repeated. Schema theory specifically addresses this particular practice condition.

As we have previously noted, many of the current ideas about the neurophysiology of motor control and learning are speculative, and no specific theory for explaining variability of practice phenomenon has been attempted by neuroscientists. But given what is known about perceptual, memory, and motor mechanisms in motor control and learning, it would seem intuitively reasonable that the adaptations that occur while practicing a variety of responses for a given movement class will facilitate the generation of a unique movement pattern within that same movement class when necessary.

Summary

Motor learning is dependent upon a variety of conditions, practice being one of the most important. Four of the most obvious effects of practice are increased speed of performance, increased accuracy, increased adaptability, and decreased attentional demands while executing movements.

Instructions before practice typically take the form of verbal instructions and demonstrations. Providing demonstrations and requiring learners to observe models have proven to be particularly effective in enhancing motor learning.

Once practice has begun, skill improvement will be most efficient only if conscientious attempts to improve are made. Mere practice will not produce proficiency; practice with the intention of learning will, and the more one practices, the higher the level of proficiency that will be obtained.

The two basic variables with which practice schedule studies have been concerned are the time of continual practice and the interval between practice trials. In general, distributed practice schedules produce superior performance compared to massed schedules, but there is very little difference in the two schedules with respect to learning. Several theoretical positions have been advanced to explain the differences in performance under massed and distributed schedules.

A substantial literature demonstrates that fatigue induced before performance or interpolated between practice trials hinders performance on a variety of motor tasks. The research results on the effects of fatigue on motor learning are equivocal, but practicing under conditions of severe fatigue does seem to impair motor learning.

It is possible to facilitate the learning of a motor skill by mental practice. Mental practice is effective regardless of when it is done between practices. This form of practice has been found to be effective for novices as well as the highly skilled. Three to five minutes of mental practice at any one time seems to yield the best results.

One prediction of schema theory for motor skill acquisition is that variable practice on a given class of movements will produce better schemata for these movements and will result in better performances on any unique variation of that same class. Research has provided moderate support for variability of practice when male adults have been the learners, while stronger support for variable practice has been generated when children and females have been the learners.

18

Feedback and Motor Behavior

Key Terms and Concepts
Augmented feedback
Closed skills
Concurrent feedback
Feedback
Interresponse interval
Intrinsic feedback
Knowledge of results
Knowledge of performance
KR-delay interval
Open skills
Post-KR-delay interval
Reinforcement
Terminal feedback

We have repeatedly emphasized that numerous factors affect the efficiency of motor skill learning and performance. Certainly one of the most critical of these factors is feedback, and at various points in this volume we have already described some of the ways in which feedback functions in motor control and skill acquisition.

Feedback is the information an individual receives as a result of some response. The positive influence of feedback on learning and performance is one of the best-established findings in motor behavior research literature. The noted British psychologist Sir Frederick Bartlett once said: "It is not practice but practice the results of which are known that makes perfect." Bilodeau and Bilodeau (1961), two of the eminent researchers of this topic, say:

> Studies of feedback . . . show it to be the strongest, most important variable controlling performance and learning. It has been shown repeatedly, that there is no improvement without [feedback], progressive improvement with it, and deterioration after its withdrawal.

Research consistently shows that feedback increases the rate of improvement early on a new task, enhances performance on tasks that are overlearned, and increases the frequency of reports that tasks seem less fatiguing and more interesting with feedback than under conditions in which feedback is withheld. Furthermore, the benefits of feedback apply to a wide variety of tasks.

As noted in previous chapters, motor skill acquisition is essentially the learning of appropriate motor programs that correspond with proper task execution. In this view, the learner first estimates the movement pattern to be performed, executes the movement, and then stores the feedback characteristics of this response in memory. Following the feedback from the response, the learner makes a comparison between the stored representation of the last response and the feedback that was received, then formulates a strategy for the next response. As the feedback comes to match the desired result, the motor program can be employed again with little or no modification—the correct movement response has been learned (Schmidt 1976b).

In previous chapters our emphasis has been on how central and peripheral mechanisms of the nervous system served feedback roles. In this chapter we shall further elaborate on this type of feedback, but give greater attention to the role instructors play in providing feedback.

Research on Feedback for Motor Behavior

Research on the effects of **feedback** on motor learning and performance has employed a wide variety of motor tasks with subjects performing under various conditions. But the vast majority has employed discrete, rather than continuous, tasks and fine, rather than gross, motor skills. The tasks have required subjects to position levers, draw lines, turn knobs, and aim guns. Much of the research on the effects of feedback on motor behavior has been limited to simple, discrete motor responses. Studies using gross motor tasks have been conspicuously few, presumably because of the rigid control necessary when feedback is the critical variable.

Terminology and Feedback

The variety of terms employed in the feedback literature is truly bewildering, and as yet we do not have complete agreement on the terminology appropriate to describe the various aspects of this topic. Feedback terminology and the various modifiers have been classified by several schemes (Holding 1965; Bilodeau 1969; Del Rey 1971). Since the selection of terms is arbitrary, we shall adopt the terminology shown in figure 18.1, except when reporting a specific investigator's research; at that time the researcher's own terminology will be used.

Feedback refers to all of the information one receives during or after a movement. It may be either intrinsic or augmented. **Intrinsic feedback** is information that is supplied to the performer as an inherent consequence of the performance. **Augmented feedback** is the provision of special information that is ordinarily not present in a task; it is extrinsic to the individual and takes the form of either verbal information by an instructor or an external stimulus, such as a machine, that supplements the feedback obtained from the senses. The jump shot can be practiced with only intrinsic feedback, or the performer might receive augmented feedback as a supplement. When learners execute a jump shot, they receive proprioceptive feedback regarding their body movements during the shot. They also see the results of their movements—the ball either goes into the basket or misses in some direction. These are examples of solely intrinsic feedback; all the feedback is inherent in the task. Augmented feedback might be provided by an instructor who can give specific information about why errors in shot direction occurred, or who might simply compliment the learner on a made basket.

Feedback can be supplied while the performer is moving, in which case it is said to be **concurrent feedback.** Or it can be supplied after the performance is completed, in which case it is called **terminal feedback.** One form of intrinsic

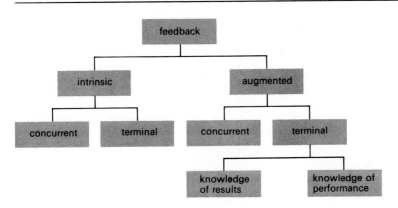

Figure 18.1 *Feedback terminology.*

concurrent feedback is that which the performer receives from the sensory systems during execution. Concurrent augmented feedback can be provided during a tracking task performance by a system of lights or sounds as a constant indication to performers that they are on or off target. Intrinsic terminal feedback is information that individuals receive as a normal consequence of their actions—the ball goes in the basket or the serve goes into the appropriate service area. Augmented terminal feedback can be supplied by some mechanical device, such as a light, that indicates the consequence of the movement, or it can be communicated by an instructor or other observer.

When an instructor gives feedback about the consequences of a movement, such as the extent to which the intended goal was achieved, this is called **knowledge of results** (KR). On the other hand, if the instructor gives feedback concerning the movement pattern itself—the temporal, spatial, sequential, or force aspects of the movement—rather than the outcome of the movement, this is called **knowledge of performance** (KP).

A gymnastics instructor may tell the learner of a particular stunt that the intended goal of the stunt was not accomplished (KR) or explain that certain body segments were employed too early or too late (KP). Obviously, skillful instructors use both KR and KP. Learners need KR to know if the movement execution was successful in attaining the intended goal, and they need KP in order to correct the spatial, temporal, and force

organization of the movements. The effectiveness of using KR and KP in teaching a skill is related to the type of skill (Gentile 1972). More will be said about this in a later section of this chapter.

Intrinsic Feedback and Motor Behavior

Fortunately, many motor tasks supply intrinsic feedback during and immediately after the response is made. Such tasks as kicking a soccer ball or serving a tennis ball provide feedback as a consequence of the actions. When a soccer ball is kicked, it either goes into the goal or misses. Proprioceptive feedback supplies data regarding the body movements that are associated with varying degrees of deviation from the target, and visual feedback provides information about directional deviations. The tennis serve either hits the net, goes out of bounds, or lands in bounds. The learner can feel and see immediately what the consequences of the movements are.

Although the precise roles that the various sensory systems play in providing intrinsic feedback have not been ascertained, there is good evidence that they play a prominent role. Learners commonly receive visual and auditory information about the success of their responses, but they also receive feedback about amount of force applied, locations of limbs, body postures, and pressure exerted via the somatosensory receptors. Two earlier chapters dealt with the role of visual and kinesthetic perception and motor behavior.

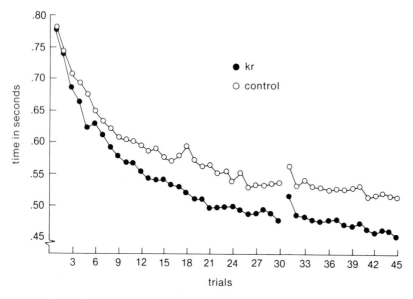

Figure 18.2   *The mean performance times of the knowledge of results and control group plotted as a function of practice.*

Intrinsic feedback is rich and varied during movement. Recent theories of motor learning propose that this form of feedback acts in conjunction with a reference of correctness to produce an error-detection mechanism (a recognition schema) that is acquired as a result of practice (Adams 1971; Schmidt 1976b). It also supplies information about the extent to which the response specifications that were generated actually achieved the intended goal.

Augmented Feedback and Motor Behavior

The first thing to realize about augmented feedback is that many motor tasks can be learned, and even a high proficiency attained, without it. Many of the motor skills we acquire have been learned by trial and error, using only the intrinsic feedback we received from each performance. However, one major difficulty with learning in this way is that it is not very efficient. Learning the same task with a judicious application of augmented feedback often speeds up the learning

rate, making the acquisition of proficiency much more efficient. Moreover, some motor tasks provide intrinsic feedback that is fragmentary and incomplete. An instructor or training aid can serve to provide performers with augmented feedback to enhance performance and learning. With instructors, this typically takes the form of verbalization and demonstrations of instructions. For training aids, videotapes, films, and other mechanical paraphernalia are often used.

In general, both concurrent and terminal augmented feedback have been found to enhance learning and performance. Even if the task itself supplies feedback about the learner's performance, supplemental information frequently enhances learning. The results of one study will be used to illustrate the effects of KR on both performance and learning (figure 18.2). Subjects were required to learn a serial arm movement response. Each subject sat at a table, a finger depressing a response key. When a stimulus light was illuminated, the subject released the response key and made several prescribed arm movements as fast as possible before depressing a key to end the trial. The time elapsed for performing the task was recorded for each trial. One group of subjects received augmented KR throughout the training trials, one through thirty, while a control group did not receive augmented KR during the training trials. Figure 18.2 shows quite clearly that the group receiving augmented KR performed better than the other group. After a rest period, both groups were switched to augmented KR. The original KR group retained its superiority, illustrating that augmented KR is effective for enhancing learning (Stelmach 1970). In another study, Robb (1968) found that learners who received the greatest variety of feedback produced the most efficient learning pattern.

The studies described above may convey the impression that augmented feedback always enhances motor learning and performance, but, in fact, this is not the case. There is some evidence that when sufficient feedback is inherent in the task itself, the use of additional feedback does not further affect the acquisition of skill on the motor task (Bilodeau 1969; Haywood and Glad 1974).

Most studies of KR have dealt with some type of accuracy on a discrete, fine motor task, rather than gross motor skills. But those that have used gross motor tasks generally corroborate the studies done with simpler tasks. Howell (1956) studied the effect of providing feedback to subjects by showing them force-time graphs on their sprint start after each practice trial. Another group of subjects did not receive this information. The first group successfully learned the desired force-time pattern and improved their speed and momentum; the second group made very little improvement. Malina (1969) studied the effects of different KR practice conditions on the speed and accuracy of overhand throwing performance. He reported marked differences in the patterns of throwing performance under the various feedback conditions: Groups receiving speed and speed-and-accuracy KR were superior to a no-KR group on throwing velocity; accuracy and speed-and-accuracy KR groups were superior to the no-KR group on throwing accuracy.

As with fine motor tasks, there have been reports that augmented feedback does not enhance motor learning for certain gross motor tasks. Bell (1968) had subjects practice the badminton long serve under four different conditions. She reported that no differences that could be attributed to the different KR conditions were found between groups. She concluded that "where sufficient knowledge of results is inherent in the task, the direction of practice through the use of additional knowledge of results does not further affect the acquisition or retention of gross motor skill at the beginning levels of performance."

It appears, then, that augmented feedback is a potentially powerful factor for enhancing motor learning and performance. Despite the findings of some studies showing little beneficial effects of this form of feedback, an instructor would be wise to use a variety of augmented feedback techniques. Augmented feedback has been shown to be effective in many studies, and it has not been shown to be detrimental in any studies. Even when it has not been shown to be especially beneficial, only a very limited type of augmented feedback has been employed. So it seems appropriate to employ this form of feedback when possible.

Augmented Feedback for Open and Closed Skills

In chapter 2 it was noted that motor skills can be classified as either open or closed, depending upon the extent to which (1) a performer must conform to a prescribed standard sequence of movement during execution, and (2) effective performance depends upon environmental events. In **closed skills,** environmental conditions are stable or stationary, and the learner is trying to become consistent in producing the most efficient and effective movement. Examples in sports are shot-putting and diving. On the other hand, **open skills** demand the absence of stereotyped movements; there is a variety of responses, each response being a match to a particular set of requirements in the environment. Here a unique movement pattern

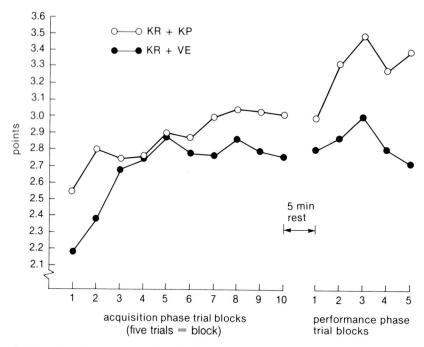

Figure 18.3 *Performance points of both groups over acquisition and performance trial blocks.*

must be constructed for each execution; a different response is required for each situation. In an open skill, no single movement pattern will accomplish the goal in all situations. There is not one single instep kick in soccer, but rather numerous responses, all called the instep kick. Each one is different, depending upon the speed to be imparted and where the ball is meant to go, yet all are called instep kicks.

The instructor may augment information available to the learner by providing KP or KR. As noted previously, KP provides information about the performer's movement patterns, about the spatial, temporal, and force employment of the body's parts. KR provides information about the consequences of the performer's movement, the results or changes in the environment that the performer's movement produced.

Gentile (1972; Gentile et al 1975) suggested that for closed skills, in which environmental conditions are stable or stationary and the learner is trying to become consistent in producing the most efficient movement, KP is the more powerful and appropriate form of augmented information. Further, knowledge of KR is the more appropriate for learning open skills, where a variety of motor patterns is the goal. The limited research on this proposal supports this contention (Del Rey 1971; Wallace and Hagler 1979). Wallace and Hagler had subjects shoot a basketball (a closed skill, since the ball was shot from the same spot on the floor each time) with their nondominant hand. One group was given both KP and KR, while the other group was given KR and verbal encouragement (VE) after each shooting trial. Significant improvement in performance for both groups occurred in the first phase of the study (figure 18.3). In the second phase KP and verbal encouragement were withdrawn. Here the group that had practiced with KP + KR in the first phase showed a significantly higher level of performance, suggesting that KP was a strong feedback source in the acquisition of this closed motor skill.

Cooper and Rothstein (1981) found that a combination of KP and KR is superior to one or the other form of feedback for both open and closed skills. This makes intuitive sense because if learning consists of correcting response selection *and* response execution errors, then feedback information focusing the learner's attention on both has greater potential than either one by itself.

Frequency of Augmented Feedback

How often should augmented feedback be given? Should it be administered after every performance, or intermittently? That is, is the total number of feedbacks in a set of performances (absolute frequency) more important than the proportion of performances on which feedback is given (relative frequency)? Bilodeau and Bilodeau (1958a) compared the performance scores of four groups of subjects that received feedback after every trial, every third, every fourth, or every tenth trial, while performing a positioning task when blindfolded. Performance improved only on the trials immediately following the presentation of KR. When the investigators plotted the error scores for only the responses that followed KR, the responses were almost identical for the four groups—in short, there was no performance improvement during trials without KR. The implication is that it is the absolute frequency, the actual number of KRs provided, that determines performance improvement and that relative frequency is unimportant. In other words, whatever the distribution of KR, non-KR trials neither hinder nor facilitate the proficiency produced by KR trials.

As with many early motor behavior studies, Bilodeau and Bilodeau did not use a transfer design specifically to assess learning effects. So their results focus on performance effects, making conclusions about learning somewhat suspect. Recently, Johnson, Wicks, and Ben-Sira (1981) conducted a similar study employing a transfer design. A transfer test was administered one week after the performance phase of the study. Surprisingly, the group that received KR after every tenth trial performed with the least error, suggesting that subjects in that group had learned the most. KR after every trial was least beneficial for learning. This finding clearly contradicts the Bilodeaus' interpretation of their results.

This latter finding illustrates, again, that learning may be occurring during practice, but that it is not immediately evident through performance scores. Only after a period of rest and after learners are allowed to practice under the same conditions do learning effects become salient.

Some practical applications can be drawn from this information. First, KR is important for improving performance, but as long as there is adequate time to allow the learner to have plenty of practice trials, using KR after every second or third trial might be as effective for learning as providing KR after every trial. Second, providing KR after every trial may produce a dependency that can be debilitating. Third, since in most instructional settings the instructor cannot possibly provide feedback to every student after every practice trial, Johnson, Wicks, and Ben-Sira's findings give some confidence to instructors that no great harm is done if students practice with only intermittent augmented feedback.

Withdrawal of Augmented Feedback

The evidence is rather consistent that when KR is provided during early practice trials and then withdrawn, performance deteriorates in succeeding trials. However, the extent to which this happens differs. The problem is to ascertain whether certain methods of administering KR during learning lead to better-maintained performance than do others in which KR is withdrawn.

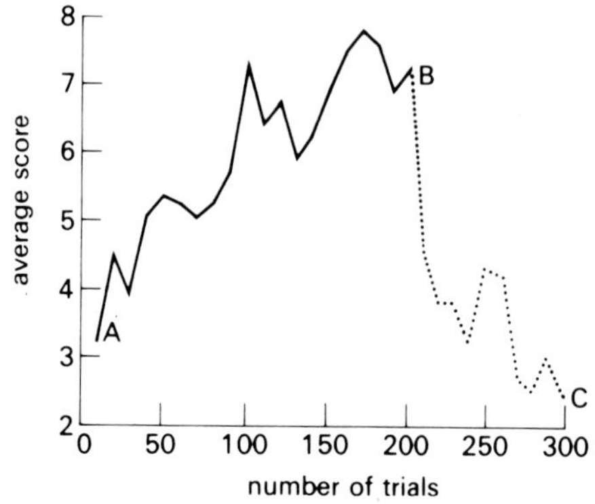

Figure 18.4   *The reduction in performance with withdrawal of knowledge of results. AB is the average curve of performance while subjects received knowledge of results. BC is the average curve after knowledge of results was withdrawn.*

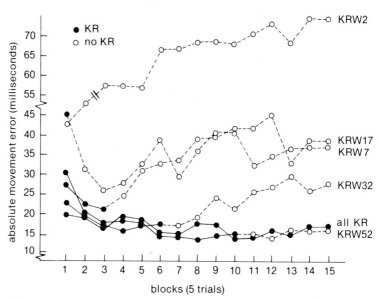

Figure 18.5   *Mean absolute movement error for KR withdrawal conditions over blocks.*

A rather dramatic example of the consequences of removing KR is the now classic study of Elwell and Grindley (1938). They used an apparatus in which subjects employed two levers to direct a spot of light on a target. In the initial stage of the experiment, the light clearly indicated where on the target subjects had landed. In the second phase of the study, KR was removed by switching off the light, so the subjects were unable to see where on the target they had landed. There was an immediate drop in performance (figure 18.4). Moreover, the subjects were annoyed by the change in conditions, they became bored and careless, and even began arriving late for practice sessions. Another frequently cited

study, this one by Bilodeau, Bilodeau, and Schumsky (1959), found progressive improvement with KR, no improvement without KR, and performance deterioration after the withdrawal of KR.

A more recent study of the effects of withdrawing KR was undertaken by Newell (1974). Subjects learned to make a rapid, ballistic arm response in a specific amount of time. They received KR in the form of milliseconds fast or slow. Five groups had KR withdrawn after a given number of trials (two, seven, seventeen, thirty-two, fifty-two trials); one group received KR for all trials. The effects of withdrawing KR at various points are shown in figure 18.5. It is evident that the withdrawal of KR adversely affected performance, and in general the decrement in performance after withdrawal of KR is an inverse function of the number of KR trials. The fewer the KR trials, the greater the performance decrement.

From these results it may be tempting to conclude that KR is important in the early phases of learning a task and unimportant in the later phases. But from a practical standpoint, Newell (1981) warns that "even though the performer can estimate his performance without KR after considerable practice, it would be advisable to ensure that outcome information is always presented to the learner, and/or that the learner always seek to ascertain the outcome of the response if this information is available directly from the environment."

Precision of Augmented Feedback

In general the efficiency of motor learning is directly related to the precision of feedback; the more precise feedback is, the more efficient acquisition of skill will be. Evidence for this statement goes back over fifty years to Trowbridge and Cason's (1932) classic study of the effect of various levels of KR precision on a line drawing task. Their findings were corroborated by Smoll's (1972) study of learning duckpin bowling speed under three levels of KR precision.

Some qualification to the notion that increased precision of feedback is beneficial to learning appears to be appropriate, based on recent research. Some investigators have found little advantage in increasing precision of feedback beyond a certain point. Rogers (1974) found that too precise KR not only was of limited value, but that it may actually inhibit learning in comparison to less precise KR. In another study of the effects of varying KR precision levels on a linear positioning task, Gill (1975) reported that KR precision level (error scores in either centimeters or millimeters) did not affect actual performance. But extremely precise KR had detrimental effects on performance evaluation and the labeling process of estimating performance by the subjects.

These studies suggest that there must be some optimal level of precision beyond which the performer cannot process and translate the information into meaningful performance improvements. From an instructional standpoint, unfortunately, the particular optimal level of precision would have to be obtained for each task. So it appears that the motor skills instructor should employ as much precision as seems reasonable. If this is done, there is little evidence that learning will be greatly deterred.

The most recent trend in the study of the effects of precision of feedback on motor learning has employed a developmental perspective. The fundamental notion is that very precise feedback is less beneficial to young children than to older children or adults. Utilizing a kinesthetic repositioning task, Thomas, Mitchell, and Solmon (1979) found that increasing the precision of feedback resulted in more errors for younger children (grade 2), while older children (grade 4) performed more accurately with more precise KR. Newell and Kennedy (1978) found evidence that the optimum level for precision of KR may be higher for older children. The implication of these findings is that one must be cautious about providing KR to children. Too much precision may overload their information-processing capabilities, or the information may be meaningless and may, therefore, actually be detrimental to learning.

Delay of Feedback

There has been a sustained interest in the effects of delaying feedback on motor behavior since research on feedback began. Because the consequences of delaying concurrent feedback and terminal feedback are so dramatically different, it is essential to treat these two feedback conditions separately.

Figure 18.6   *Various time intervals between responses.*

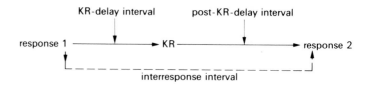

Concurrent Feedback

Some tasks lend themselves to concurrent feedback utilization; others impose limits on the feasibility of concurrent feedback because of the speed and frequency with which they must be made (such as the golf swing). In motor tasks in which intrinsic concurrent feedback can be used in task performance, any delay—even a delay as short as a fraction of a second—seriously hampers or even precludes appropriate execution. The effect of this kind of feedback lag is dramatically illustrated in delayed feedback of speech. In this condition, the average person stutters, slurs words or omits whole syllables, and speaks as if in a state of intoxication (Chase et al. 1961a, 1961b, 1961c). Similar effects have been reported for various types of motor acts.

K. U. Smith and his colleagues (Smith and Smith 1962; Smith 1962) have demonstrated the disastrous effects of delaying concurrent visual feedback on motor activities. Employing complex television camera-videotape arrangements, Smith has modified the visual feedback so that performers see themselves doing things shortly after they are actually done. Time delays as brief as one-fifth of a second produce an entire breakdown of performance. Smith (1962) writes:

Various studies of delayed sensory feedback, both visual and auditory, have produced strikingly similar results. Delays of even a small fraction of a second cause serious disturbances of behavior organization, often accompanied by emotional effects. . . . All evidence indicates that there is little, if any, effective adaptation to conditions of delayed feedback.

Terminal Feedback

As noted above, terminal augmented feedback is information provided the learner after a trial or performance, commonly taking the form of KR or KP. When considering the application of KR, there are three time intervals involved in the time between response 1 and response 2 (figure 18.6). First is the **KR-delay interval**, which is the period following the end of the response until KR is presented to the learner. Second, the time interval that follows the presentation of KR until the learner must make the next response is called the **post-KR-delay interval.** The third interval is the total amount of time from the end of one response to the next response. Called the **interresponse interval** (IRI), it incorporates the first two intervals.[1]

KR can be delivered immediately after a movement is completed, or it can be delayed; after KR has been given the next movement can be executed immediately, or it can be delayed. A basic question for investigators has been how varying these two periods and/or the interresponse interval affects motor behavior.

In addition to the question of the effects of simple delay of KR on motor behavior, there is also the issue of introducing into either the KR-delay interval and/or the post-KR period some intervening (usually called interpolated) task for the learner to perform. The question at issue is whether the interpolated task performed during one or both of the delay intervals influences motor behavior.

---

[1] The emphasis in this section will be on KR rather than KP because most research on delay of feedback has involved KR. The reason is that motor performance outcomes can be more readily measured and can be delivered more accurately than KP.

The KR-Delay Interval

The KR-delay interval has more often been studied over the years, but the results of this research have led to some confusion about the consequences of this type of feedback delay on human learning. There are two main reasons for this confusion: First, results of studies with lower animals have been generalized to humans. Second, there has been a mixing of results for studies in which there was no interpolated task and results of studies in which there was such a task.

Many years ago, studies with animals clearly established the fact that delay of feedback produces learning decrements (Hamilton 1929; Roberts 1930). But the classic study by Lorge and Thorndike (1935) called into question the application of animal results for humans, since delaying KR did not deter learning. Subjects performed a ball-tossing task at a target that they could not see. KR was given immediately or delayed. The results showed that delays of KR up to six seconds did not affect improvements in performance.

The Lorge and Thorndike study triggered an ongoing controversy that is still active today. In terms of sheer numbers of studies supporting one side or the other, the research is overwhelmingly in support of Lorge and Thorndike's original finding—that the mere delay of KR does not adversely affect human motor learning (see Bilodeau 1969 for a review). Perhaps Bilodeau and Bilodeau's (1958b) research provides the most convincing evidence that merely delaying feedback during the KR-delay interval does not deter learning. Five studies were undertaken, each one providing KR delay. (One used a one-week KR-delay interval!) The studies failed to show that KR-delay had any effect on the learning of the skills. In a review of delay of KR studies, Bilodeau and Bilodeau (1961) said that "to delay or to give immediate KR can be quite immaterial for learning to make relatively simple Rs [responses] when the periods between Rs are relatively free of specially interpolated Rs."

A major problem with this early research is that transfer designs were not used to assess the relative amount of learning for the various KR-delay groups. But in a recent study, in which a transfer design was employed, the investigators found no evidence that KR-delay was relevant in learning the task (Schmidt and Shea 1976), thus corroborating Lorge and Thorndike's original study.

The evidence is not completely unequivocal (see Simmons and Snyder 1980 for a recent report that longer KR-delay intervals produced greater errors than shorter KR-delay intervals). But the evidence strongly supports the conclusion that KR-delay alone does not affect the learning of motor tasks. However, despite the fact that delaying KR has not been found detrimental to rate of skill acquisition, it would seem wise for instructors to provide KR as soon after the completion of a performance as possible. From an instructional standpoint, there is no compelling reason for delaying feedback. The principle that information about the correctness of performance should be provided quickly has been used successfully in teaching a wide variety of verbal and motor tasks. It appears that KR should be provided as soon as possible after a response is completed, but, if a delay must occur, the instructor need not be overly concerned because the delay will not have disastrous results.

From a theoretical viewpoint, the consolidation memory theory would suggest that the unfilled KR interval would not adversely affect, and may enhance, learning because the short-term trace of the response could be well maintained. Thus, from what has been said about short-term memory, we should expect lapse of time, as such, to have either no effect or an enhancing effect.

Studies concerned with the effects of interpolated activity on the KR-delay period are not numerous, and the findings do not lead to definitive conclusions. Research on this subject has used two basic interpolated activities: In the first, the interpolated activity is some kind of verbal or motor task performed during the KR-delay interval. In the second, KR is given a number of *trials* after the response to which it actually refers. For example, a one-trial delay is: response 1, response 2, KR for response 1, response 3, KR for response 2. . . .

Boulter (1964) found that the interpolation of a motor task, a verbal task, or a combination of these in the KR-delay interval, while subjects were attempting to learn a positioning task, did not interfere with skill acquisition. On the other hand, Shea and Upton (1976) had subjects learn two positions on a linear positioning task, with one group performing interpolated positioning movements (not the same ones as they were attempting to learn) during the KR-delay interval, while a second group that was learning the same positions merely rested during the KR-delay interval. Figure 18.7 shows the results of their study. The performance curves on the left side of the figure indicate quite clearly that the interpolated activity had a negative influence on performance. The curves on the right side display the measures on a transfer test of twelve trials during which KR was not given to either group. The curves indicate that the interpolated activity also interfered with learning the task.

Shea and Upton (1976) interpret the differences between their findings and previous research as follows:

Failure of previous studies . . . to find interference effects of interpolated resonses during the KR-delay interval on skill acquisition might have been due to the failure to require the subjects to remember the interpolated responses. The interpolated responses may not have been stored in memory and thus would not have been expected to interfere with the stored representation of the subjects' last estimate of the criterion position.

The evidence is not overwhelming. But with regard to the practical implications of requiring verbal or motor activities during the KR-delay interval, the evidence suggests that this period should be kept free of these types of activities if

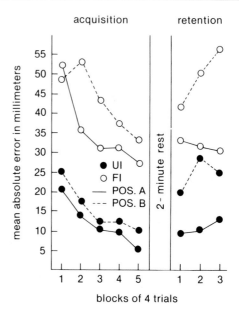

Figure 18.7 *Mean absolute error scores computed over trial blocks for acquisition (KR trials) and retention trials (no KR trials). (UI=unfilled interval, FI=filled interval.)*

possible. They have the potential for retarding performance and skill acquisition. From a theoretical viewpoint, it would seem that intervening activities and the shifts in attention that accompany them would be disruptive to short-term memory processes. If they are, long-term memory will not be formed.

KR given one or more trials after the response to which it actually refers is called the trials-delay procedure. Lorge and Thorndike (1935) and Bilodeau (1956) reported that when KR was given following the response to which it referred, it produced decrements in performance. The Lorge and Thorndike subjects tossed balls at a target they could not see and received KR after an interval filled by another throw that referred back to the previous throw. Bilodeau (1956) studied the effect of delay of knowledge of results in an experiment in which additional responses had to be made during the delay. For example, in a two-trial delay condition, knowledge of results of the first trial was given only after the third trial had been completed, knowledge of results of the second trial were given after the fourth trial was completed, and so on. She reported that with one-, two-, three-, or five-trial delays, level of accuracy achieved with thirty KR trials decreased with the number of trials by which KR was delayed.

This basic finding has been replicated for performance, but when a transfer design has been employed (which Lorge and Thorndike and Bilodeau did not use) to assess the relative amount of learning, the results have been surprising. Lavery (1964) and Lavery and Suddon (1962) reported performance results very similar to previous results. However, when they administered a series of transfer trials in which no KR was provided, the differences in the groups disappeared. In fact, the groups that had practiced under the trials-delay condition were slightly better than the group that had not experienced the trials-delay condition.

From a theoretical standpoint, the trials-delay procedure would appear to disrupt learning mostly through the information confusion that it creates by having KR for a prior movement presented at the time the STM processes are active for the just completed movement. That the brain can make use of this form of feedback illustrates the marvelous capabilities of the brain.

The Post-KR-Delay Interval

The theoretical significance of the post-KR delay interval is that it is primarily during this period that the learner presumably makes a comparison between the stored representation of the just completed movement and the KR just received. Then the learner formulates a strategy for the next response. In the view of current motor program theories, the learner uses KR to compare it with centrally stored representations of both previous sensory feedback and KR to update the recall and recognition memories (Schmidt 1976b).

The post-KR-delay interval has not attracted the degree of research interest that the KR-delay interval has. In general, however, the limited research suggests that the various lengths of unfilled post-KR-delay intervals have little effect on motor learning, provided that they are not extremely short (less than a second or two) or long (days or weeks).

Since the learner needs time to process KR and incorporate it into a plan for new response strategies for future movement execution, it has been proposed that there is an optimal post-KR period. According to this view, if the post-KR-delay interval is too short, the necessary processing and planning do not occur; if too long, forgetting results. Adams (1971) states that "increasing the post-KR interval up to a point will improve performance." Although this notion is intuitively and theoretically appealing, there is little empirical evidence to support it.

It does appear that if the post-KR-delay interval is extremely short, such as less than a second or two, performance is hampered. This interval was varied at one, five, ten and twenty seconds by Weinberg, Guy, and Tupper (1964) with subjects who were learning a positioning task. The one-second interval resulted in the least accurate performances, while the other intervals produced about equal accuracies. Similar effects were reported for children by Gallagher and Thomas (1980). The younger the children, the more detrimental were short post-KR-delay intervals. When children are allowed to choose their own post-KR intervals, they chose intervals of two or three seconds (Barclay and Newell 1980).

There appears to be little need for the motor skills instructor to be overly concerned about post-KR-delay interval, provided its duration is neither less than a second or two nor extremely long (days or weeks), and provided it is not filled with interpolated tasks. We turn to this latter issue now.

Research of the effects of post-KR intervals that are filled with interpolated verbal or motor activities has produced equivocal results; at present no firm conclusions may be made. Several investigators have reported that post-KR activity adversely affects motor performance, but others have found interpolated tasks to have no affect on performance. Boucher (1974) reported that the pronunciation of difficult multisyllabic words during the post-KR-delay interval adversely affected motor performance early in practice but not later in practice. Magill (1973; 1977) reported results indicating no effect on performance when the verbal activity was counting backward.

In the post-KR interval, the learner is assumed to process the information by developing new strategies and hypotheses about the nature of the task and how to accomplish it, resulting in the selection of appropriate motor programs. In relation to consolidation memory theory, an unfilled period should facilitate consolidation, provided that the period is not too brief for neural processing. An interval with interpolated activity should disrupt short-term neural processing. But there is some evidence that motor short-term memory processing may be somewhat different from verbal short-term processing, since several investigators have found kinesthetic-distance forgetting to be unrelated to interpolated activity (this issue is discussed in detail in chapter 14).

Given the incomplete nature of the research at this time, it seems intuitively clear that learners need time to process KR and to generate appropriate new responses (assuming previous responses were not perfect). Thus it seems appropriate for the instructor to try to provide an uninterrupted period during the post-KR interval.

The Interresponse Interval

The interresponse interval (IRI) has typically not been held constant in the studies of KR-delay and post-KR-delay. This lack of consistency may account for much of the equivocal nature of the findings in the KR-delay research. However, the

findings with respect to the effects of the IRI itself on motor skill acquisition are also equivocal. Bilodeau and Bilodeau (1958b), on the basis of the results of two of their studies, suggested that the IRI is the critical variable for learning motor skills and that the KR-delay and post-KR-delay intervals had little or no effect on motor learning. More recent research by Magill (1973; 1977) and Shea (1975) does not support the importance of the IRI in learning.

The issue of the effects of IRI on motor behavior is, of course, related to the issue of retention of motor skills. Both consolidation memory theory and recent motor learning theories consider that the strength of a motor program for response execution is dependent upon the IRI. According to the latter, the internal standard of correct movement is weakened through forgetting during the IRI, causing a performance decrement. From a consolidation memory theory standpoint, decay of neural mechanisms that constitute long-term memory has the same consequence.

It appears that the motor skills instructor need not be overly concerned about adversely affecting motor learning, provided that the IRIs are not too short, which might produce the performance decrements described for massed practice, or too long, which might produce memory loss.

Modes of Augmented Feedback

Augmented feedback can be presented to learners through a variety of modes, but the most desirable type of augmented feedback for motor tasks remains to be identified. Aside from the work on KR and KP for open and closed skills, there is virtually no other research to provide guidelines. Still, the most appropriate form of feedback is an important question since there may be a great deal of variance in the consequences of different types of augmented feedback.

Table 18.1   *Types of augmented feedback*

Form
Auditory augmented feedback
  Feedback provided orally
Auditory-tactile feedback
  Feedback provided orally and by manual assistance
Auditory-visual feedback
  Feedback provided orally and by teacher demonstration
	Explicative feedback
	  Feedback intended to provide an interpretation or explanation of the performance of a motor skill
	Prescriptive feedback
	  Feedback intended to provide instructions for the subsequent performance of a motor skill
	Affective feedback
	  Feedback intended to provide an attitudinal or motivational set toward the performance of a motor skill

Direction
A single student
  Feedback directed to only one student, although it may be seen or heard by other students in the class
A group of students
  Feedback directed to more than one student, although it may be seen or heard by all students in the class
All students in the class
  Feedback directed to the entire class
	General referent
	The whole movement
	  Feedback provided about multiple components in the performance of a motor skill
	Part of the movement
	  Feedback provided about one component other than the outcome or goal of the performance of a motor skill
	Outcome or goal of the movement
	  Feedback provided about the result of the performance of a motor skill

Time
Concurrent feedback
  Feedback provided during the performance of a motor skill
Terminal feedback
  Feedback provided some time after the performance of a motor skill
	Specific referent
	Rate
	  Feedback provided about the time or duration of the movement involved in the performance of a motor skill
	Force
	  Feedback provided about the strength or power expended in the performance of a motor skill

Intent
Evaluative feedback
  Feedback intended to provide an appraisal of the performance of a motor skill
Descriptive feedback
  Feedback intended to provide an account of the performance of a motor skill
Comparative feedback
  Feedback intended to provide an analogy related to the performance of a motor skill
	Space
	  Feedback provided about the direction, level or magnitude of the movement involved in the performance of a motor skill

Source: Based on Fishman 1974.

One of the most complete lists of augmented feedback classifications was developed by Sylvia Fishman (1974) and is shown in table 18.1. This nicely illustrates the numerous ways in which augmented feedback can be delivered.

In addition to the most common form of feedback—verbal—other forms of augmented feedback that have been studied are the use of videotape replays and kinematic or kinetic movement feedback. The use of videotape replays would seem to be particularly useful since the replay is available very shortly after the performance and provides a vivid and accurate form of information of the movement itself and perhaps the outcome as well. Unfortunately, for all of the apparent appeal of videotape, there is little evidence that this technique of providing feedback is very effective. Recent research on this topic indicates that the effectiveness of videotapes for feedback is very disappointing (Rothstein and Arnold 1976; Rikli and Smith 1980).

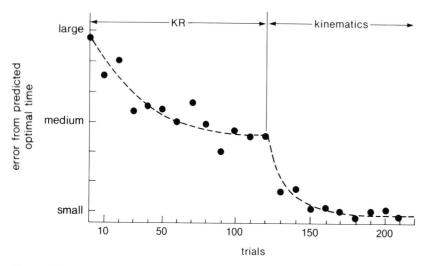

Figure 18.8   Timing error from predicted optimum for leg raise as a function of form of feedback over trials.

Studies in which learners are cued to examine specific aspects of a movement during replay consistently produce the most positive effects, suggesting that if an instructor uses videotape replay the learner should be cued to focus on only a few relevant dimensions of the execution (for example, arms or legs) and ignore the less relevant aspects of the response. As learning progresses, and form or style becomes more important, such as in preparing for competition in gymnastics or ice skating, the student may be encouraged to focus on the entire movement sequence.

Little use has been made of kinetics of the movement (the patterns of forces that were applied) or the kinematics (relations between displacement, velocity, and acceleration) of the movement. But the few studies that have been reported using these techniques as feedback show promising results. Howell (1956) provided feedback to subjects who were learning the runner's sprint start by showing them force-time graphs after each trial. Learners were able to modify their force-time patterns so as to achieve a criterion that the investigator imposed.

A study by Hatze (1976) illustrates the potential of kinematic information as feedback. The subject learned to lift the right leg through a specific range of movement as rapidly as possible. In the first phase of the study, KR in the form of time to complete the movement was given. At the point where little improvement was occurring, the investigator showed the subject a time-velocity curve of performance in conjunction with a derived time-velocity model of optimal performance. This resulted in a rapid reduction in movement time, approaching the optimum for the subject (figure 18.8). This shows the potential value of using kinematic information as a feedback mode.

Functions of Feedback

While the evidence is quite clear that learners need feedback about their responses to assist their acquisition of a motor skill, one major issue is not so obvious concerning the role of feedback in learning and performance: What exactly is the function of feedback? Ammons (1956) was one of the first psychologists to identify and discuss the three functions that feedback can serve: information, motivation, and reinforcement. According to this view, feedback may inform individuals about what they should or should not do, or be doing; it may motivate individuals; and it may reward individuals for correct performance or punish them for incorrect performance.

Although feedback can certainly serve these three functions, it is practically impossible to establish exactly how and why feedback is working—whether the main effects are informational, motivational, or reinforcing. The nature of the interaction of these variables is not clearly known and few investigators have thrown any significant light on the problem.

Information Function

The informational function of feedback is given a prominent place in current motor program theories (Adams 1971; Schmidt 1976b) because the feedback derived from the movement is viewed as the critical information source enabling the learner to abstract the relationship between the response and its outcome. It is the abstracting of these relationships that enables the learner to decide what response modifications are needed to improve performance on the next response. Feedback, from this standpoint, is primarily a source of information, which results in corrections that eventually lead the learner to the correct response. Advocates of the information function of feedback do not insist that feedback is not used as reinforcement or motivation, but they assert these are not the primary functions served in human learning. In chapter 14 four functions of feedback described by Keele (1973) were discussed. Since these functions are all basically informational, the reader is urged to review these at this time.

Motivation Function

Many types of feedback can serve both informational and motivational functions. The manner in which feedback functions to motivate learners is quite complicated. Any type of feedback that serves a cueing function may indirectly affect motivation, but the converse is not necessarily true. Some types of feedback could not be used to correct errors or to improve one's method of performing a task. Examples of ways of providing feedback that do not give the learner information about a better *method* of performing are total time-on-target scores on a pursuit task, total score on some task after several trials, and total score after several throws on a target-throwing task (Locke 1967). Any effects on performances from these types of feedback can be attributed to motivational factors since, presumably, only the learner's level of effort is affected.

Smode (1958) hypothesized that a higher feedback-of-information schedule would produce superior performance than a lower information-feedback schedule due to motivational effects. He found that high information feedback facilitated performance and that interest level increased as a function of increased information feedback. He concluded that "the effect of the higher information feedback was mediated by an increase in motivation."

Gibbs and Brown (1955) attempted to isolate and measure the purely motivational function of KR. Their subjects worked at an extremely dull and repetitive task (copying pages from difficult scientific reports, encyclopedias, and historical reviews). In the experiment, KR was casual and incidental. In half the trials, subjects could see a counter that tallied each page as it was copied. In half the trials the counter was covered; the subjects were given no incentives or rewards for the work completed. Nevertheless, the findings showed that when the subjects could see the counter, their output was significantly higher than it was when the counter was covered.

Undoubtedly, feedback functions as an incentive and aids performance, even after a task has been well learned. It has been found that if two well-trained groups perform a task, with one group receiving KR and the other group not receiving KR, the group receiving KR will consistently give the better performance.

The way in which feedback exerts its motivational effects is not yet fully understood. One suggestion is that certain types of feedback affect the goal the performers set for themselves; it may motivate the learners to try harder and persist longer at the task (Locke 1967; Locke, Cartledge, and Koeppel 1968).

An increase in arousal state, which is one aspect of motivation, may also mediate the effects of feedback on motor behavior. Arousal states have been found to be related to performance and learning; up to a point, increases in arousal results in increased learning and performance. Why this is so is not clear. A moderate level of arousal presumably strengthens the consolidation process for long-term memory and perhaps strengthens the memories already there. This topic will be discussed more fully in chapter 20.

Reinforcement Function

In the **reinforcement** view, feedback is rewarding or punishing, and a rewarding result preserves the behavior that preceded it (Skinner 1969). Obviously, reinforcement can be intrinsic or augmented. The satisfaction of seeing the basketball go into the basket, the feel of the baseball against the bat, and the feel of a solid tackle all provide intrinsic feedback to the learner. When a movement pattern is executed, two stimulus events occur in close temporal proximity. First, we experience (feel, see, hear) what our bodies have just done, and then we experience either satisfaction or dissatisfaction with the performance. Since the two stimulus events are paired in rapid succession, we have the basic reinforcement paradigm, in that the feedback of a pattern of stimuli becomes conditioned to an emotional reaction of satisfaction or dissatisfaction. Put another way, feedback indicating that one's performance matches personal goals sustains effort by producing feelings of self-satisfaction about the achievement, thus raising goals for subsequent performance.

As with the motivational function of feedback, it has been suggested that reinforcements may stimulate the arousal system and thus lead to a higher level of firing in appropriate cells. It is assumed that the more often the appropriate neurons are fired, the more robust the memory trace.

Augmented feedback as reinforcement can come in the form of rewards or punishment. Rewards may be verbal praise or some material gift. Punishment may take the form of verbal reproof or physical chastisement. (Some writers refer to rewards as positive reinforcement and punishment as negative reinforcement.)

Experiments comparing rewards and punishment as feedback generally show rewards to be more effective for learning and performance. (However, punishment has been one of the more widely used feedback techniques.) Studies by numerous investigators show that, with humans, punishment frequently has unpredictable and varied consequences, and is generally not nearly as effective as rewards. Of course, in some cases punishment is effective as feedback. A person touching a burning match is not likely to repeat that behavior. A badminton player hitting a clear shot too short and having it smashed back is likely to stop this behavior and attempt to hit the next clear shot deep to the opponent's baseline.

It has been suggested that in instructional situations punishment says "Stop doing what you did," but it does not indicate what should have been done. Punishment may merely suppress the behavior without reducing the strength of the drive that gave rise to it. For undesirable behavior to be eliminated, appropriate alternative behavior must be taught and rewarded. One additional weakness of punishment in instructional situations is that interpersonal conflicts between instructor and student may arise, causing emotional stress and reduction in learning and performance efficiency.

Shaping Behavior and Reinforcement

Many times in the early phases of learning the ultimate goal may be a long way from present performance levels. If the goal is the only criterion used to obtain reward, the behavior leading to it may be impossible for the present—and no reward occurs. What is required is a systematic application of reinforcement contingencies to gradually shape the behavior toward the ultimate goal. In the shaping procedure subgoals are established, and reaching them elicits rewards. At the same time instructions are provided to the learner as to what to do.

Schedules of Reinforcement

The basketball player does not make a basket with every shot, nor does the batter hit the ball with every swing. Reinforcement in dynamic motor tasks does not occur every time. Does it make any difference how frequently reinforcement is given to the learner? A very similar topic was discussed earlier in this chapter under the heading "Frequency of Augmented Feedback."

Generally, but depending upon the task, schedules of partial reinforcement[2] with both animals and humans produce slower rates of learning, but learning continues long after reinforcement stops. Also, a task learned under partial reinforcement is more resistant to extinction.[3]

---

[2] The two basic partial reinforcement schedules employed in the laboratory are interval and ratio schedules. In the first, the subject is given reinforcement after specific time intervals. The time intervals can be fixed (constant) or varied. In a ratio schedule, subjects are given reinforcement after making a certain number of responses. Here, too, the ratio can be fixed or variable.

[3] Extinction is the gradual diminution in magnitude or rate of a response upon withdrawal of the reinforcement.

The Instructor as a Movement Diagnostician and Prescription Expert

It should be obvious from information presented in this and the previous chapter that practice and repetition without feedback are very ineffectual. One of the critical tasks of an instructor of human movement is to make the learning of motor skills more efficient than trial-and-error or learn-by-yourself approaches. To do this, the instructor needs to be a movement diagnostician and a manipulator of feedback. First it is essential to be able to diagnose which are the correct and the incorrect movements learners are making. Then it is necessary to provide feedback to learners in the form of movement prescriptions so as to enhance the correct response and eliminate the incorrect responses. The better instructors are at accomplishing these tasks, the more effective they are as teachers since efficient and effective learning and performance are the outcomes.

Summary

Feedback is the information an individual receives as a result of some response, and the positive influence of feedback on learning and performance is one of the best established findings in motor behavior research. Feedback can be concurrent or terminal and intrinsic or augmented. Feedback by an instructor about the consequences of a movement is called knowledge of results (KR), while feedback concerning the movement pattern itself is called knowledge of performance (KP).

Since many motor tasks supply intrinsic feedback during or after a movement, this form of feedback is a rich and varied source of movement information. Both concurrent and augmented feedback have been found to enhance motor learning and performance. KP appears to be more effective with closed skills and KR more effective with open skills.

KR and KP should be supplied to learners as frequently as possible to enhance learning. But in cases where this is not possible, no great harm is done if only intermittent KR and KP are given. The complete withdrawal of feedback will produce a deterioration in performance and learning. In general, the efficiency of motor learning is directly related to the precision of feedback, but extremely precise feedback may be meaningless and actually detrimental to learning.

Delays of even a fraction of a second seriously degrade intrinsic concurrent feedback, but delaying KR during the KR-delay interval is not detrimental to motor learning. However, if interpolated activities must be performed during this period, learning may be adversely affected. The post-KR-delay interval is the period when the learner is presumably comparing the stored representation of the just completed movement and the feedback just received, so it would seem to be an important interval. Research suggests that the lengths of unfilled post-KR-delay intervals have little effect on motor learning, provided they are not shorter than a second or two or extremely long. The same principle appears to hold for interresponse intervals.

Feedback can be provided in a variety of ways. Research on the effectiveness of videotape for feedback is very disappointing. The use of kinetic and kinematic feedback appears to have good potential for enhancing motor learning.

The three main functions that feedback can serve are information, motivation, and reinforcement. These three functions are interrelated.

19

Transfer of Motor Learning

*W*hen an individual has learned some particular skill, the capability acquired by that learning can affect to some extent the subsequent learning of that individual. The effects of the original learning are said to "transfer" to subsequent activities. **Transfer of learning** refers to the effects of learning one skill on prior or future learning. The effect that learning to play tennis has on learning to play badminton would be considered a case of transfer of learning.

Transfer of learning plays an important role in a wide variety of human behaviors. Our society assumes that school experiences will have transfer value for out-of-school activities. It is an article of faith that skills learned in school will transfer to the occupational world. A basic belief of many instructors of motor skills is that movement patterns learned for one task will transfer to other tasks, that is, will facilitate learning similar tasks. Many teachers of motor skills take transfer of learning for granted. For example, general coordination or agility exercises are frequently used by physical educators and coaches with the expectation that practice of these movement patterns will transfer to improved performance and learning of specific sports skills.

In view of the fact that instructors of motor activities desire and expect their programs to promote transfer of learning, it is essential that instructors in these programs understand the conditions that govern transfer of learning. Directors of motor skill learning can inhibit or enhance students' acquisition of skills, depending on their knowledge and use of transfer of learning research findings. This chapter examines the various conditions that affect transfer of learning.

The Study of Transfer of Learning

Experimentation on transfer of motor tasks has been conducted primarily in research laboratories and has been limited primarily to fine motor tasks. Most of the studies investigating motor skill transfer have used the same fine motor tasks (such as rotary-pursuit, tracking apparatus, and mirror tracing) that have been used for practice and feedback studies. Relatively few studies involving transfer effects on gross motor skills have been undertaken.

Transfer of Learning Concepts

Transfer of learning can be positive, negative, or absent. The influence of learning a task may be such that the learning of that task facilitates the learning of a second task; this is called positive transfer. Positive transfer of learning means that individuals are able to learn a second task more readily than they could prior to learning the original task. When the learning of one task impairs or inhibits learning a second task, this is called negative transfer; individuals are able to learn something less readily than they could prior to the original learning. If the learning of one task has no measurable influence on learning a second task, zero transfer is said to have occurred.

Both positive and negative transfer can exist in components of a complex motor task, and the net transfer will be a function of the relative amounts of positive and negative transfer from the components to the entire task. Mixed transfer effects might occur, for example, by learning to play baseball after having learned to play softball. Basic movement patterns developed for positioning to catch and throw the ball and other components of the task of playing the game would probably show positive transfer, but batting the ball and actually fielding and throwing the ball may show negative transfer initially because of the differences in the size of the ball and the distances of the pitcher and the bases.

Transfer Experimental Designs

Many experimental designs have been used to study and measure transfer, and it is beyond the scope of this book to discuss all of them. The two basic designs are called "proactive" and "retroactive" designs. They can be illustrated as follows:

Proactive design

Experimental group:	Learns task 1	Learns task 2
Control group:	Rests	Learns task 2

In this situation, the experimental group learns task 1, while the control group is given no special training, so it is said to rest. Then both groups learn task 2. This type of design is called a proactive transfer design, meaning transfer effects that are the result of previous experience. Thus, if learning task 1 facilitates the learning of task 2, proactive facilitation, or positive transfer, is said to have occurred. But if learning task 1 inhibits learning task 2, proactive interference, or negative transfer, is said to have occurred. If both groups learn task 2 at equal rates, this represents zero transfer.

Retroactive design

Experimental group:		
Learn task 1	Learn task 2	Test task 1
Control group:		
Learn task 1	Rest	Test task 1

In this design, both groups learn task 1; then the experimental group learns task 2, but the control group does not. Both groups are then tested on task 1. This type of design is called a retroactive design because task 2 may have a retroactive effect on task 1. If learning task 2 enhances the performance on task 1, there is retroactive facilitation, or positive transfer. If performance on task 1 is inhibited, retroactive interference, or negative transfer, has occurred.

Transfer Measures

A number of transfer formulae have been developed to ascertain the amount and direction of transfer that occurs in a given experiment. The amount of transfer of learning is often expressed as a percentage of transfer. One percentage-of-transfer formula is as follows:

$$\text{Percentage of Transfer} = \frac{E - C}{E + C} \times 100,$$

where E represents the mean average performance of the experimental group on the transfer task and C represents the mean performance of the control group on the transfer task. The maximum amount of positive transfer that can be obtained is 100 percent, and the maximum amount of negative transfer is -100 percent.

This formula is appropriate if the measure of performance is such that the larger the value of the measure, the better the performance. For example, if the measure of performance is the number of correct responses, then the formula is appropriate because the number of correct responses becomes larger with better performance.

This transfer formula can be illustrated as follows: If we employ a group that practices a left-hand task for a given amount of time and then is tested on a right-hand task, and a control group that is tested on the right-hand task without practicing the left-hand task, we can obtain a percentage of transfer score. Assume that the experimental group (E) averages a score of 25 on the right-hand task, while the control group (C) averages 15. Applying the formula, we obtain:

$$\frac{25 - 15}{25 + 15} \times 100 = \frac{10}{40} \times 100 = 25\% \text{ transfer}$$

The E group shows 25 percent transfer from the left-hand task to the right-hand task.

This formula must be modified by reversing the positions of the experimental and control group scores in the formula if the measure of performance is such that the smaller the value of the measure, the better the performance. The formula must be modified to read:

$$\text{Percentage of Transfer} = \frac{C - E}{E + C} \times 100.$$

This formula is appropriate with measures such as errors, trials to reach some criterion, or time. As errors, trials, or time are reduced in value, performance improves.

A less popular method of measuring transfer is the savings method. With this technique, the number of trials the experimental group uses to reach an equivalent level of proficiency with the control group on a motor task is counted. If the experimental group requires fewer trials than the control group, it is said that learning the task that the control group did not learn (such as task 1 in the proactive design above) produced a savings. Thus, if a control group has reached a certain level of performance after twenty trials on task 2, and the experimental group, having learned task 1, reaches this level of performance on task 2 after ten trials, this means that ten trials on task 2 were saved by learning task 1.

The measurement of transfer of learning is plagued by the problem that the various formulae that can be used do not yield identical results. So the importance of knowing which transfer formula was used in a given study becomes obvious, especially if one wishes to compare the magnitude and direction of transfer obtained in different studies. Moreover, several variables might affect the transfer results, such as conditions under which the subjects were tested.

Transfer and Similarity

We employ two basic approaches to explaining transfer of learning. The first is called the task similarity hypothesis and the second the general factors hypothesis. The former will be examined in this section. The general factors view will be discussed in the next section.

A basic notion in transfer of learning is that the amount of transfer depends upon the similarity between two tasks. This principle of task similarity is an outgrowth of Thorndike's (1903) "identical elements" theory of transfer. One of the first theories of transfer, it was formulated as a response to the theory of formal discipline.

Figure 19.1 *Effects of task similarity on transfer. When tasks 1 and 2 are identical or highly similar, performance on task 2 is facilitated. When the tasks have opposite stimulus-response elements, performance on task 2 is hindered. When the tasks are completely dissimilar, performance on task 2 is unaffected.*

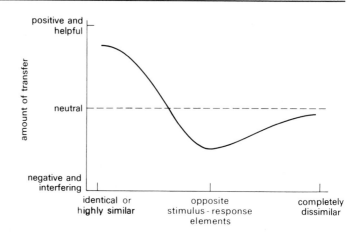

Thorndike said, "A change in one function alters any other only insofar as the two functions have as factors identical elements." His **identical elements theory** proposed that transfer of learning occurs to the extent that identical components exist in the two specific tasks. If learning a given task is effective in producing improvement in learning efficiency in a second task, it is because the components, or elements, of the specific tasks are identical.

A rough guide for describing the effects of task similarity on transfer of learning was proposed by Robinson (1927) as a way of making the identical elements theory more operational (figure 19.1). In essence, this idea proposes: As responses become increasingly dissimilar for similar task stimuli, the transfer effects shift from positive to negative. Positive transfer occurs when the successive responses learned to identical or similar stimuli are associatively related, and negative transfer results when new, unrelated responses to old stimuli are learned.

One of the persistent problems of Thorndike's notion of identical elements is that it is difficult to ascertain whether *identical elements* refers to the simplest components of a whole or to the general "set" toward the task.

Transfer and Similarity for Motor Learning

The evidence that has accumulated over the past fifty years suggests rather clearly that, in general, when responses to identical task stimuli are required, positive transfer occurs; on the other hand, learning different or incompatible responses to identical stimuli usually results in initial negative transfer. When different responses are required for different stimuli, there is usually little or no transfer. These findings are congruent with the work described in chapter 16 dealing with the issue of specificity of motor learning. As you recall, there is strong support in the motor skills literature for the idea that learning motor skills is not based on a few general motor abilities. Rather, it is based upon the possession of specific motor abilities that are related to the demands of a particular task.

Motor skill transfer studies have been concerned with transfer of learning from one task to another, such as from tennis to badminton, as well as from one variation of a task to another variation of the same task. The first is often called intertask transfer; the second, intratask transfer.

Intertask Transfer

Studies of motor skill transfer from one task to another are not numerous, but they do consistently support the notion that there is little **intertask transfer.** Motor task studies in which the stimulus and response variables are quite different between tasks confirm the expectation that little transfer takes place. Nelson (1957) investigated the transfer effect of swimming upon learning and performance of two gross motor skills (volleyball tap for accuracy and high-hurdle skill). He attempted to determine whether swimming while learning other gross motor skills results in transfer. He found no transfer effect from swimming to the other skills. Lindeburg (1949) measured the transfer effect of practicing table tennis and "quickening exercises" (tasks requiring rapid action and decision making) upon reaction time and peg-shifting (moving pegs from one location on a board to another as quickly as possible). He found no transfer of learning from the table tennis and quickening exercises to reaction time or peg-shifting. He concluded that quickening exercises that involve many rapid, skillful movements do not improve performance on other motor tasks. He stated that "the results agree with the theory that transfer is highly specific and occurs only when the practiced movements are identical."

Movement education is an approach to education in which the underlying components of movement (such as time, force, and space) become the content. It has received a great deal of interest in elementary physical education over the past twenty years. Those who advocate adoption of a movement-education approach propose that transfer of this learning will facilitate performance and learning of new motor skills. Unfortunately, there is little empirical evidence for this idea. Toole and Arink (1982) specifically designed a recent study to assess transfer of movement-education training to new skill performance and to evaluate skill improvement as a result of movement education and traditional instruction.

They reported that traditional instruction was better than movement education for acquiring several specific skills, and movement-education students were no better than traditional-instruction students in performing two new skills that were introduced after a twenty-week program. The investigators concluded that a traditional-instruction approach is better than movement education, if one's objective is to teach a specific skill.

In a related issue, there has been some popularity among high school and college physical educators in recent years for courses in movement fundamentals or basic skills. The assumption behind offering these courses is that the movements learned will transfer to enhanced learning of specific sports. There is little evidence for this assumption; from that which does exist, it would appear that such transfer is negligible. For example, Coleman (1967) found no significant differences in bowling performance between groups that experienced a movement-education course prior to a bowling course and a group that enrolled only in bowling. In another study, Burdenshaw and her colleagues (1970) assessed the effectiveness of a basic skills course as a prerequisite for learning badminton skills. The group that experienced a basic skills course before enrolling in the badminton course performed about the same as a group that enrolled initially in the badminton course.

The findings of these studies are in agreement with research on specificity versus generality, which was discussed in some detail in chapter 16. Rather than reintroduce these findings here, the reader is encouraged to review these studies at this time.

In summarizing data on intertask transfer with motor tasks, it appears that there is typically little transfer of any kind. There is almost never negative transfer, and any positive transfer tends to be minimal. Thus, the motor skills instructor need not worry about producing negative transfer with students as long as they do not have to learn contradictory responses.

Intratask Transfer

Intratask transfer refers to transfer from one variation of a task to another variation of the same task. One way of varying a task is to speed up or slow down the rate of performing it. Studies of this type have examined the effect of emphasizing speed or accuracy during practice trials on performance of the task when performed at normal speed. Other studies have been concerned with the transfer effect of practicing parts of a task on performance or learning the whole task. Finally, a few studies have varied the task in a way to make it easier or more difficult and have assessed the transfer effect when the task is performed normally.

Speed versus Accuracy. In 1928 Agnes Poppelreuter published a study in Germany in which she stated that speed should be retarded until a reasonable level of accuracy was attained. This sparked a controversy in physical education and psychology that still exists today. The controversy has centered around the appropriate time and place in motor learning to emphasize speed and accuracy. (In motor skill instruction the teacher may impose a set for action, the instruction being for either speed or accuracy or both in combination.)

Studies over the past fifty years have indicated that Poppelreuter's formulation was much too simple. Using a variety of motor tasks, investigators have found that if speed is a predominant factor in subsequent performance, an early emphasis on speed is desirable, allowing accuracy to be acquired in time. But if both speed and accuracy are important, an early emphasis on both is most appropriate.

Several investigators have used the rotary-pursuit apparatus to study the effects of practicing at a faster or slower speed of rotation (forty rpm or eighty rpm) on subsequent performance at a criterion speed (sixty rpm). The design of these studies typically calls for one group to practice at forty rpm, another to practice at eighty rpm, and a third to practice at sixty rpm. After the practice trials, all groups are tested on a series of transfer trials at sixty rpm.

In most of these studies, more positive transfer is observed when the practice conditions are similar to the criterion speed. In studies using various practice speeds, transfer task performance tends to reflect a response generalization gradient. The concept of response generalization is based on the notion that while a given response to a stimulus is being learned, this stimulus also tends to evoke other responses that are similar to the learned response in force, direction, distance, and rate of movement (Baker, Wylie, and Gagne 1950). Thus, the closer the practice speed is to the criterion speed, the greater the positive transfer.

One major weakness of all these studies, from the standpoint of actually learning motor skills, is that the practice speed for each group has been constant throughout the pretransfer practice. As Jensen (1975; 1976) has correctly observed, most motor skills would be taught and learned more naturally on a gradual build-up of speed if one wished to employ an accuracy-to-speed methodology. Research designs employing one constant speed of practice for each treatment group seem inappropriate if one wishes to make application for motor skill acquisition. Jensen (1975) included three different combinations of rates of speed on the pursuit rotor during the pretransfer practice period: twenty-twenty-forty rpm; thirty-thirty-forty-five rpm; and thirty-forty-fifty rpm. These treatment groups were compared with a control group that used the criterion speed (sixty rpm) throughout the practice and transfer trials. Jensen found only one overall difference in transfer performance of the groups: The control group performed better than the experimental group that trained at the slowest speed.

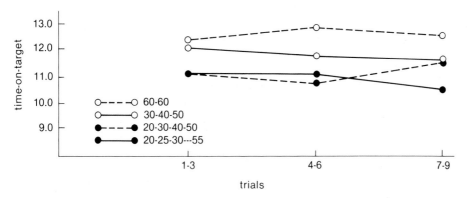

Figure 19.2   *Mean time-on-target scores for transfer trials.*

Since very little is known about the acquisition of motor skills when a gradual and progressive increase in speed is employed as the practice technique, Sage and Hornak (1978) examined more fully the transfer effects of response variation along the dimension of rate. The progressive increase in speed was an attempt to simulate more accurately the methodology emphasizing gradually increasing speeds that is frequently used to teach and learn motor skills. Various schedules of progressively increasing speed were employed, with one group practicing at the criterion speed (sixty rpm) throughout the practice trials. After thirty-five practice trials, all subjects were transferred to sixty rpm for nine transfer trials (figure 19.2). There were no significant performance differences during transfer trials between the various experimental groups that employed progressive and gradual increases in speed during the pretransfer practice and the control group, which practiced at the criterion speed throughout the pretransfer practice period.

These results suggest that a progressive speed buildup is as effective as beginning at the criterion speed. That is, the appropriate spatial and temporal organization of a motor task can be acquired efficiently if the speed with which the learner practices is gradually increased and is increased to approximate the criterion speed. This is in agreement with the response generalization theory described above (Baker et al. 1950).

In a further effort to design research that is more like the learning of sports tasks, Siegel and Davis (1980) proposed that since people performing sports skills rarely execute responses at only one speed over the course of performing a skill, a more relevant method of examining the effects of practicing a skill at certain speeds on subsequent performance is to provide for multiple speed transfer conditions among learners. Accordingly, they examined the effects of practicing the rotary pursuit at specific speeds on performing over a range of speeds. One group practiced at thirty rpm, a second practiced at sixty rpm, and a third divided practice over three speeds, thirty, forty-five, and sixty rpm. On the transfer trials, all groups were tested at thirty, forty-five, and sixty rpm. The group that had practiced at the three speeds performed equal to or better than the other groups across the range of speeds during the transfer trials (figure 19.3). Thus, the group that distributed its practice over three

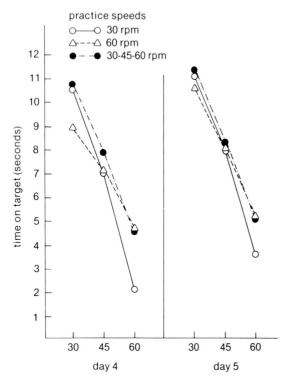

Figure 19.3   *Mean time on target for groups over transfer days*

speeds performed equal to groups that had had three times as much practice at those speeds. The investigators suggest that although one might expect from the principle of similarity that more practice at a particular speed would result in better performance at that speed, it is possible that subjects got to a point at which additional practice at one speed did not improve proficiency to any great extent.

Using sports skills, Woods (1967) assessed the effect of varied instructional emphasis on speed and accuracy on the acquisition of the forehand tennis stroke. The most desirable results were obtained by equal instructional emphasis on speed and accuracy simultaneously; an accuracy emphasis followed by a maximum velocity emphasis proved least beneficial. Hornak (1971)

found that a teaching sequence of speed, accuracy, and then a combination of the two was a better method of teaching the soccer instep kick, when considering both accuracy and speed scores. Other investigators have found that sports skills that require both speed and accuracy are most efficiently learned by equal emphasis during practice.

The question of whether speed or accuracy or both should be emphasized in learning motor skills has generated a great deal of research interest, but little definitive findings. In general, it appears that if a task is to be performed at a given speed, it should be practiced at that speed. Good basketball players, for example, get their jump shot off in less then two seconds. When learning to shoot, players may take longer than two seconds as they attempt to develop an effective movement pattern. Then during a game, since they must shoot the ball quickly to prevent its being blocked, they speed up the movement. This alters the habit they learned in practice, and the result is a poor performance. During practice drills, therefore, performers should be executing their skills at "game speed" in order to gain optimal transfer from practice habits to game habits. Thus, the teaching method of requiring beginners to practice a task at a slower tempo than is actually needed for effective execution of the task must be viewed with suspicion. On the other hand, a progressive practice schedule of gradual increases in speed does not seriously retard the acquisition of skill. Moreover, if the eventual performance on a task will require movement at various speeds, practice under variable speed conditions will be more beneficial than practice at a single speed.

Level of Difficulty and Transfer. Some transfer studies have examined the effect of modifying a task to make it easier or more difficult, having learners practice under the modified conditions before performing the task under normal conditions. The question under consideration here is whether it is harmful or beneficial to practice an easy or difficult modification of a task when attempting to learn that task. Investigations of this type have usually made a task easier or more difficult by decreasing or increasing the size of targets to be followed or hit, changing the speed of the target, or increasing or decreasing the distance of the target (for example, pistol shooting and archery).

Regardless of whether the modification is in target size, target distance, or speed of target, the findings are equivocal; some studies show a superiority of practice with an easy modification, others show a superiority with a difficult modification. But in general, practice on the actual task to be learned in a normal manner appears to be as valuable as practicing modifications of the task. For example, in one of the few studies where a sports skill was used, Singer (1966) used archery accuracy as the skill to be learned by the subjects. An easy-to-difficult group practiced archery ten yards from the target; a difficult-to-easy group began at forty yards from the target; and a control group started at twenty-five yards from the target. All groups were then tested at twenty-five yards. Singer reported no significant differences in transfer effects from easy-to-difficult compared with those from difficult-to-easy conditions. Ultimate success, measured by the Columbia Junior Round, was not influenced by the distance at which initial practice occurred.

In another study involving gross motor skills, Scannell (1968) studied transfer of accuracy training, using a dart throw and a softball throw, when the difficulty was controlled by varying target size during practice. He found no significant difference in the effects of practice with targets equal to, smaller than, or larger than the test target. The study showed that easy-to-difficult or difficult-to-easy conditions did not make any difference on performance of the test skills. Scannell suggested that "attempts to enforce, in practice, degrees of precision greater than those required in the test situation, while not deterring the subject's progress, will not enhance the progress."

Several writers have suggested that the task, as well as other factors, may make one condition more favorable than the other. Some tasks may transfer better with an easy-to-difficult arrangement, while the reverse may be true for other tasks. It seems that optimal conditions must be established for each task. Holding (1962) echoes this viewpoint. In summarizing over twenty-five articles on this topic, he concluded that "difficulty is not a useful category for the prediction of transfer efficiency, and . . . the solution lies in examining the skills involved."

Variability of Practice. The review of speed-versus-accuracy and level-of-difficulty topics has focused on traditional research approaches. An entirely new theoretical orientation to the study of these topics has been opened up with the formulation of schema theory. One of the most salient predictions of this theory of motor learning is that an increased amount of variability of practice *within a response class* will enhance skill acquisition. Typically, in studies designed to test this prediction, a variability group practices several variations of a task, while a control group practices only one variation of a task constantly. After a set of practice trials under the respective conditions, the groups are transferred to a novel variation of the task within the response class. According to schema theory, the group receiving variability of practice should perform the novel variation more effectively than the group that did not undergo variability of practice. This is because variability of practice should lead to greater schema strength. Therefore, performance on the novel variation within the same response class should be superior for this group.

As we noted in chapter 17, this prediction of schema theory has been examined extensively over the past few years (for a review see Shapiro and Schmidt 1982). In general, the results of these studies with male adult subjects provide minimal support for variability of practice. On the other hand, childrens' and females' motor skill acquisition seems to be more favorably affected by variability in practice. Newell (1981) cautions that although some of the findings about the value of varied practice "are supportive of the schema position, none of the data are terribly convincing and it has to be concluded that the benefits of variable practice have yet to be unequivocally established."

Whole-Part Transfer. Another intratask transfer variable related to practice methodology concerns whether a motor task should be practiced in its entirety with each practice trial or whether it should be divided into component parts and the parts practiced separately, being combined to perform the entire task only after the parts have been mastered. Or should some combination of these two methods be employed? This is the issue of **whole-part transfer.**

A task that is capable of being divided into parts can be practiced in two basically different ways. First, it can be practiced as a whole, that is, practiced from beginning to end at each trial until it is learned or until a certain level of proficiency is attained. Second, it can be separated into two or more parts. Each component of the task is practiced as a separate unit and then connected with other units to form the whole movement pattern. This second method, called the part method, can be further divided into three variations: (1) a pure-part method in which each part of the task is learned separately, then all the parts are performed in sequence to produce the whole task; (2) a progressive-part method in which the learner practices the first two components of a skill, combines these to form a whole, practices a third component, chains it to the first two, and so forth, continuing by progressive addition of components until the whole task has been learned; (3) the repetitive-part method is accomplished by practicing and mastering the first component, then doing the same for components one and two together, then components one, two, and three together. This continues until all the parts are mastered.

Much of the early research into the relative effectiveness of whole versus part learning was done with verbal material. We shall not review these studies, but rather focus on studies involving motor tasks. The findings on motor task studies have fairly consistently (considering the inconsistency in this area) replicated the findings of studies that used verbal materials.

In an integrated motor task the performance of a single component by itself is different from the performance of the same component when it is embedded in the entire task. When analyzing the findings of research on tasks that have a great deal of integration and interaction among components, it appears to be inefficient to practice on the components first (Lewellen 1951; Niemeyer 1959; Lersten 1968).

A general rule for whole versus part learning might be: Whole practice increases in effectiveness as the integration of the component parts of the skill increases in importance. For example, tasks that lend themselves to the whole method are those in which timing and speed are critical in order not to destroy the total movement pattern. In such tasks, the proper timing and coordination of the whole task might be destroyed if isolated parts of the total task were practiced. Skills such as the tennis serve and the jump shot are composed of almost inseparable links—one link blends into and provides the cue for the next link in a sequential manner. The real value of the whole method is that it enables the learner to realize the relationships of the component parts to the entire task.

Some motor tasks are actually composed of several relatively independent components, or movements. When the total task involves separate, independent movements, it seems that dividing the task into parts for practice may facilitate learning the whole task. Adams and Hufford (1962) reported that learning a series of separate movements that were a part of a larger task, flying an airplane, showed a great deal of transfer to the performance of the whole task. While others have reported similar findings with tasks involving separate, independent movements, there have been contrary findings as well.

It appears that the effects of whole-part practice on tasks of this type need to be established for each task. In lieu of doing this, the following proposal suggested by Fitts and Posner (1967) might be applied:

If the components of the skill are independent of each other . . . , then it is better to practice each component separately. . . . When, however, the task involves synchrony between the components . . . , much of the learning is concerned with the overall integration of the components and thus is best learned as a whole. A practical exception to this may arise if the components are too complex to allow the beginner to practice the task as a whole. The best plan here is to program practice so as to develop some proficiency in the separate components, choosing component processes that are as nearly independent of each other as possible and alternating between part and whole.

Some motor tasks are very complex or are composed of various components, each of which can be identified as a complete unit. For tasks of this kind, the part method of practice may be more efficient and effective than the whole method. For example, the offensive motor tasks of basketball shooting, dribbling, and passing, offer a complex task with several subtasks. Many team sports fall into this category. Individuals can profitably practice the subtasks separately. As skill improves, they can learn to use these tasks in combination and in relation to teammates and opponents, and in reference to the rules of the sport. So for complex tasks, the whole method might be employed for connecting the components together *after* the components are learned by the part method.

Even when the part method is used, it must be used with reference to a concept of the whole task. The most important characteristic of a motor task is its wholeness. Learners must know what the entire task consists of (a general idea of the whole) if they are going to learn the whole task. It is only after learners achieve a general idea of the whole complex task that they should isolate the subtasks and practice them.

Traditionally, research on whole-part methodology has focused on the classification of tasks to be learned. Recently, Murray (1979) suggested that individual differences in learners' cognitive style might be relevant to whether whole or part practice is most effective. She classified subjects as either holistic or sequential information processors on the basis of cognitive style tests. Subjects learned to juggle with either whole or part teaching methods. Sequential learners using the part method and holistic learners using the whole method took significantly less time to learn to juggle than sequential learners using the whole method and holistic learners using the part method. It appears that motor skills instructors might consider the cognitive styles of the learners when organizing whole or part practice. Some learners may acquire a skill better under whole practice, while others may be more efficient with part practice.

Transfer and General Factors

We now turn our attention to the second major explanation for transfer of learning. Up to this point, our emphasis has been on specific transfer, but we must differentiate between specific and general transfer. When we learn a task, we acquire not only the specific movements of the task, but also many other aspects of it that make for enhanced performance. These can include such varied things as learning how to fixate attention on certain stimuli, how to organize the task demands into meaningful parts, and how to use certain devices to form associations. These general skills, strategies, and other habits acquired for a task can in turn influence learning of quite different tasks. Research suggests that there is indeed the potential for general transfer when learning motor tasks.

Judd (1908) was the first to take exception to the extent and nature of Thorndike's theory of identical elements. He reported that boys who had been given instruction on the principles of light refraction were more accurate at hitting a target submerged in water than were boys who had not received this instruction. He proposed that the learner can use principles and laws as well as general strategy to transfer learning from one task to another. Obviously, this theory allows for the potential for a great deal more transfer than Thorndike's theory, and has therefore been called a **general factors** theory.

A related concept that has arisen in the transfer literature of the past thirty years is *learning to learn.* In tests of verbal material, people tend to improve their ability to master lists of nonsense words by experience with lists of such words. Learners are said to have learned how to learn; they perceptually organize general features common to the two tasks and use the successful strategy of one task to solve the problems of mastering a different task.

Transfer of Principles

Beginning with Judd's paper, numerous studies have examined the transfer effect of presenting information about principles underlying motor tasks. Judd (1908) extended and reported a study, started by Scholckow, that demonstrated transfer of principles. As noted in the previous section, the specific principles were those of refraction of light. In this study, subjects threw darts at a target submerged in water. When the target was four inches under water, the group that had been given knowledge of the principles of refraction adapted quickly to the situation and produced superior performance over the group that lacked knowledge of refraction principles.

Hendrickson and Schroeder (1941), in an attempt to make a general replication of Judd's study of target accuracy and transfer of knowledge of principles on a target submerged in water, had subjects shoot an air gun at a submerged target. Experimental groups were given an explanation of the theory of refraction prior to shooting. With targets at a water depth of six inches, experimental groups performed better than a control group, and essentially the same results occurred when the target was raised to two inches below the water surface.

In the past two decades several investigators have reported that providing learners with certain biomechanical principles related to the motor tasks they were attempting to learn enhanced the rate of skill acquisition. Mohr and Barrett (1962) reported that a group of swimmers who had received instructions on the biomechanical principles involved in swimming made significantly greater improvement in their swimming proficiency than a group not receiving the instruction. They concluded that "exposing students to an understanding and application of biomechanical principles will effect greater improvement than instruction without reference to those principles." Papcsy (1968) reported that eighth-grade boys learned a handball skill at a faster rate after having been taught the mechanical principles involved. They also performed better on a bunting skill. Finally, Werner (1972) showed that teaching four science concepts (levers, Newton's first law of motion, Newton's third law of motion, and work) to fourth-, fifth-, and sixth-grade students enhanced their performance on a variety of gross motor tasks.

The studies cited above may give the impression that every study has demonstrated a facilitation of learning when biomechanical principles are employed, but this is not the case. Several investigators have reported no advantage to the mechanical principle instruction group (Coville 1957). However, the fact that instruction in biomechanical principles has been found to enhance the learning of a number of motor tasks and that it is typically fairly easy to incorporate this type of information into verbal instructions suggests that instructors might use this technique to some advantage. Providing a variety of examples when employing biomechanical instruction and actively emphasizing similarities between movement patterns of different motor skills is one way to maximize transfer potential of biomechanical principles (Gallahue, Werner, and Luedke 1975).

Other General Factors Phenomena

Learning for optimal positive transfer effects might include experiences that permit the learner to form generalizations applicable to a new situation, while at the same time helping the learner to distinguish basic components in each task so as to recognize the differences in the tasks. A verbal explanation often attempts to utilize transfer from one skill to another. References such as "the serve in tennis is just like the overhand throw in baseball" attempt to cause learners to transfer their baseball-throwing pattern to the tennis serve. Broer (1958) gave an experimental group instruction emphasizing problem solving and biomechanical principles of learning volleyball, basketball, and softball basic skills. Also, the experimental group was given one-third, two-thirds, and the same amount of specific instructions on volleyball, basketball, and softball, respectively, as the control group. The experimental group surpassed the control group on all skills tests for the various sports given at the completion of each unit.

A few studies show positive transfer between small-pattern motor practice and large-pattern learning. For example, Cratty (1962) studied the transfer effect of prior practice on three small-patterned mazes on large-patterned maze-learning efficiency. He concluded that prior practice on a similar small-patterned maze resulted in initial positive transfer of traversal time on the large-patterned maze and that prior reverse pattern practice caused initial negative transfer.

In a unique study, Vincent (1968) classified two criterion motor tasks (a hop-and-jump task and a static balance task) by their perceptual components and their motor components. Experimental group subjects then practiced to a high level of competence in the perceptual components of the criterion tasks through the use of practice tasks similar to the criterion tasks in perceptual makeup, but not similar in motor demands. He hypothesized that subjects who practiced tasks with perceptual components similar to the criterion motor tasks would exhibit higher proficiency on the criterion tasks than a control group that practiced unrelated exercises. His results confirmed the hypothesis; the experimental groups were significantly superior to the control group on both criterion motor tasks. Vincent suggested that the transfer resulted from the similarity in perceptual components of the practice and criterion tasks, and that perceptual abilities are subject to improvement through practice.

Summary of General Factors

It can be seen from the discussion above that the identical elements theory of transfer of training is incomplete. Although it is not possible to identify the stimulus and response characteristics of most tasks, it is fairly obvious that a good deal of transfer cannot be accounted for by an identical elements theory. The more contemporary view is that transfer effects are best explained as the result of a combination of elements, both specific and general.

Some psychologists, on the basis of their research, have advanced what has been called a "two-factor theory of transfer of learning." Two-factor theories propose that individuals not only transfer identical stimulus-response elements from task to task, but they also transfer general elements, such as principles of problem solving, learning to learn, and insight.

Additional Conditions and Transfer

Several other transfer conditions have been studied, such as inter-limb transfer, degree of initial learning, variety of previous experiences, and effects of learning two tasks simultaneously. The results of these studies have implications for motor learning and performance.

Bilateral Transfer

When people practice a motor skill, such as throwing a ball, with their right hand, there is usually some positive transfer to their left hand even though they have not practiced with the left hand. Transfer from a limb on one side of the body to the limb on the opposite side is called **bilateral transfer.**

Perhaps the earliest report of bilateral transfer with a motor task was a study by Swift (1903). He studied the transfer of learning on a juggling skill where the subjects attempted to keep two balls going with one hand, receiving and throwing one while the other was in the air. He found unmistakable evidence that "practice with one hand trains the other." In an extensive review of the literature on bilateral transfer of learning in the late 1950s, Ammons (1958) concluded that investigators had consistently found that skill acquired in practice with one limb transfers to the unpracticed limbs. Further, this transfer occurs from hand to foot as well as hand to hand or foot to foot, but the greatest transfer is in the corresponding limb on the opposite side of the body.

In spite of the continued interest in bilateral transfer, there are many bilateral transfer conditions on which little or no research has been done. For example, does more transfer occur from the dominant to the nondominant hand? or is the reverse true? or is the transfer effect due more to the proficiency of the limbs? Answers to these questions cannot be made with any confidence because of the limited research.

Several explanations to account for bilateral transfer have been proposed, but the three most cited notions are: (1) the motor overflow, (2) motor programming, and (3) cognitive learning. The motor overflow explanation is based on neuroanatomical and neurophysiological evidence of motor transmission. While the motor signals over the pyramidal and extrapyramidal tracts are primarily contralateral, there is considerable ipsilateral transmission. Motor output from the left motor cortex will have its primary effect on the spinal motoneurons controlling limbs on the right side of the body, but there will be some overflow of motor signals ipsilaterally that will stimulate spinal motoneurons controlling the limbs on the left side of the body (Davis 1942).

One consequence of motor overflow that has been rather well documented in exercise physiology is a gain in strength and endurance in an untrained limb as a result of training the contralateral muscle group (Moritani and deVries 1979; deVries 1980). A behavioral manifestation of the motor overflow is that when performing a two-hand task simultaneously (such as writing your name at the same time with both hands), the moving limbs seem to be locked together, producing a very similar pattern. Over eighty years ago, one of America's pioneer psychologists, Woodworth (1903), commented on this phenomenon: "It is common knowledge that movements with the left and right hands are easy to execute simultaneously. We need hardly try at all for them to be nearly the same."

The motor program explanation draws on the notion of generalized motor programs proposed by Schmidt (1976b), namely, that programs developed through practice with one limb can be used when the same task must be performed by the contralateral limb. Evidence for the notion that in executing a particular movement the two hands can be controlled by the same motor program has been provided by several investigators (Kelso, Southard, and Goodman 1979; McGown and Schmidt 1981), and a recent study by Shapiro (1977) supports the idea that bilateral transfer is a result of the motor program used for one limb simply being employed with the contralateral muscles.

The cognitive learning explanation for bilateral transfer is based on the well-known principle that the early learning phase in skill acquisition involves such cognitive activities as understanding the goal of the task, thinking about which movements will bring about accomplishment of the goal, and cognitively formulating the techniques that will work best to produce successful movements.[1] Thus, when a task has been learned with one hand, much of the cognitive understanding important for performing the task is already acquired and does not have to be reacquired when practice begins with the opposite limb.

Since so many sports skills involve the use of one or more limbs, what are the implications of bilateral transfer for teaching sports skills? In sports where a ball must be thrown, caught, or kicked, it is obvious that most of the practice must be done with the limbs that will carry out these tasks most frequently. Quarterbacks whose right hands are dominant can more efficiently improve their passing accuracy by practicing with their right hands. However, in situations in which fatigue or injury to the dominant limb exist, practice with the other limb may facilitate performance with the dominant limb. Sports skills that require ambidextrous use of the limbs, such as kicking in soccer and dribbling in basketball, can be taught with the understanding that extensive practice with one limb does not necessarily mean no change for the other limb. Indeed, it may facilitate rate of improvement when the second limb is used to practice.

Initial Learning

In situations wherein positive transfer is known to occur, the transfer effect increases with increasing practice on the original task. This finding has been reported by numerous investigators. A critical deterrent to securing positive transfer, when it is expected or known to occur, is incomplete initial learning on the original task. Theoretical explanations for this are plentiful. In schema theory, schemata are assumed to develop with continued practice on a task. Assuming that schemata developed for one task can be employed in performing others, the more fully the schemata are developed for the first task, the greater the positive transfer to other tasks. Both consolidation memory theory and levels of processing would predict that the durability of the memory trace is a function of sustained experiences with a task. The more durable the memory trace for the original task, the greater the positive transfer, if indeed there is positive transfer between the two tasks.

An important implication for motor skill teaching exists here. Superficial practice on the original task is not likely to produce the intended positive transfer to subsequent tasks. A primary weakness of many school programs is that numerous sports skills are presented with provision for only superficial practice on each one. About the time students begin to learn the motor skills for one sport, the teacher moves on to a new "unit" that requires the learning of a new set of motor skills. The learner is never given sufficient time to master a set of motor tasks. The result is that any positive transfer that might occur from task to task is prevented. The overall consequence is that most students obtain virtually no mastery of any game or sports skills from their physical education classes.

Simultaneous Learning of Tasks

Is it best to learn two similar motor tasks simultaneously or at different times? The limited research indicates that tasks that involve similar movement patterns can be learned together without adversely affecting the learning of either skill. Studies based on Battig's (1979) conceptualization that increased contextual interference during skill acquisition will lead to improved retention or transfer have supported this notion (Shea and Morgan 1979; DelRey, Wughalter, and Whitehurst 1982). The concept of contextual interference and its theoretical underpinnings are too complex to describe here, but the basic notion suggests that it is actually helpful to learn and practice more than one skill at a time. Shea and Morgan's (1979) findings support this view. They say: "The results of this study suggest that instructors should teach a number of skills during each session for a number of sessions in order to achieve maximum retention and transfer."

---

[1] Kohl and Roenker (1980) have demonstrated that bilateral transfer occurs when people mentally imagine themselves performing a movement with one limb.

Variety of Previous Tasks

While there is a great deal of evidence that positive transfer is related to similarity of tasks and the initial learning of a previous task, it is also true that complex motor skills, such as those employed in sports, are dependent upon and built upon a variety of movement experiences. The learner's past movement experiences are extremely important in acquiring new skills because the motor programs (schemata) available for employment in learning new tasks are the result of previous motor learning. Thus, statements in previous sections of this chapter should not be interpreted to mean that variety of motor experiences is unimportant. Even when the transfer from one task to another is very small, the experience of a wide variety of tasks appears to be important for learning motor skills. It is a common observation of physical educators and coaches that students who have been deprived of a rich background of movement experiences have greater difficulty in learning sports skills. Teaching basketball to a student who does not have a movement background in running, catching, and throwing is quite difficult.

Summary

Transfer of learning refers to the effects of learning a task on prior or future learning, and transfer of learning plays an important role in a wide variety of human behaviors. Two basic designs are used in the study of transfer. One is called a proactive design and the second a retroactive design.

We have two basic approaches to explaining transfer of learning. The first is called the task similarity hypothesis and the second the general factors hypothesis. Transfer of learning is greatest when two tasks are highly similar. When a task requires the learner to make different, incompatible responses to identical or similar stimuli that appeared in the original task, some initial negative transfer will likely result. When a second task is quite dissimilar to the original task, little or no transfer usually results.

If the eventual performance on a task will require movement at various speeds, practice under variable speed conditions will be more beneficial than practice at a single speed. If the components of a skill are independent of each other, part practice is appropriate; but when the task involves an integration and coordination of components of the task, whole practice is more efficient.

Practice with one limb usually results in positive transfer to all the other limbs. Positive transfer increases with increasing initial mastery of the original task, provided there is positive transfer between the two tasks. An understanding of the general nature and biomechanical principles that are important to task performance produces positive transfer. Several motor skills can be learned together without adversely affecting the learning of any one of them.

The learner's past involvement with movement experiences is extremely important in acquiring new skills, and experience with a wide variety of tasks is important for learning new skills.

20

Motivation and Motor Behavior: Arousal Considerations

Key Terms and Concepts
Activation
Adrenal medulla
Arousal
Biofeedback
Cue utilization
Exercise-induced activation
Hypothalamus
Inverted-U hypothesis
Limbic system
Meditation
Motivation
Progressive relaxation
Reticular formation
Social facilitation
State anxiety
Trait anxiety
Yerkes-Dodson law

*H*uman behavior of almost any type is affected by motivation. In hitting a baseball or running a 100-yard dash, performers must be motivated if they expect to achieve effective and efficient performance. If they are not, they may go through the motions, but the result is likely to be a poor performance. It is as though no power had been supplied to the machine. It is entirely possible, then, for performers to possess a high level of skill and yet perform poorly. Indeed, performance is rarely commensurate with skill level. Bringing individuals' performance to the maximum of their capabilities requires that they be motivated.

Motivation is an important topic and its dimensions are so varied and complex that two chapters have been devoted to it in this volume. Even so, only selected aspects of the subject will be discussed, and no claim is made for a comprehensive and in-depth coverage of motivation here. The amount of literature on this subject is awesome, and there is a wide variety of theoretical approaches that could lead us far astray from our main focus—motor behavior. The criterion used to assess what information to include in this book was the extent to which it seemed important for basic understanding of motivation and application to motor behavior.

Definition and Function of Motivation

Like so many other concepts used in the study of human behavior, there is no precise and uniformly accepted definition of motivation. There are even some psychologists who feel that it is not a useful word or, better, that the concept is unnecessary. This, of course, is an extreme position and, since the word is so firmly embedded in the popular vocabulary, it is unlikely that it could be abolished by some researcher's dictate. Moreover, most psychologists feel it is a useful concept, notwithstanding the definitional problem.

For our purposes, **motivation** will be defined as the internal mechanisms and external stimuli that arouse and direct behavior. All complex human behavior takes place in the presence of a certain level of arousal and it is goal directed. The combination of arousal and direction toward a goal are integrated into what is called motivated behavior.

It can be seen, then, that motivation involves two basic functions: One is an arousal, or energizing, function that is involved in the mobilization of the bodily resources for vigorous and intense response. The second is a directive function that guides behavior to specific ends. This involves why individuals select a particular behavior at a particular time and why they choose certain goals and not others. Of course these two functions are not mutually exclusive. Certainly, behavior at any one time is the result of the integration of both aspects of motivation. Since arousal is such a key element in motivated behavior, in this chapter we shall review the physiological mechanisms underlying this state and examine the relationship between this physical state and motor behavior.

The Concept of Arousal

Arousal (**activation** is synonymous[1]) is a concept that attempts to order the intensive aspects of an individual's functioning. When we say that people are motivated, we mean, at least partly, that they are aroused. Elizabeth Duffy (1962), perhaps the most renowned of arousal theorists, defines **arousal** as being "the extent of release of potential energy stored in the tissues of the organism, as this is shown in activity or response." This notion that arousal refers to the degree of neural activity and behavior manifested by an individual is common to arousal theorists.

An individual's state of arousal can be viewed as a continuum, with deep sleep at one end of the spectrum and intense excitement at the other end. Every person goes through a daily cycle of deep sleep (low arousal), awakening and engaging in normal behavior throughout the day (average arousal), becoming sleepy (diminished arousal), and sleep again (low arousal). While this daily cycle holds fairly constant, wide variations occur throughout each day, especially in the waking hours. For example, you have to take an important examination—arousal level goes up. You have to sit through a boring lecture—arousal level goes down (sometimes so low as to cause sleep!). You have to play an intramural basketball game—arousal goes way up. Variations of arousal are different each day, and the arousal level, it can be seen, is changing moment by moment.

Two basic tenets underpin arousal theory. First, there is the notion that people are motivated to seek levels of stimulation that are optimal for general function. The underlying notion is that for a given person there is a level of arousal that is normal or appropriate for that person.

---

[1] *Arousal* and *activation* are used interchangeably by most motivation theorists, although there are some who have attempted to make distinctions between the two concepts. In this text, the two words will be considered to be synonymous. *Emotional, tense,* and *anxious* are other adjectives that are frequently used to express the same idea, and in sports *"psyched up"* conveys the same notion.

Behavior is motivated toward achieving and maintaining that normal state of arousal. The individual will engage in behavior to decrease the arousal level when it is too high and increase it when it is too low (Schultz 1965; Korman 1974).

A second major tenet of arousal theory is that there is an optimal state of arousal for best performance, and performance is impaired when arousal is too high or too low; the greater the distance from the optimal point, the greater the impairment of performance. In brief, the hypothesized curve relating performance to arousal is that of an inverted U. Direct and indirect evidence for this relationship has been thoroughly reviewed by Duffy (1972). In this chapter we shall focus on this second aspect of arousal theory rather than the first tenet, since the latter seems more pertinent to understanding motor learning and performance.

Neurological Basis of Arousal

Fundamental to arousal theory is the notion that specific structures in the nervous system are responsible for arousal states. One of the primary structures, the reticular formation, was discussed in some detail in chapter 7. But the "arousal system" is composed of several structures, each of which makes a unique contribution to the arousal response.

The Cerebral Cortex

As noted in a previous chapter, the brain emits characteristic wave patterns, depending upon the state of the organism. When the individual is awake but relaxed, the wave pattern tends to be characterized by high amplitude, low frequency waves in the range of eight to twelve Hertz, which are called alpha waves. The effect of an environmental or internal stimulus is to disrupt the alpha activity and produce a wave pattern characterized by a rapid, low amplitude, asynchronous pattern, known as beta waves. Thus, the neural correlate of arousal in the cortex is an increase in neural discharge characterized by rapid, asynchronous bursts of impulses.

The Reticular Formation

The primary location of arousal structures is in the brainstem and midbrain. The **reticular formation** has probably received the most attention with respect to the arousal function. As you will recall, this structure extends from the medulla up to the lower thalamus, with branches into the posterior hypothalamus. This vast network of neurons seems to function by sending diffuse axons throughout the nervous system, especially throughout the cortex. Impulses over these fibers facilitate neuronal centers throughout the brain and spinal cord. This network is the so-called reticular activating system.

The input to the reticular formation comes from collaterals from the various sensory modalities. Also, the cortex projects axons to the reticular formation, so cortical activity is capable of activating reticular neurons as well as vice versa. Finally, there are cells in the reticular formation that are sensitive to epinephrine (also called adrenalin), a hormone secreted by the adrenal medulla[2] during emergencies that flows throughout the body. The secretion of this hormone has the effect of heightening activity in the reticular formation.

The Hypothalamus

The **hypothalamus** is also part of the arousal system. This structure consists of a series of nuclei that lie on the floor of the diencephalon behind the optic chiasma and between it and the pons (see figure 4.10). This structure receives input from higher-brain centers as well as from other internal organs of the body. It is thus in a critical position for integrating messages from the higher nervous centers as well as those from the internal organs.

The posterior area of the hypothalamus plays a critical role in maintaining wakefulness. Lesions in this area produce sleep and drowsiness,

---

[2] The adrenal medulla is the inner portion of the adrenal glands. The adrenal glands rest on the superior surface of the kidneys.

Figure 20.1 *Schematic diagram of the limbic system.*

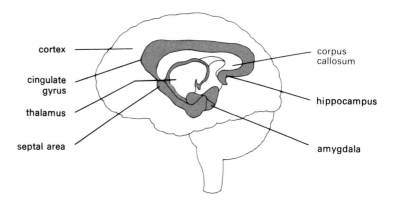

while electrical stimulation applied to the posterior hypothalamus causes alertness and excitement. In addition, electrical stimulation to this portion of the hypothalamus causes the secretion of hormones by the adrenal medulla, which in turn produces all of the responses associated with arousal, such as increase in heartbeat, respiration increase, and sweating. In this context, hypothalamic influence on the adrenal gland emphasizes the biochemical component of arousal.

The Limbic System

In recent years, neurophysiological studies using selective lesions and electrodes implanted in subcortical areas of the brain have led researchers to claim that areas in the **limbic system** are involved in the arousal process. The exact way in which this limbic system subserves motivation is unknown, but it seems to be involved with the development and elaboration of emotions.

The literature is inconsistent in the identification of the structures of the limbic system, but the structures usually listed are seen in figure 20.1. These subcortical structures are located in the medial and ventral parts of the forebrain, between the diencephalon and cerebral cortex, and this system has a complex network of fiber connections with these latter structures. Moreover, limbic structures are interconnected with each other by fiber pathways. Finally, they have connections with the hypothalamus, so there is probably a functional relationship there, too.

The Adrenal Medulla

A final structure that must be mentioned in relation to the arousal system is the **adrenal medulla.** Although this structure is not located in the brain, as are the other arousal mechanisms, some of the subcortical structures activate the adrenal medulla, which through its hormonal secretions reactivates subcortical arousal mechanisms.

Arousal Integration

All of these structures interact with each other, and with other systems such as the endocrine, sensory, and musculature. All in some way play a role in regulating overall arousal. On the basis of this arousal and the specific information being fed into the brain by the sensory systems, the individual prepares to respond to a stimulus situation.

Arousal and Motor Performance

We now turn our attention to the effects of arousal on motor performance. Almost everyone has had the experience of not performing up to their capability during an important examination or competitive event. "I was too tense" or "I was too anxious" or "I was too psyched up" are common expressions after such an experience. Indeed, college counseling offices report that test anxiety is one of the most common problems among students who are having academic difficulties.

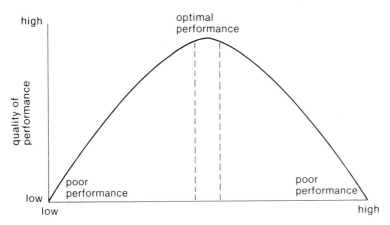

Figure 20.2 *The inverted-U relationship between arousal and performance.*

Studies of the relationship between effort and performance carried out in the first three decades of this century demonstrated that induced arousal facilitated such tasks as memorization, solving addition problems, and naming letters (Bills 1927). But as work of this type continued, it was demonstrated that not all degrees of arousal were equally effective at enhancing performance. Of special interest was the finding that behavioral efficiency increased to a maximum as arousal rose to an intermediate level and then began to decline as arousal continued to increase (Freeman 1933; 1938).

This work became incorporated into arousal theory and, indeed, became one of the major propositions of it under the name of the **inverted-U hypothesis.** The inverted-U hypothesis simply proposes that increases in arousal are accompanied by increases in the quality of performance up to a certain point, after which additional increases in arousal result in a deterioration in the quality of performance. The level of optimal arousal lies somewhere in the middle range of the arousal continuum (figure 20.2).

A number of studies have provided support for the inverted-U hypothesis, but only a few will be mentioned here. Perhaps the best-known study in which arousal was directly manipulated via reticular formation stimulation is the one by Fuster

(1958). He studied the effects of electrical stimulation of the brainstem reticular formation on tachistoscopic perception[3] of monkeys. First, the animals were trained to discriminate between geometric objects presented in pairs, with a food reward under one of the objects in each pair. Then the animals were subjected to a series of trials where the objects were briefly exposed and the number of correct responses and reaction time were measured. Finally, with electrodes implanted in the brainstem, different intensities of electrical stimulation were applied shortly before the presentation of the discrimination task trial. Moderate intensities of stimulation increased the animal's efficiency at discrimination by improving percentage of correct responses and shortening reaction times, compared with controls. Higher intensities had a deleterious effect on the responses and reaction times. Others subsequently reported findings with reticular stimulation that supported the notion that there are intensities of reticular activity that are associated with optimal performance.

---

[3] Tachistoscopic perception is assessed by a slide projector that exposes pictures to subjects for very brief durations of time (fractions of a second).

Stennett (1957), in another frequently cited study, examined the relationship between auditory tracking performance of human subjects under four conditions of increasing incentive and two physiological measures of arousal (skin conductance and electromyograph [EMG] recordings). The incentive conditions varied. At one extreme subjects were under the impression that their scores were not even being recorded; at the other extreme subjects' scores determined whether or not they avoided a strong electric shock and earned bonus money from $2 to $5. The most efficient tracking performance was associated with intermediate EMG gradients and intermediate levels of palmar skin conductance. Performance on tracking associated with very high or lower levels of physiological functioning was inferior to tracking performance associated with moderate levels of physiological functioning.

Motor behavior studies testing the inverted-U hypothesis have not produced consistent results, but several have provided support for this notion. In a study that manipulated arousal level through **exercise-induced activation** (EIA), Sjoberg (1968) showed a clear-cut inverted-U relationship. Human subjects pedaled a bicycle ergometer at work loads of 150, 300, 450, 600, and 750 kilogram-meters (kgm) per minute for five and one-half minutes and then performed choice reaction time trials while continuing to pedal. The work loads produced mean heart rates of 84 beats per minute (bpm) at rest to 147 bpm at the highest work load. Thus, the EIA levels ranged from low to moderately high. Best performance occurred at the 450 kgm per minute, with the mean heart rate at 121 bpm at this work load.

More recently, Weinberg and his colleagues (Weinberg and Hunt 1976; Weinberg 1978; Weinberg and Ragan 1978) have provided support for the inverted-U hypothesis with motor

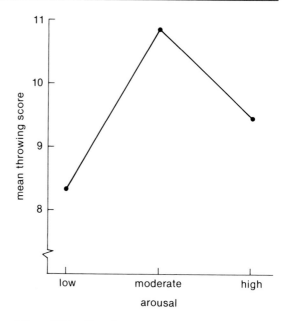

Figure 20.3 *Throwing accuracy as a function of three arousal levels.*

tasks. Weinberg and Ragan (1978) tested the hypothesis using three levels of stress while subjects were performing a throw-for-accuracy task. Figure 20.3 illustrates a clear inverted-U curve.

In one of the few field studies, Klavora (1979) assessed the arousal-performance relationship with high school basketball players. Figure 20.4 shows the performances at different arousal levels. Although there are slight differences, a clear inverted-U curve is present.

Klavora states:

The most important finding of this investigation is the fact that the two curves confirm the inverted-U model. . . . Various clusters of pre-game arousal scores on both poor and average levels of performance indicate that indeed a basketball player may be performing poorly (or only at an average level) because of two quite different reasons: either he is psychologically not ready for the upcoming competition, or he is too excited about it.

(a) <u>player 1 profile</u>

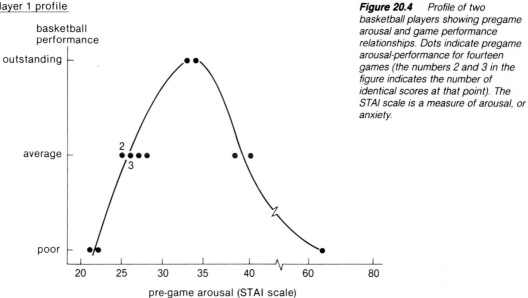

Figure 20.4 *Profile of two basketball players showing pregame arousal and game performance relationships. Dots indicate pregame arousal-performance for fourteen games (the numbers 2 and 3 in the figure indicates the number of identical scores at that point). The STAI scale is a measure of arousal, or anxiety.*

(b) <u>player 2 profile</u>

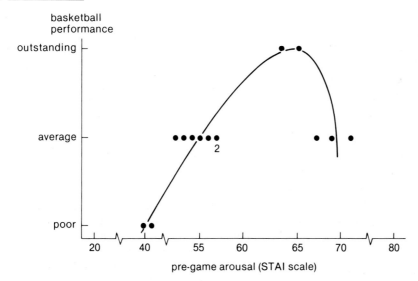

Figure 20.5 *A model illustrating the Yerkes-Dodson law. As tasks increase in difficulty, peak performance is achieved with less arousal.*

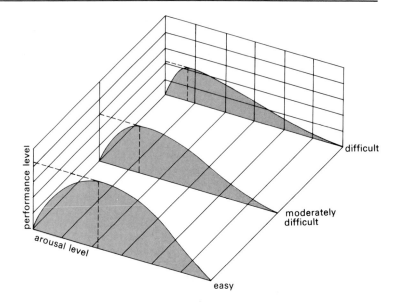

Even though a number of studies demonstrate an inverted-U relationship in motor behavior, this relationship is not clear and simple, and evidence for it is far from conclusive. Nevertheless, there is something to it, and the inverted-U appears to be a useful concept when attempting to maximize the performance of people engaged in motor activities (see Landers 1980 and 1982 for reviews of this topic).

Optimum Levels of Arousal

Since motor activities must frequently be performed under conditions of varying arousal levels, a fuller examination of the effects of arousal upon skilled performance is necessary. The optimal degree of arousal for efficient and effective performance is probably a fluctuating one, depending upon a wide variety of factors. We shall describe four factors that seem to be important when considering optimal levels of arousal.

The Nature of the Task

The oldest notion concerning an optimal level of performance was first formulated over seventy years ago by two comparative psychologists, and it carries their names as the **Yerkes-Dodson law** (1908). Simply stated, it proposes that optimal

arousal for behavioral efficiency decreases with increased task difficulty or complexity (figure 20.5). Yerkes and Dodson found fewer errors in performance when an electric shock of medium intensity was applied to mice than when shocks of low or high intensity were applied. When tasks were made more difficult, the optimal shock for the most efficient behavior was found to be progressively weaker.

Although several lines of research have confirmed this hypothesis in the intervening years, it has several problems. The chief ones are the questions of what is a "difficult" or "complex" task and what is a "simple" task. In recent years several scholars have advanced proposals that attempt to classify tasks in an information-processing framework and in the degree of inhibition and precision required during performance. The first classifies tasks by the perceptual and cognitive demands; the greater these requirements, the more complex the task. The second classification proposes that motor tasks can be thought of in terms of the degree of inhibition and precision required for appropriate performance. Thus, to the extent that a task involves a great

Table 20.1 The complexity of motor performance

Perception	Decision	Motor Act
Number of stimuli needed	Number of decisions necessary	Number of muscle actions
Number of stimuli present	Number of alternatives per decision	Amount of coordination of actions
Duration of stimuli	Speed of decisions	
Intensity of stimuli	Sequence of decisions	Precision required
Conflicting stimuli	Number of items needed from memory	Other?
Other?	Other?	

Note: No attempt is made to list the items by priority since this varies with the nature of each act
Source: Based on Billing 1980.

deal of information processing or inhibition-precision, high levels of arousal result in poor performance. One example of classifying factors that contribute to task complexity is shown in table 20.1.

It can be inferred from the above that motor tasks requiring concentration, judgment, discrimination, and fine muscle control, such as in tracking, aiming, and steadiness, are performed best under rather low to moderate states of arousal. Conversely, motor tasks demanding strength, endurance, speed, or in which ballistic movements dominate necessitate rather high arousal levels.

The manipulation of task complexity or difficulty and arousal has not been a popular research topic, so there is very little empirical work on this topic, especially for motor tasks. One approach, though, that has generated some interest makes use of exercise-induced activation (EIA) for manipulating arousal. Arousal levels can be influenced by various stimuli, including exercise, since the proprioceptors are known to supply a rich input to the reticular formation as well as influencing other parts of the arousal system. Thus, movement activity presumably affects arousal.

When tasks have been classified for the inhibition required for their performance, the effects of EIA on tasks at either the very high or very low ends of the inhibition continuum have resulted in rather consistent and clear-cut findings: High EIA facilitates tasks demanding little

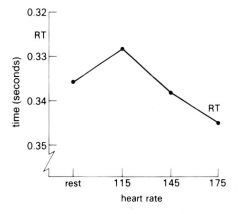

Figure 20.6 Five-choice reaction time as a function of heart rate.

inhibition and disturbs performance of tasks requiring inhibition (Phillips 1963; Gutin et al. 1974). Similarly, Levitt (1972) assessed the effects of various arousal states, induced by exercise, on tasks of varying information-processing demands. He exercised subjects on a treadmill at heart rates (HR) of about 80, 115, 145, and 175 bpm. A clear inverted-U curve was found, with optimal performance at HR of 115 and 145 bpm. Performance was poorer at 80 and 175 bpm. Under similar HR conditions Levitt and Gutin (1971) found that a five-choice reaction time task was performed best at 115 bpm, which can be interpreted as a rather low to moderate level of arousal, and worst performance was at 175 bpm (figure 20.6).

Table 20.2 *Optimum arousal level for some typical sports skills*

Level of arousal	Sports skills
5 (high arousal)	Football blocking and tackling Running (100 yards to 440 yards)
4	Running long jump Shot put Swimming short races Wrestling
3 (moderate arousal)	Basketball skills Most gymnastic skills Soccer skills
2	Baseball pitchers and batters Fencing Football quarterback Tennis
1 (slight arousal)	Archery and bowling Basketball free throw Pistol shooting Golf putting and short irons

The effects of "psyching up" to produce high levels of arousal for performing a simple task have recently been investigated by Shelton and Mahoney (1978). Weight lifters were instructed either to "psych up" or merely count backwards before performing a static strength task (squeezing a hand dynamometer). Lifters who were instructed to psych-up showed dramatic increases in performance, while those counting backwards showed no improvement in performance. Weinberg, Gould, and Jackson (1979) extended those findings by examining the effects of psyching-up on the performance of three different motor tasks. Their findings indicated the psyching-up effects were task specific, facilitating performance on a simple dynamic strength task (isokinetic leg extension), but having no effect on a balancing task or a speed-of-arm movement task.

One implication for the motor skills instructor is that in order to regulate arousal for optimal performance, an analysis of the information processing and inhibition demands of the task should be made. On the basis of this analysis, a decision can be made as to whether procedures should be taken to produce low, medium, or high states of arousal in performers. Some speculation of the relationship between arousal and sports performance as a function of task characteristics is shown in table 20.2

Skill Level of the Performer

Optimal arousal level seems to be sensitive to the skill level of the performer. A given level of arousal that might disrupt performance when the performer is a beginner may enhance performance when the task is well learned. Put another way, the greater the level of skill, the higher the arousal can be without causing disruption in performance. Typically, the poorly skilled athlete does poorly under pressure when arousal is high, while the highly skilled athlete excels when the pressure is greatest.

Research on social facilitation provides the most complete literature on the effects of arousal on performers of different proficiency. **Social facilitation** examines the consequences upon individual performance of the sheer presence of others. The first research on social facilitation goes back to just before the beginning of this century, but the mid-1960s Zajonc, a social psychologist, made a careful analysis of the previous research, drawing upon the rather extensive literature that shows that arousal enhances dominant responses and upon the evidence that the presence of others increases an individual's arousal state. He combined this information with the results of previous social facilitation results and proposed the first general theory of social facilitation (Zajonc 1965; 1966).

Zajonc's theory can be explained in this way: In the early stages of learning, performers' dominant responses are mostly incorrect ones. They will emit more wrong responses than right ones; wrong responses are dominant and strong during early learning. However, when individuals have mastered a task, correct responses become dominant. Assuming that an audience has arousal consequences for a person and that arousal enhances the emission of dominant responses, it can be seen that if the dominant responses are the wrong ones, as is the case during early learning, the wrong responses will be enhanced in the presence of an audience, and poor performance will be the result. But if dominant responses are the correct ones, which is the case after mastery of a task, an audience will enhance an individual's performance.

A flurry of research testing Zajonc's formulation followed in the next few years. While support was found by some investigators, others did not find such support (see Landers and McCullagh 1976 for a review). A refinement of Zajonc's original theory was proposed by Cottrell (1968) to account for results of studies that do not support the theory that the mere presence of others is sufficient for social facilitation to occur. Cottrell proposed that the mere presence of others is not the source of arousal in social facilitation research. Instead, the source of arousal resides in the anticipation of positive or negative

reactions from performing in the presence of others. Notice, though, that both Zajonc and Cottrell imply that the effects of arousal will be the emission of dominant responses on the part of the performer. The result is that novice performers will perform poorly under the arousal produced by the presence of others (their dominant responses are incorrect ones), while skilled performers will perform well in the presence of others (their dominant responses are correct ones).

This topic has taken a new turn recently, with a focus on attention as a mediating factor in the arousal-performance relationship. According to this view, the presence of others is distracting and creates attentional conflict. The arousal created in performers who experience distraction and attentional conflict leads to a loss of attention to relevant environmental cues (Baron, Moore, and Sanders 1978; Kushnir and Duncan 1978). The problem for a performer, then, is inadequate reception of information, rather than inappropriate output after the information has been processed. The novice experiences these attentional problems acutely, while the experienced performer's responses to relevant task cues are automatic, with less chance that the experienced performer will not process the relevant input.

Individual Differences

Individuals vary considerably in what might be called their "normal arousal state." Everyday observation confirms this; some people seem constantly to operate in a state of hypertension, anxiety, and "hustle bustle," while others go about their daily tasks in a relaxed, lethargic manner.

Instruments for assessing this general arousal state, such as Spielberger's state-trait anxiety inventory (Spielberger et al. 1970), confirm that indeed there are great individual differences in what Spielberger (1966) calls **trait anxiety,** which is a "motive or acquired behavioral disposition that predisposes an individual to perceive a wide range of objectively nondangerous circumstances as threatening and to respond to these with **state anxiety** reactions disproportionate in intensity to the magnitude of the objective danger." Accordingly, Spielberger indicates that people high in trait anxiety respond to evaluative situations with greater amounts of arousal than people low in trait anxiety.[4]

The potential effect of this differential reactivity on the arousal-performance relationship proposed by the inverted-U hypothesis is that since high and low trait-anxious people respond with different amounts of arousal to identical stress situations, these different levels of arousal lead the two types of people to perform differently in similar situations. In general, research tends to support this notion. Individuals high in trait anxiety tend to perform better than individuals with normally low arousal levels on very simple tasks. High trait anxiety tends to enhance performance when the task is simple. On the other hand, these high-anxious individuals tend to do worse on complex tasks, especially if novel responses are required.

---

[4] Suggestive evidence that differences in trait anxiety are related not only to general arousal, but also to arousal responses to specific situational stimuli and ultimately to performance, comes from the British personality theorist Hans Eysenck (1967). He has identified what he believes are two independent dimensions of personality: (1) extraversion-introversion, (2) stable-neurotic. Extraversion refers to the outgoing, uninhibited, impulsive, and sociable person, while the typical introvert is quiet, introspective, and somewhat "nervous." There is some evidence indicating that level of arousal is related to degree of introversion, with the introvert being higher in "normal arousal" and responding with higher levels of arousal to stimuli. Moreover, according to Eysenck, high neuroticism scores are indicative of emotional lability and overreactivity. People who are high in this dimension of personality "respond more strongly to stimuli, show greater variability of response, and take much longer to return to their prestimulation baselines."

Two or three examples of this research will suffice to illustrate the findings. Carron (1968) reported differential performance of high-anxious and low-anxious subjects on the stabilometer when an electric shock stresser was introduced early in the learning. High-anxious subjects were significantly inferior to other groups. More recently, several studies by Weinberg and his colleagues (Weinberg and Hunt 1976; Weinberg 1978; Weinberg and Ragan 1978) have demonstrated that high-anxious people perform less well under stress while low-anxious people perform better. In one study, three levels of stress were produced. Results showed that high-anxious subjects performed best in the low-stress situation, while low-anxious subjects performed best in the high-stress condition (Weinberg and Ragan 1978) (see Martens 1977 for information about performance of high- and low-anxious people in competitive situations).

Physical Fitness

Various studies have shown that when tasks are performed during or immediately after an exercise bout, the groups in better physical condition are somewhat less fatigued as a result of the exercise and tend to perform the tasks better (Gutin and DiGennaro 1968; Stockfelt 1970; Reynolds 1976). Stockfelt found that "well-trained" subjects performed arithmetic computations better at 25, 65, and 85 percent of previously determined maximal aerobic capacity than did "poorly trained" subjects. The well-trained group maintained a higher level of performance under physiological stress than the other group did.

In a series of studies Weingarten (1973; Weingarten and Alexander 1970) tested subjects on an abstract reasoning task during physical exertion. As with other studies, he found that fit and unfit subjects performed the same under relaxed or relatively mild physical exertion, but during severe physical exertion the fit subjects performed significantly better. Weingarten (1973) summarized work on this topic in this way: "When relatively complex problems were to be solved by physically fit and nonfit persons under stress, the fit consistently out-performed the non-fit."

Presumably, the differences in performances that have been noted during or immediately after physical exertion by physically fit and unfit subjects are related, at least in part, to the effects of the exercise on arousal levels. During physical exertion the physically fit person is probably closer to an intermediate level of arousal than the less fit, whose level of arousal is probably quite high, because the exercise does not alter the physiological mechanisms of arousal as dramatically for the fit person as for the unfit. One of the consequences of a conditioning program is physiological adaptation that makes a given amount of exercise less stressful.

Explanations for the Arousal-Performance Relationship

Attempts to explain the inverted-U function relating arousal and performance have been formulated by several psychologists. We shall make only a very brief examination of this literature.

Hebb (1972) proposed that "with low arousal cortical transmission is poor and with high arousal it is too good, permitting the occurrence of irrelevant and conflicting cortical activities; with very high arousal, too many messages get through and prevent the individual from responding selectively to any one set of stimuli." Similarly, Welford (1976) proposed that when arousal is very low the nervous system will be inert and signals are likely to be "lost" in either the perceptual

system or at some later point in the chain leading to a response. The deterioration in performance at high levels of arousal, according to Welford, is due to the cortical cells not only being facilitated, but actually being fired, when the stream of impulses impinging on the cortex becomes intense. The cortex becomes "noisy" when this occurs, and signals from external stimuli or impulses from one part of the nervous system to another tend to become blurred.

Using a slightly different perspective, Esterbrook (1959) proposed a "range of **cue utilization**" to relate arousal and performance. At low levels of arousal, irrelevant cues are being attended to. An increase in arousal reduces the attention to irrelevant cues and increases attention to relevant ones, resulting in improved performance. But very high levels of arousal tend to narrow the utilization of relevant cues, resulting in a decrement in quality performance. Figure 20.7 illustrates this notion. Others have also related the inverted-U relationship to attentional mechanisms (Bacon 1974; Nideffer 1976).

In summary, the hypotheses relating arousal and behavior suggest that moderate arousal tends to have an organizing effect on behavior by enhancing transmission throughout the brain. On the other hand, high levels of arousal can activate the brain centers so completely that all selectivity of transmission is lost. The result can be an inability to integrate and coordinate sensory inflow and motor outflow. Viewed another way, the ability of specific sensory data to guide behavior is very poor if the arousal level is low or very high. When arousal is low, the cortical activity is low and sensory data are not fully processed in the brain; when the arousal level is too high, the selectivity of the integrative functions of the brain is disturbed. Thus, brain function is best during periods of medium arousal.

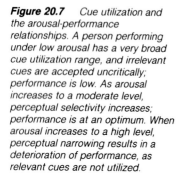

Figure 20.7 *Cue utilization and the arousal-performance relationships. A person performing under low arousal has a very broad cue utilization range, and irrelevant cues are accepted uncritically; performance is low. As arousal increases to a moderate level, perceptual selectivity increases; performance is at an optimum. When arousal increases to a high level, perceptual narrowing results in a deterioration of performance, as relevant cues are not utilized.*

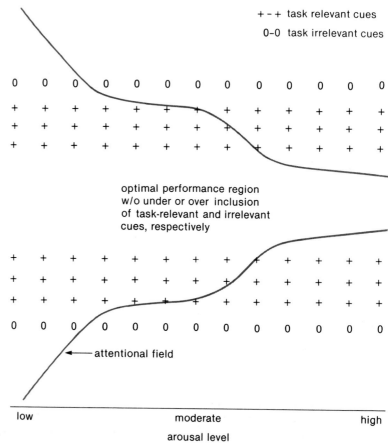

Arousal and Motor Learning

Throughout this chapter, emphasis has been on the effects of arousal on performance. No mention has been made of the effects of arousal on learning. This has been intentional because the effects of arousal on motor learning are more confused than the effects on motor performance, despite considerable interest in this topic extending over the past five decades. Over fifty years ago Bills (1927), Freeman (1931; 1933), and others found that the learning of various tasks was improved if, during performance, tension was induced in irrelevant muscles of the body—for example, squeezing a hand dynamometer improved the rate of learning. More recently several investigators have found that enhanced arousal states facilitate learning rate. They propose that consolidation memory theory can be employed to explain the underlying mechanism of this phenomenon (Walker and Tarte 1963; Weiner 1966; 1967; Weiner and Walker 1966). Walker and Tarte (1963) suggest that the neural memory trace established by practice will be more robust under high arousal, and, since this neural trace is essential for the production of a structural modification in the nervous system (represented as long-term memory), the higher arousal during practice will produce greater long-term memory. Weiner (1966) suggests that differences in memory under motivational and nonmotivational conditions "are not caused by differential rehearsal of stimuli." For Weiner, learning effects are attributed to some as yet unspecified arousal func-

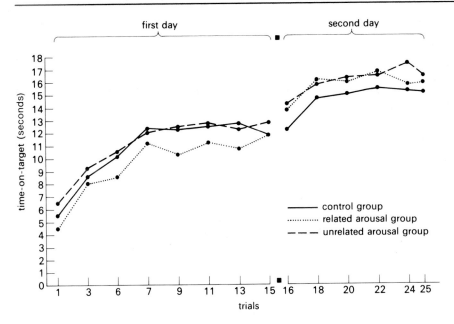

Figure 20.8   Mean performance scores for three groups over two days of practice. Twenty-four hours of rest were interpolated between trials 15 and 16.

tion so that "augmented motivation during memory trace formation makes . . . the trace more resistant to interference" or, possibly, more resistant to decay.

The effects of arousal on motor skill learning have been studied by several investigators (Marteniuk and Wenger 1970; Sage and Bennett 1973; Pemberton and Cox 1981; Cox 1982). The studies by Marteniuk and Wenger (1970) and Sage and Bennett (1973) provided support for enhanced states of arousal for learning in the motor domain. In both studies, subjects practiced a rotary-pursuit task under conditions of induced arousal (the experimental groups) or without induced arousal (control group), and were tested for learning after a period of twenty-four hours. Learning scores were significantly higher for the subjects who practiced under the aroused conditions than for the control subjects (figure 20.8). On the other hand, investigations by Cox (1982) and Pemberton and Cox (1981) have failed to find support for a facilitating effect of induced arousal on motor learning.

For now, we can say only that the exact relationship between arousal and motor learning will have to await further research for clarification. As with other conditions related to learning, a variety of environmental and personal differences undoubtedly combine with arousal states to influence the learning that occurs.

Measurement of Arousal

Since the concept of arousal is closely related to nervous system function, it is obvious that assessments of such functions as the activity of the brain, muscle tension, skin conductance, heart rate, blood pressure, respiration, temperature, and catecholamine[5] responses would be used in measuring arousal. Indeed, a great deal of work has gone into assessing arousal by these various physiological methods, singularly and in combinations. Unfortunately, physiological measures are

---

[5] Catecholamines are compounds that are secreted by the adrenal medulla and certain neurons during periods of arousal.

cumbersome to employ, and their interpretation encounters many problems. Moreover, the various physiological measurements are only moderately successful in assessing arousal states, and there are only moderate correlations, at best, between different measures of physiological arousal. This suggests that whatever each of these measures is measuring, each one is measuring something separate from the others in addition to measuring the commonality that exists. The best generalization seems to be that there is some degree of generality in physiological responses and some degree of particularity with respect to the stimulus situation and the individual.

One solution to the problem posed by imperfect validity of any one physiological measure is a composite index of several physiological variables. It has been proposed that this may yield a more accurate measure of arousal than any single measure. While the simultaneous measurement of several physiological arousal variables does provide a somewhat more accurate means of measuring arousal, it certainly restricts activation assessment to laboratory situations. This limitation of arousal assessment to circumstances that require the use of elaborate and bulky measurement apparatus seems especially unfortunate to the motor skills instructor—who would like to make assessments in dynamic situations.

Another method of assessing arousal makes use of a simple self-report of arousal. Thayer (1967; 1970) developed the activation-deactivation adjective check list (AD-ACL) and reported that it correlated more highly with a physiological composite of heart rate and skin conductance than these two physiological measures correlated with each other. The trait-state anxiety inventory of Spielberger et al. (1970) is a frequently used self-report instrument, and Martens (1977) has developed a competitive anxiety self-report inventory that is often used to assess arousal toward competitive athletic participation. These instruments provide alternatives to the physiological assessment procedures for measuring arousal, but valid measurement of arousal remains a problem. Indeed, it has been called "the

severest limitation to the utility of arousal as a psychological or physiological concept" (Martens 1974).

Manipulating Arousal

Controlling or manipulating arousal levels is more of an intuitive art form than a science at this time, but nevertheless motor skills directors have at their disposal a number of ways to deal with arousal phenomena.

Determining Arousal

In the previous section of this chapter it was noted that the measurement of arousal states is difficult, especially if one is seeking a precise assessment. On the other hand, if one is seeking a rough measure of arousal, several indices can be used. Observation of the following provides an indication of arousal: hand tremor, body perspiration, eye dilation, and restless and random fine and gross body movements. Another assessment that can be made without elaborate equipment is heart rate. Self-report inventories, such as the State-Trait Anxiety Inventory (Spielberger et al. 1970) or the Sport Competitive Anxiety Test (Martens 1977) can be used.

Increasing Arousal

A state of high arousal is best attained and sustained under conditions of stimulus variety and intensity. In situations where stimuli are monotonous and unchanging, arousal level wanes and, if alertness is needed to perform in this situation, performance will decline. For example, numerous studies have shown that if subjects work at monotonous, boring tasks for long periods of time, their performance deteriorates in direct proportion to the time spent on the task. If individuals must monitor a radar scope or watch for defective parts on an assembly line, their chances of making correct responses decline in proportion to the time spent on the job.

Visual stimulation, such as bright, blinking, and moving lights, will enhance arousal, as will intense and varying auditory stimuli. The pro-

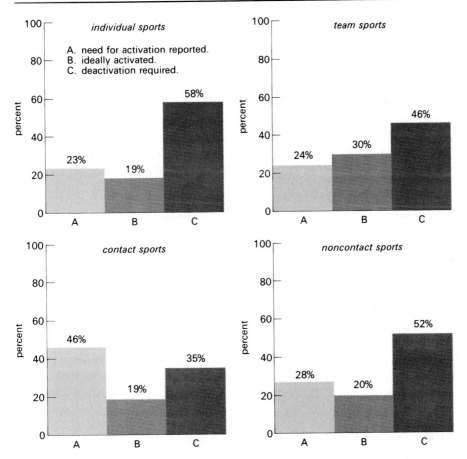

Figure 20.9 *Athletes were asked for an opinion of their typical psychological state just before competition.*

prioceptors provide a rich source of input to the reticular formation, so movement increases arousal.

Since cerebral cortical impulses activate the arousal system, cognitive content, such as appeals to survival, pride, self-esteem ("Get this one for the Gipper!") increases arousal, as do incentives, rewards, and punishment.

Reducing Arousal

Very little attention has been given to reducing arousal in motor behavior. Coaching manuals are filled with ways to motivate athletes, but motivation in this context invariably refers to increasing the arousal level. The fact that overarousal

can disrupt performance does not seem to be known or appreciated by most physical educators and coaches, which is unfortunate. In a study of over 380 athletes representing twenty-four sports and ranging from youth to professional competitive levels, the technical director of the coaching association of Canada, Lloyd Percival (1971), asked the athletes for an opinion of their psychological states just before competition. The athletes indicated that in a great many cases they felt that they were too aroused (figure 20.9). Percival's study implies that pep talks and other techniques commonly employed before athletic events in an effort to motivate athletes can be counterproductive. In many cases, the athletes might need to have their arousal states reduced.

Just as sensory variety and stimulus intensity are useful in enhancing arousal, low levels of stimuli are effective in reducing arousal. **Cognitive content** designed to distract the performer from arousal-inducing content and content aimed at placing competition and performance in the context of the "larger picture" of the world may also reduce arousal. One coach before an important contest told his athletes: "Less than one percent of the entire world's population knows we are even playing today!"

We have some techniques for systematically developing arousal control. Several of these are used in medicine and psychotherapy, but they are capable of being employed in other situations. Over forty years ago Edmund Jacobson (1938) developed a method of relaxation, which he called **progressive relaxation.** This technique has been used extensively in clinical settings.

The basic principle of this method rests upon people's developing a kinesthetic awareness of tension in their various muscles. The method requires the individual to learn to tense and relax specific muscle groups, gradually relaxing the entire musculature of the body. Since the proprioceptors play a prominent role in activating the arousal system via their collaterals that innervate the reticular formation, Jacobson's method of neuromuscular relaxation does provide a means for reducing arousal. Once having learned to relax, the person is capable of relaxing in arousal-inducing situations. A similar technique called "autogenic training" was developed in Europe and has been frequently used by athletes on the continent (Schultz 1956).

Biofeedback training provides a potential technique for teaching people to reduce arousal. **Biofeedback** is the instantaneous presentation of information to an individual about ongoing physiological processes such as muscle tension, heart rate, temperature, and brain waves. The physiological processes are typically recorded by specially designed electrical equipment and fed back to the individual by visual or auditory means, such as lights or sounds. With this immediate and objective feedback, a person can learn to regulate these normally involuntary processes.

Biofeedback research has demonstrated that people can be taught to self-regulate numerous physiological processes, especially the processes that control arousal states. Having learned to regulate these processes with the aid of the biofeedback equipment, the individual retains the ability to control them without the equipment, and upon command (Brown 1978; Danskin and Crow 1981).

Although biofeedback training has been employed primarily in medicine and psychotherapy up to now, there is every reason to believe that its use will become quite widespread. Its potential for use in teaching motor activities is already being explored (Zaichkowsky and Sime 1982).

The notion of reducing arousal has occasionally been promoted by mystics and oriental religions. Usually the approach is to some kind of mind-over-matter concepts. Transcendental Meditation (TM) is currently the most popular of the various **meditation** techniques. As described by Maharishi (1969), TM is a systematic procedure of "turning the attention inwards towards the subtler levels of thought until the mind transcends the experiences of the subtlest state of thought and arrives at the source of thought. This expands the conscious mind and at the same time brings it in contact with the creative intelligence that gives rise to every thought."

TM meditators report improvement in tension reduction in stressful situations and increased psychomotor function. Much of the TM research is still in its infancy but that which has been published is sufficient to establish that the psychophysiological effects during and after TM are real and unique in their degree of integration (Wallace and Benson 1972; *Fundamentals of Progress.* 1974; Smith 1975).

Although the idea of using **hypnosis** to control arousal states may strike some as being far out, this technique has been frequently employed in medicine and dentistry. Few people realize that it is also occasionally used in motor behavior. Mitchell (1972) has discussed in some detail the use of hypnosis in sports. The competence of the hypnotist and the ethical and legal issues of using this technique with motor performers are beyond the scope of this text. Suffice to say that these considerations should be fully explored before hypnosis is employed.

Because of the inherent ethical questions, little use has been made of depressants or tranquilizers with motor performers. With the increasing use of drugs, though, the coming years may witness their use to control arousal. The uncertain effects of these pharmaceuticals make their use undesirable in industry and education at this time.

Summary

Human behavior is greatly affected by motivation, which has been a central topic among those interested in motor behavior. Motivation is the internal mechanisms and external stimuli that arouse and direct behavior. The arousal aspect of motivation is concerned with energizing the body's resources for vigorous and intense responses. The directive aspect guides behavior toward specific ends.

Fundamental to arousal theory is the notion that specific structures in the nervous system are responsible for arousal states. The cerebral cortex, reticular formation, hypothalamus, limbic system, and adrenal medulla are the most salient structures of the arousal system.

The inverted-U hypothesis is the most noted proposition regarding the relationship between arousal and motor performance. The inverted-U hypothesis proposes that increases in arousal are accompanied by increases in the quality of performance up to a certain point, after which additional increases in arousal result in a deterioration in the quality of performance. There is considerable support for the inverted-U hypothesis, but the relationship is not clear and simple, and evidence for it is far from conclusive.

The so-called optimal level of arousal for efficient and effective performance is a fluctuating one, depending upon a wide variety of factors. Four of these are: the nature of the task, skill level of the performer, trait anxiety, and physical fitness. These factors and others affect the actual point of optimal arousal for best performance.

Several explanations for the arousal-performance relationship have been proposed. These theories suggest that arousal influences the nervous system in such a way that the perceptual, cognitive, and motor mechanisms are influenced. The result is poor performance during under and overarousal states and best performance at intermediate states.

Research on the effects of arousal on motor skill acquisition is inconclusive. Consolidation memory theory proposes that learning under highly aroused states should facilitate learning, and some studies show support for this prediction; other studies have failed to demonstrate support. As with other conditions related to learning, a variety of environmental and personal differences undoubtedly combine with arousal states to influence the learning that occurs.

The two main techniques for assessing arousal are physiological measures and self-report measures. Both have strengths and limitations, and valid measurement of arousal remains a problem.

Controlling and manipulating arousal levels is more an intuitive art form than a science, but several techniques are available. Some of the most commonly used are cognitive strategies, progressive relaxation, biofeedback, meditation, and hypnosis.

21

Motivation and Motor Behavior: Directive Aspects

*W*e have examined the arousal function of motivation. Now we shall consider the second basic function of motivation, which is the integrative and directive function. In the arousal function, the individual is prepared for action—energized. In the directive function, specific behavior is selected and sustained.

As we noted in chapter 20, the subject of motivation is too immense for us to enter into a full examination of its literature. Entire books are devoted to this single topic. Thus, only selected parts of the directive aspects of behavior are discussed here.

The Direction of Behavior

The direction of behavior can be viewed as either moving toward or away from a stimulus situation. The directional aspect of motivation derives from the fact that behavior typically exhibits selectivity; the individual approaches certain objects, situations, people, or certain aspects of them, and withdraws from others. Behavior, therefore, could be described as directed toward or away from various stimuli. Behavior can occur at any of many possible degrees of intensity, frequency, and duration.

Behavior is normally channeled toward a goal. The goal of motivated behavior is the meeting of some need or needs of the individual. The individual approaches or withdraws from certain persons, objects, or situations as they are interpreted as a means to achieving a goal and meeting a need.

While it seems fairly simple and straightforward to say that behavior is directed toward achieving some goal, and thus meeting or satisfying **needs,** the "need structure" of an individual cannot be directly viewed. Any effort to describe a certain behavior as meeting a specific need or attempting to structure conditions so as to induce a person to behave in the service of meeting a need is fraught with difficulties. In the first place, individuals vary considerably in their need structure; second, need structures are constantly changing, although there are underlying persistent needs. Third, individuals themselves may not be consciously aware of their own needs. Finally, sometimes behavior is not immediately need satisfying. For example, the soldier who goes into battle and risks being killed is certainly not gratifying some immediate need. Things that bring immediate pleasure are not necessarily need satisfying, while things that bring immediate pain are not necessarily dissatisfying or punishing. A person gives meaning to an event or behavior, and thus it takes on need-meeting characteristics.

Neural Basis of Directed Behavior

Basic physiological processes can go a long way toward explaining certain types of human motivated behavior. But they fall short of providing an adequate account of normal human motivation, especially as it is manifested in complex games, sports, dance, and occupational behavior. Much is known about such aspects of motivation as hunger, thirst, aggression, and sex partly because it is easy to observe and measure their behavioral expressions—eating, drinking, and so forth. However, there is little useful work linking brain structures to specific types of motor behavior found in games, sports, and other complex motor skills.

Categories of Needs

For many psychologists it has seemed essential to catalog needs. Once this is done it is believed that greater understanding of human behavior will emerge, and for those who are interested in influencing the behavior of others, conditions might be manipulated in such a way that persons will behave in the service of meeting needs.

Human needs have been classified into two general categories: biological and social. Although there is considerable disagreement in the psychology literature as to exactly how many needs exist in each category and in which category certain needs fit, there is agreement that the biological needs are unlearned, that they fulfill a survival function, and that the social needs are learned by particular interactions with the environment. It is further agreed that, although social needs would not occur in the absence of learning, once they are learned they can be as essential to the maintenance of the normal health of an individual as biological needs. A state of motivation, then, can be triggered by biological needs, such as hunger, thirst, need for oxygen, temperature regulation, and elimination, or by acquired needs, such as achievement, self-respect, security, and recognition.

In the process of fulfilling both biological and social needs, we learn to associate specific responses with those needs. For example, going to a restaurant and ordering food is a learned response for the hunger need. Working on a job to earn money is a learned response for security and other social needs. Every need has various learned responses associated with it. The presence or absence of something in the body or in the environment acts as a stimulus to a tendency to respond.

Motivation Techniques

Regardless of the need structure, various manipulations and controls can be administered to get an individual to perform or behave in a certain way to satisfy a need. Commonly used motivational techniques are the employment of incentives and reinforcements (sometimes called "motivators").

In the motivation literature, complex semantic problems surround the concepts of incentive and reinforcement, and some writers have written elaborate explanations differentiating the two. As we shall use the term here, **incentives** are objects, conditions, or stimuli, either material or symbolic, that produce a state of arousal in individuals so that they will be energized to approach or withdraw from an object, condition, or stimulus.

Incentives can be divided into positive incentives, which the individual tends to approach, and negative incentives, which the individual tends to avoid. In humans, since symbolic processes are so well developed, incentive objects, situations, or states, both positive and negative, can be imagined. In this case, the incentive is internal rather than external.

Incentives have two basic functions. One is to evoke a state of arousal so that the individual will approach or withdraw from the incentive. The second is to instigate directive actions toward it or withdraw from it. In both cases, incentives motivate partly through their effects on personal goals and intentions. The final point, with regard to an incentive, is that it is in some sense the *promise* that produces changes in behavior before any reward or other reinforcement is given (Bandura 1977). Thus people will work hard to obtain food (an incentive) to satisfy a need.

Any event that modifies the strength of some response is called a reinforcer, and the operation of providing for the occurrence of the reinforcer is called **reinforcement.** Like incentives, reinforcers are either positive or negative. Any event that increases the probability of a recurrence of some response is a **positive reinforcer,** while any event that decreases the probability of recurrence of some response is considered punishment or a negative reinforcer.[1] The reinforcing effect refers to the role of a reinforcer in producing more or less permanent behavior changes (Bandura 1977). The critical temporal aspect of reinforcement is that it is administered *after* the behavior, and its application is contingent upon specific, appropriate behavior.

Effectiveness of Motivators

Incentives and reinforcers are both powerful means for influencing behavior, but before discussing the application of incentives and reinforcers, it may be well to examine a number of well-known factors that influence the effectiveness of these motivators. First, the person who is employing the motivators is known to be important. Incentives and reinforcers successfully used by coaches are frequently ineffective when used by parents and classroom teachers. In general, motivators are more effective when used by people who are highly esteemed and respected by an individual or a group.

---

[1] This definition of negative reinforcement differs from that commonly used in operant psychology, but there is a great deal of confusion in the psychological literature on this issue. Throughout this chapter we shall use the word *punishment* instead of *negative reinforcement* because we have a clearer general understanding of *punishment*.

Second, receptiveness to motivators varies with age. Young children are more receptive to verbal incentives and reinforcements than older ones. What is effective for one age group may strike another as "corny." There are also sex differences; several studies have found that females are more responsive to verbal exhortations than males are, which is probably related to parental socialization practices in which girls are talked to more than boys, beginning in infancy (Lewis 1972).

Third, since lower social class child-rearing practices differ from those of the middle and upper classes, differential responses to incentives and reinforcements can be expected, and have been documented. This same notion probably cuts across racial and ethnic backgrounds.

These are only a few of the numerous factors that influence the effectiveness of motivators. Recognizing this, one principle of human motivation should become quite clear: Individuals cannot be treated alike if one wishes to motivate them! What will be effective for one person will not be effective for another; what may have been effective at one time for an individual may not be effective at another time. The extreme complexity of motivating factors makes it impossible to set forth definite statements about which motivating techniques are the "best." Successful instructors must be aware of all these factors and use techniques that fit the different needs of the students as well as their own personalities. We shall now describe some of the motivational methods that have been studied.

Incentives

Although an incentive is viewed as a promise of a reward, previous experiences that involved reward affect present behavior because, after rewards have been employed, the individual acquires an *expectancy* that certain responses will be followed by a reward. The expected reward provides an incentive to perform those responses that will lead to the reward, or expected goal. Incentive theories assume that behavior is primarily energized by anticipation of reward or punishment consequences.

Many incentives have been used to induce people to perform. In industry, workers are constrained to work by the promise of more money or better working conditions. In school, students are enticed by the promise of good grades for high performance. Athletes may be promised medals, trophies, or public recognition for outstanding performances. In all cases, though, it appears that an essential condition for incentives to affect behavior is that the individual recognize and evaluate the incentive and generate goals or intentions in response to the evaluation.

Verbal Exhortations

Perhaps the most frequently used incentive in motor skills instructional settings is **verbal exhortation.** The verbal learning literature is replete with studies showing that verbal exhortation is useful in bringing about enhanced verbal performance and learning, but there is a scarcity of research on the incentive effects of verbal exhortation in motor behavior; consequently there are wide differences of opinion regarding this topic. It seems likely that verbal exhortation will be effective as an incentive, if the performers are not exerting maximum effort.

Research in the fields of industrial and sports psychology suggest that the urgings of supervisors and coaches can bring about enhanced performance, but the effects on learning are still inconclusive. Urging for greater effort will have a more beneficial effect when the task being performed involves strength, speed, or endurance than if the task is complex; in the latter case verbal exhortation may push the arousal level of the performer beyond the optimal state for best performance.

Competition

Competition has been found to be a powerful incentive, and physical educators, coaches, and employers have used it as a favorite incentive technique. Competition serves as an incentive because its outcomes meet a variety of individual needs, especially in a society whose core value orientation is the exaltation of the successful competitor—the winner. Studies of the effects of competition upon motor performance have shown that competition between individuals and groups tends to enhance performance in a variety of tasks and for various age groups (Scanlan 1978; Carron 1980).

These results have led to a general assumption that competition is a reliable means of improving performance, but the disturbing fact is that in some cases competition does not improve performance (Lloyd and Voor 1973). There are a number of possible reasons why competition may not enhance performance and may even reduce performance efficiency. Neurophysiological evidence indicates that competition tends to increase arousal; whether the competition enhances or decreases performance will depend on the level of arousal it produces. If the increased arousal produces a state near the optimal level for performance of that task, performance will be enhanced. If it pushes the arousal state beyond optimal for performance on that task, a decrement in performance will occur.

Competition is an effective incentive if the participants believe that they have a chance to win. If they do not believe they have a chance to win, it frequently is not an effective incentive—the participants may either refuse to compete or compete in a halfhearted fashion. Competition among people or groups of nearly equal skill produces better peformance than among those of unequal skill. If winning is a matter of skill, interest and effort decline rapidly when the same person or group wins consistently. Moreover, persistent losing in a competitive situation may be reflected in a significant decline in both positive self-concept and favorable body image (Rosenberg 1979).

The incentive effects of competition have complex dimensions to which we cannot devote space in this volume. But one final aspect of competition as an incentive deserves note. Competition in a sport setting often takes the performers' attention from the main purpose of performing a task well and focuses it upon an outside goal—winning at any cost. Documentation for this can be seen in many organized sports programs.

Threats of Force

There is little question that threats of force serve as a powerful incentive, and there are situations wherein they may have to be used. But while immediate performance may be enhanced by threats of force, it may also be impaired if the fear and anxiety created by the threats excites the performer to an extremely high arousal state. Moreover, two potential long-term adverse outcomes of this method of incentive are frequently evident. First, it often creates an overdependence on the instructor. Some people may function in such a state of fear of the instructor that they cease to show initiative and imagination for fear that the leader may disapprove and punish them. These students rarely perform with a spontaneous enthusiasm for the activity. Second, threat tends to create resentment. Invariably, individuals who are threatened believe that they are being treated unfairly, and cooperation is difficult to obtain. So if threat of force is to be used, it must be used wisely and discreetly.

Goal Setting

Goals serve as incentives, and people will expend great effort to achieve them. There are two basic ways in which **goal setting** is accomplished: Goals can be set by someone other than the person performing the task, in which case they are called "other-identified performance goals," or goals can be set by the performer, or a group of performers, in which case they are called "self-identified performance goals." In both cases there is considerable evidence to support the view that goals and intentions are important determinants of task performance (see Mitchell 1979 for a review).

The initial theory and research of goal setting was done by Locke and Bryan (Locke and Bryan 1966a; 1966b; Bryan and Locke 1967; Locke 1968). In one study, subjects performed a complex hand-eye coordination task and were either allowed simply to "do their best" or given a goal corresponding to their previous best score plus a fixed increment above the subjects' best

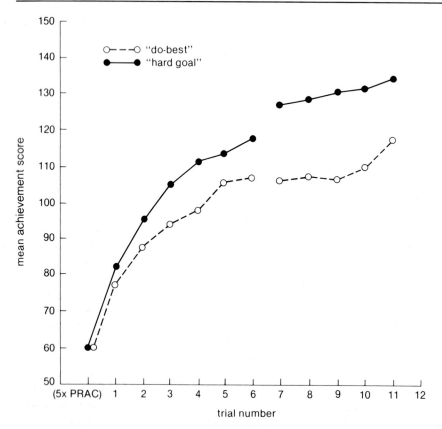

Figure 21.1 *Performance curves for two groups provided with different goals for performing a complex hand-eye coordination task. Subjects in the Do Best group were just told to "do your best." Subjects in the Hard Goal group were given a goal that was an increment above their best previous performance.*

previous score. The findings showed that setting a specific standard ("hard goals") led to both a faster rate of improvement and an overall higher standard (Locke and Bryan 1966a) (figure 21.1). A number of subsequent studies have shown that having goals results in higher performance than not having goals (Mitchell 1979). In general, also, it appears that setting difficult goals results in higher performance than setting easy goals (Campbell and Ilgen 1976; London and Oldham 1976; Yukl and Latham 1978).

Evidence from industrial psychology shows that when workers are asked to establish their own goals, they set higher goals than management expects, and they reach those goals at a better rate than management-established goals (Gyllenhammar 1977; King, Streufert, and Fiedler 1978). If, for example, an individual or group is encouraged to establish a suitable goal for itself, striving toward that goal seems to spur the individual or group toward improved performance. The goal serves as an incentive for better performance, and when the goal is achieved it is quite rewarding.

In terms of meeting needs, participation in goal setting seems to involve two of the strongest social needs—self-esteem and social approval. Self-esteem comes into play when individuals feel that they are respected enough to be consulted about group decisions. Social approval acts through people feeling that their roles are important in the group's activity.

Using participation in self-identified and group-identified goals sometimes conflicts with the traditional viewpoints of many teachers and coaches regarding their assigned role and that of their students; teachers and coaches often want students to do as they are told rather than use their initiative. But the implications of work on self-identified and group-identified goals suggest that if individuals choose their own goals, they may produce better performance than when goals are set for them. Moreover, studies suggest that when people perceive themselves as voluntarily undertaking arduous tasks in order to achieve a goal, they tend to evaluate the tasks more highly than if they feel themselves to be coerced into performing the tasks.

Level of Aspiration and Self-Efficacy

Closely related to the topic of goal setting is level of aspiration. Here self-identified performance goals are set by the performer, but the unique concern is with previous performance on subsequent performance goals. A great deal of the incentive that motivates people comes from the consequences of their own behavior. When performance leads to successful accomplishment of a goal, or at least closely approaches the goal, it can serve to sustain, even improve, the same behavior at a subsequent time when the task must be performed.

Level of aspiration refers to the goal level individuals or groups set for themselves on a particular task—the belief that people have concerning their potential for performance. Investigations of level of aspiration usually involve two basic considerations: first, comparisons of the

effects of success or failure on estimations of future performance; second, comparisons between individuals' or groups' estimation of their performance and their actual performance.

Although it is not always possible to predict how success and failure will affect a person's aspiration about future performance, Cofer and Appley (1964) have proposed the most generally accepted generalizations. Simply stated, aspiration level is affected by past experience; successful performance tends to lead to an increase in the level of aspiration, or standard of excellence; failure tends to lead to a decrease in aspiration level; and people with high aspirations perform at high levels. These generalizations have been confirmed with individuals on a wide variety of motor tasks (Clawson 1965; Harari 1969) and with selected groups (Zander 1971).

More recently, Bandura (1977) has proposed a theory of self-efficacy to account for cognitive variables in performance. According to this notion, behavior change is mediated by a cognitive mechanism—**self-efficacy**—that is considered to be the strength of conviction that the performer can successfully execute a behavior required to accomplish a particular task. Accordingly, efficacy expectations "determine how much effort people will expend and how long they will persist in the face of obstacles and aversive experiences" (Bandura 1977). Self-efficacy theory proposes that actual performance will be predicted by the belief in the individual's own personal competence. Of course, the importance of skill level or other factors is not discounted by Bandura. Several studies have demonstrated support for self-efficacy in the area of motor behavior (Feltz, Landers, and Raeder 1979; Weinberg, Gould, and Jackson 1979; Weinberg, Yukelson, and Jackson 1980).

The implications of the works on aspiration level and self-efficacy for teaching motor skills are rather clear. It is apparent that an important job of the motor skills instructor is to manipulate the environment so that successful experiences can regularly be achieved by the performers. These kinds of experiences are most beneficial in developing self-confidence, which in turn leads to enhanced performance.

Reinforcement

The basis of reinforcement theory goes back to E. L. Thorndike's (1911) proposal known as the "law of effect." This idea postulates that those responses that occur in a situation and that lead to "satisfaction" will tend to be repeated when the situation recurs, whereas those responses that do not lead to satisfaction will not be strengthened. Other psychologists refined reinforcement theory during the first half of this century. But it was B. F. Skinner of Harvard who extended and elaborated Thorndike's law of effect into what has become known as operant psychology, a modern reinforcement theory.

The basic notion behind reinforcement theory is that reinforcement of a response produces a repetition in the response on subsequent occasions. When this happens, the reinforcer is said to be a positive reinforcer. When the reinforcement produces a cessation of a response, it is said to be a punisher. Thus, in the sense that positive reinforcements lead to meeting certain needs, they have a positive or attractive influence and lead to satisfaction. Punishment satisfies needs in the sense that the body has a need to escape painful or unpleasant stimuli. Since we tend to move toward positive reinforcers and away from punishment, we might view ourselves as being drawn toward certain behaviors and pushed away from others. There are, then, two ways of influencing behavior with reinforcers, one associated with reward and another with punishment. Reinforcers are either material or symbolic and are given *after* certain behavior has been emitted.

Positive Reinforcers

It is necessary to note at the outset of this section that no effort will be made to discuss the reinforcement effects of feedback on motor behavior. This was covered in chapter 18.

One of the most frequently employed types of reinforcement is positive reinforcers, which can be social (praise, smiles) or material (money, candy, trophies). They are commonly referred to as rewards. Typically, the reinforcer is applied immediately after a response and it is, of course, contingent upon appropriate behavior. Extensive programs employing reinforcement techniques have been employed in clinical psychology, schools, mental hospitals, and prisons under the label of "behavior modification" programs. Many remarkable stories have been recounted about the successes in using various kinds of positive reinforcers. Several publications have introduced behavioral modification techniques into the teaching of motor activities (Rushall and Siedentop 1972; Siedentop 1976; Dickinson 1977).

Both social and material reinforcement research on verbal behavior has been much more prevalent than studies examining the effect of reinforcement on motor behavior. Of those studies that have been done with motor behavior, positive social and tangible reinforcement of various types has been found to be effective in enhancing the response rate of subjects performing tasks that emphasize speed, rate, and other quantitative responses. However, studies in which tasks emphasizing accuracy, fine motor control, and other qualitative responses were used have found that reinforcement had little influence on the early performance trials of these tasks (Martens, Burwitz, and Newell 1972; McCaughan and Gimbert 1981). In physical education and sport settings, several studies demonstrate that positive operant reinforcement is a viable instructional technique for developing and maintaining motor skill proficiency (see Donahue, Gillis, and King 1980 for a review of this topic).

Early studies with sport performers in which systematic programs of reinforcement were employed dealt with competitive swimming and employed social reinforcers such as attention and praise to increase attendance and the number of laps swum each day (McKinzie and Rushall 1974). Others have extended the use of reinforcement to a number of sport settings. In general, the studies demonstrate that positive reinforcement is a successful technique for enhancing sports skills performance (Komaki and Barnett 1977; Buzas and Ayllon 1981).

Even though there is empirical support for positive reinforcement in motor behavior settings, one must be cautious about its usefulness in any specific situation. Nevertheless, it seems clear that supportive and encouraging signs (as reinforcers) by an instructor create a favorable interpersonal atmosphere among participants and instructor. This social environment is rarely measured in laboratory studies, but it is present, and important, in dynamic settings where motor tasks are performed. And there is evidence that where a favorable social climate exists, participants enjoy their experiences and wish to continue their relationship with people in that group.

Positive reinforcers seem to be effective in producing feelings of satisfaction and pleasure on the part of the recipient of these rewards. However, there is always the danger that when the reinforcers that have been employed to reward appropriate behavior are withdrawn, the appropriate behavior may cease. This will be discussed in more detail in a later section of this chapter.

Reward techniques may also lead to resentment. When individuals are performing in response to rewards that are manipulated by a leader, they frequently come to understand that they are actually being tricked into performing—much like the dog who sits up for a morsel of food. Although dogs never seem to resent this trickery, humans do because they perceive this form of behavior control as an insinuation that they are unintelligent and naive. Many instructors fail to understand this phenomenon and are completely at a loss to understand why individuals or teams sometimes suddenly lose enthusiasm or fail to perform at all in response to rewards that are being offered.

Punishment

Conceptual confusion exists throughout the literature on reinforcement about the distinction between negative reinforcement and punishment. Rather than getting bogged down in this definitional issue, we have used only the word punishment and use it to mean the application of an aversive stimulus or event after a response, which decreases the frequency of the behavior that preceded it. Punishment can be social (reproof, frowns) or material (physical assault, shock). Punishment is a commonly used technique in behavior control, but it is also the most controversial and complex of the reinforcement methods and is generally disavowed.

Research on the effects of punishment on behavior indicates that it is usually an effective means of stopping unwanted behavior. It is effective in the short run, but it tends to produce various undesirable by-products. In an extensive review of the literature some fifteen years ago, Parke (1969) stated:

Punishment can be an effective means of controlling behavior. The operation of punishment, however, is a complex process and its effects are quite varied and highly dependent on such parameters as timing, intensity, consistency, and affectional and/or status relationship between the agent and recipient of punishment, and the kind of cognitive structuring accompanying the punishment stimulus.

More recent reviews have come to essentially the same conclusions (Walters and Grusec 1977).

Aside from the issue of the effects of punishment on learning and performance, this form of reinforcement has the potential for a number of unintended consequences. Fear and phobias may be produced by punishments that produce a great deal of pain, for example. In addition, a regular program of punishment is likely to foster resentment on the part of the recipient of the punishment against the person doing the punishing. In this case, while remarkable behavioral control can be maintained by an instructor through the employment of punishers, this may produce dislike on the part of the performer, not only for the administrator of the punishment, but also for the entire activity or situation in which it occurs. Thus, motor skills instructors who resort to frequent use of punishment to control performers' behavior may indirectly produce a general dislike for the instructors as well as an abhorrence for the motor skills they are teaching.

While positive reinforcers are typically employed in a rational way, punishment is frequently employed irrationally without consideration of its potential effects. In an instructional situation it is often employed when instructors are frustrated because the students have not performed up to the instructor's expectations. Frustration often leads to aggressive behavior, and punishment is a form of aggressive behavior that people use to alleviate their frustrations. Unfortunately, when punishment is used this way it can merely frustrate and anger the people being punished, rather than motivate them toward appropriate behavior.

Of course, there are occasions when punishment may have to be used. People of all ages continually explore limits; if there are none, behavior can get out of hand. Rushall and Siedentop (1972) suggest a guideline for the application of punishment: "When punishment must be used it should be specific, have minimal emotionality attached to it, should be relatively severe, and should always be applied consistently." It might also be added that punishment highlights what *not* to do. When punishment is used, a good teaching procedure is to describe an alternative response that would be appropriate, since punishment itself does not specify what is the appropriate behavior.

Vicarious Reinforcement

Vicarious reinforcement occurs when the behavior of an individual is influenced as a result of observing someone else's behavior and the reinforcement that follows. This kind of social influence has been found to be important in influencing behavior of the observer. People, especially young people, model their behavior after others, and a number of researchers have shown that children and youths imitate the behaviors of adults. It is common to see, for example, youngsters imitate the techniques of successful performers.

One of the critical factors that affects the degree of imitation of a model by young observers is the consequences of the model's behavior. In general, if the model is given positive reinforcement for certain behaviors, young observers tend to emulate these same behaviors when given the chance; when the model receives punishment, these behaviors are suppressed by those witnessing them. Another important factor affecting the influence that an adult model has on a young observer is the perceived power and prestige of the model. In general, the greater these perceived characteristics, the greater the imitation that takes place (Gould and Roberts 1981).

Instructors of motor skills need to be aware that their own behavior is being observed closely by those whom they are instructing. Since they are perceived as powerful and prestigious people by young people, their behaviors will be emulated. While the cliche, "Don't do as I do, do as I say," may give an instructor a convenient excuse for not setting a good example, it is not likely to be heeded. "Teaching by example rather than by precept" seems to be a more appropriate teaching model in terms of what is known about vicarious reinforcement.

Summary

Behavior is normally directed toward a goal, and the goal of motivated behavior is the meeting of some need or needs of the individual. Human needs have been classified into two general categories, biological and social. Biological needs are unlearned and fulfill a survival function, while social needs are learned through interactions with the environment. Once learned, social needs can be as essential to the maintenance of normal health as biological needs.

Regardless of the need structure, various manipulations and controls can be administered to induce an individual to behave in a certain way to satisfy needs. Commonly used motivational techniques are the employment of incentives and reinforcements. Incentives are objects, conditions, or stimuli, either material or symbolic, that produce a state of arousal in individuals so that they will approach or withdraw from the object, condition, or stimulus. Any event that modifies the strength of some response is called a reinforcer. A number of factors influence the effectiveness of incentives and reinforcers.

Several of the most frequently used incentives are verbal exhortations, competition, threats of force, goal setting, aspirations, and self-efficacy. Each has been found to be effective with individuals and groups.

Reinforcers are given after certain behavior has been emitted. Positive reinforcers produce a repetition in a given response on subsequent occasions. There is considerable evidence that positive reinforcement is an effective means for enhancing motor learning and performance. Punishment is an aversive means of controlling behavior. Research indicates that it is usually an effective means of stopping unwanted behavior, but it tends to produce various undesirable side effects.

A great deal of learning is the result of observing others' behavior. Young people are particularly susceptible to the influence of older people, whose behavior they will model, especially if an older person's behavior is seen to lead to positive reinforcement.

22

Phases of Motor Skill Acquisition and Instructional Techniques

The main focus of this text has been on helping the reader understand the mechanisms, processes, and factors involved in motor control and learning. An underlying assumption is that understanding a subject must precede applying the subject to specific situations. One of the very obvious applications of motor behavior subject matter is teaching motor skills to learners. But understanding the processes and factors involved in learning and performance simply is not the same as knowing how to *help* people learn and perform. As one of America's first notable psychologists, William James, said over eighty years ago:

> You make a great mistake if you think psychology . . . is something from which you can deduce definite programs and . . . methods of instruction for immediate . . . use. Psychology is a science, and teaching is an art; and sciences never generate arts directly out of themselves. An intermediary inventive mind must make the application by using its originality (James 1899).

Although great advances have been made in psychology, and specifically in understanding motor behavior, James' comments are as valid today as they were in his time.

An understanding of motor behavior does not automatically lead to knowing how to apply this knowledge to an instructional situation, and, although this is not a "methods of instruction" text, it seems appropriate to devote this last chapter to a discussion of instructional techniques, since many readers aspire to be instructors of motor activities.

General Principles of Instruction

The primary job of an instructor is to optimize learning. This is done by creating optimal conditions for learning. Having said this, it is important to emphasize at the beginning of this discussion that there is a "first principle" that must be etched in the mind of every instructor: There is no such thing as *the* way to teach; there is no *best* methodology in teaching. This is true for at least two reasons. First, there are at least four components to the teaching-learning process: the learner, teacher, task, and situation. It has become increasingly evident that learners do not all respond to the same methodology equally well. Like individual differences of other kinds, there are important differences in learning styles (Gregorc 1979; Hunt 1979). To say that learners differ in **learning style** means that certain instructional approaches are more effective than others for certain individuals.

Not only are there differences in learning styles, but there are differences in **teaching styles** consisting of personal behaviors and media used to transmit data to the learner (Gregorc 1979). Variations in teaching style affect the learning process. There is also an incredible variety of motor tasks, everything from fine, manipulative to gross, ballistic tasks; obviously, instructional techniques must be adapted to these variations. Finally, motor learning situations vary from swimming pools to gymnasiums to assembly lines to physical therapists' offices. Instructional techniques must be modified to take into account the learning environment.

A second reason why there is no one way to teach is that there are immediate consequences and long-term consequences in the use of particular instructional techniques. An effective instructional technique for one may not be effective for the other. For example, the use of artificial guidance appliances, such as harnesses and golfers grooves, that force the learner through a correct movement pattern may produce rapid initial performance increments but actually hamper learning.

Facilitating Motor Learning

Instructional strategies must be adapted to variations in learning and teaching styles, the task(s) being taught, and the environment in which the teaching-learning is occurring. While no specific recipe for skill instruction will be universally appropriate, the various responsibilities of the skills instructor have been enumerated by Arnold (1981):

The responsibilities of the teacher include identifying the goal of the activity and the environmental constraints on performance, structuring the practice situation, directing the learner's attention to critical environmental cues, assisting in movement organization, and providing augmented feedback to assist the learner in evaluating the effect of the selected response. As learning progresses, the teacher must guide the learner toward developing larger units of movement, achieving appropriate timing within and among components of movement, refining anticipatory skills, and effectively using proprioceptive feedback as well as visual information to evaluate the outcome of a response.

From the standpoint of learners, they typically go through several general phases as they acquire a motor skill. Each phase presents particular problems and challenges to learners and each has unique implications for the employment of instructional strategies. Several motor behavior scientists have identified certain phases of motor learning, but the actual number has varied.

The late Paul Fitts (1965), a pioneer in the development of the study of motor behavior, identified three phases of skill learning: An early (or cognitive) phase, an intermediate (or associative) phase, and a final (or autonomous) phase. These phases were derived from a study by Alfred Smode, who interviewed physical educators and coaches and asked them questions about the acquisition of sports skills. Gentile (1972) proposed that motor skill learning involves two stages, an initial skill-acquisition stage and a fixation/diversification stage. Adams (1971) also proposed two stages, a verbal-motor stage and a motor stage. Finally, Welford (1976) enumerated five stages in the motor learning process. It can be seen that the *actual* number of phases is somewhat arbitrary. In this chapter the three phases identified by Fitts will be used as a model, but a synthesis of ideas from the others will be incorporated into the description.

Phases of Motor Skill Learning

Before describing the three phases of motor learning identified by Fitts, it must first be noted that skill learning is a continual process; it is a mistake to assume independent and distinct phases in skill learning. There are gradual shifts in the movement patterns of skills, and in the nature of the processes employed, as learning progresses. The movement pattern is gradually organized into larger units and toward hierarchical organization.

The term **hierarchical organization** implies that certain higher structures have overall responsibilities for the functions of the entire system, with lower structures serving subordinant roles in carrying out specific functions. It has already been noted that the nervous system can be viewed as a hierarchical system, with the lowest levels in the peripheral and spinal cord areas and the higher centers in the brain. Each level can act independently of other levels, but this is normally not the case; behavior initiated by the higher centers usually requires activity of the lower centers for its completion. There is, therefore, anatomical support for the notion of hierarchical organization of motor skills.

The Initial or Cognitive Phase

In the **cognitive phase of motor learning,** the novice must first understand the task and its demands. Three broad aspects of understanding are (1) the goal of the task, (2) the movements that will bring about accomplishment of the goal, and (3) the strategy that will work best to produce the desired movements. The learning of a skill does not begin when actual practice starts, but before, with a cognitive understanding of the motor task.

The notion that the initial step in motor learning involves the formation of some cognitive structure has been consistently proposed by motor behavior researchers (Bartlett 1932; Miller, Galanter, and Pribram 1960; Adams 1971; Schmidt 1975; Neisser 1976). The actual name for this cognitive mechanism of how the movements should look/feel/sound if the task is performed correctly has been quite varied. Some examples are: **cognitive map,** cognitive plans, cognitive model, and template.

After the first few years of life, an individual begins the acquisition of a skill with a background of many already existing and highly developed abilities and specific skills. When one learns to swim, the skill is learned against a complex of existing movement patterns. For example, a person knows how to kick, to move his arms around, and to breathe before actually going into the water. So motor skill acquisition involves building new movement patterns out of already existing skill patterns. Rarely is an entirely new skill learned; instead, it is put together out of an existing repertoire of skills.

The effects of these prior skills on the acquisition of new skills are especially important in this cognitive phase of motor skill acquisition because past experience provides the raw material out of which the learner comes to understand the new skill. The transfer of schema, methods of performance, and appropriate strategies, which are a product of previously learned skills, are related to the new skill.

Based on the cognitive understanding that is developed, the next step is the selection of an appropriate motor program, with the specific parameters for movement execution (a recall schema), which produces movement for the first practice trial. This motor program relies heavily upon previously learned tasks in ordering the execution of motor commands. Orders tend to be brief and incomplete, making movements jerky and inefficient. But as the learner obtains feedback, motor programs tend to become more complete and appropriate for task accomplishment. These programs then produce smoother and more efficient and effective movement patterns. Since the motor commands become more elaborate, producing longer and longer movement sequences, the learner has only to monitor occasionally the actions, thus being freed to perform other tasks during movement.

Once a motor program has been selected, response specifications determined, the motor command implemented, and the movement sequence executed, the next important step for the learner is to verify that the plan has been carried out as intended and that it was successful at achieving the goal. Feedback is critical here. Feedback from the movement is compared with the plan or desired outcome. When discrepancies exist between the action and the plan, the motor programs (or recall schema) can be modified to produce a more appropriate movement pattern on the next practice trial. Proficiency on a task, then, is accomplished by matching the plan of action with feedback from the movement, and learning by response consequences is largely a cognitive process.

The way in which the learner constructs the cognitive plan (or recall schema) is important. Learners who have difficulty forming an accurate plan of what is required will not be able to achieve the desired results, regardless of how much they practice. Many failures to learn are due to failures to perceive (or comprehend) what has to be learned, rather than any difficulty of registering or holding material in memory.

Several motor behavior scientists have emphasized the importance of learner verbalization in the early phase of motor learning. Motor skills learners can, covertly or overtly, verbalize with themselves in several ways. They can actually describe what they are attempting to do before practicing, they may talk themselves through a performance, and they can verbally provide feedback to themselves after a performance. This allows the learners to arrive at a conceptualization, or plan, of the task to be learned.

According to Schmidt (1975), learners acquire skills by comparing expected and actual sensory consequences of the movement and then verbally labeling the error. The labeled error is viewed as subjective reinforcement. A similar view is expressed by Adams (1971) that individuals consciously, but covertly, use verbal responses during the early phase of learning. For this reason, he called this phase the verbal-motor stage. Two lines of evidence support this view. Evidence that people who are high in verbal competence tend to perform better on certain motor tasks during the early stages of learning has been demonstrated (Adams 1969). Also, the use of verbal labels during practice results in greater motor memory for movement (Shea 1977). Thus, much of the improvement in skill during the cognitive phase can be viewed as verbal-cognitive in nature, with the major improvements being in terms of what to do, rather than in the movement patterns themselves.

The cognitive phase of motor learning can be accomplished in a few moments or a few weeks, depending upon such factors as the complexity of the task, prior experience with similar tasks, perceptual abilities, and frequency of practice. It is during this stage that various forms of instructions to the learners are most effective. Although an instructor can communicate the general strategy to be used, it remains for the learners to supply the detailed tactics of using individual muscle groups for carrying out the plan with their own muscles.

Instructional Techniques

An instructor is certainly not necessary for an individual who wishes to learn a motor skill. Many motor skills that each of us has acquired have been learned without the presence of an instructor, usually in a laborious trial-and-error manner. However, skills can be learned more expediently with effective instruction. One of the key contributions of a capable instructor is to enhance the learning rate and the ultimate proficiency level of a learner.

Just as the first step for the learner in acquiring a skill is to understand the task and its demands, the first instructional techniques employed by the instructor should be focused on clarifying the goal of the task, identifying subgoals and their relationships to the goal of task execution, and describing the environmental constraints under which the task is typically performed. There are three basic means by which these instructional tasks can be carried out: visually, audibly, and manually. Each has unique contributions to make, and each may be more or less effective with different learners. Moreover, the task to be learned may lend itself to employment of one or the other of these communication channels.

It is generally accepted that some form of demonstration is the most direct and economical technique of communicating the task to the learner. A demonstration provides a visual model—a model that can be internalized into a cognitive plan of action.

Bandura (1977) has noted:

Behavior is learned symbolically through central processing of response information before it is performed. By observing a model of the desired behavior, an individual forms an idea of how response components must be combined and sequenced to produce the new behavior. In other words, people guide their actions by prior motions rather than by relying on outcomes to tell them what they must do.

The capacity to learn by observation enables learners to acquire integrated patterns of movement without having to undergo tedious trial-and-error practice.

Observational learning studies have demonstrated that visual observation of another's performance facilitates motor learning (see chapter 17 for a detailed discussion of this topic). Skillful demonstration models motivate increased imitation by learners and direct more attentional processes toward the model's behavior. This suggests

that models who have high competence, who are purported experts, who demonstrate a high level of ability, and who possess status-conferring symbols are more likely to command attention and serve as more influential sources of behavior than models who lack these qualities. It seems, then, that demonstrations should be performed as well as possible even though a beginner will not be able to perceive all of the details, nor be able to imitate a demonstration in detail in the initial practice trials.

In some cases, a demonstration can be done through the use of loop films or videotapes. The amount of information can be controlled this way and repeated as often as the learner seems to need it. Although there is little empirical work on the speed (or tempo) at which a demonstration should be performed, some writers suggest that the demonstration should be given at performance speed. However, if the objective of the demonstration is to show the sequence of the movement pattern, the demonstrator should emphasize that the learners look for this sequence; slowing down the tempo of the demonstration may be helpful in this case. But when the spatial and temporal organization is being emphasized, a demonstration of normal speed seems appropriate.

Auditory communication with learners may be the most used and abused mode for transmitting information, especially to the beginner. Not only is there a tendency for instructors to overdo verbal descriptions, but there is also some evidence that a great deal of the verbalization is not related to task objectives. Schwartz (1972) analyzed statements made by fifteen teachers during instruction and found that only 1.3 percent of the more than two thousand statements were related to the objective of the lesson.

While verbal description has a place in assisting the learner to develop a cognitive map, we actually know very little about its effectiveness in facilitating learning. Several factors have to be considered with regard to the amount of verbalization, such as the complexity of the skill, maturity of the learners, and comprehension level of the learners. Nevertheless, verbalization is well suited for directing attention to specific aspects of the task, helping to establish a learning set, giving feedback, and motivating learning.

Another communication tool for instruction is manual guidance. When this technique is used, the learner is guided through the task by either the instructor or some mechanical apparatus. Guidance techniques are based on the notion that they prevent learning of inappropriate movements and increase the rate of learning.

It would appear that a major advantage of manually guiding learners through a motor skill is that it is a potential medium for helping them achieve a cognitive map of the task. The few studies in which this technique has been employed do not concur in their findings. Nonetheless, motor skill manuals are filled with various suggestions of where to employ this technique: only in the early learning stages, with slow learners rather than fast learners, with young students, and so on. These suggestions are merely speculations, rather than conclusions based on experimental findings.

As we noted in chapter 11, there is no evidence that manual guidance actually *hinders* motor learning. So perhaps the best generalization is that it can be used as a last resort when learners lack confidence to perform on their own, when they are having difficulty developing a cognitive map through other communication media, or when they are visually or aurally restricted.

In addition to actually communicating with the learner, the instructor has the critical task during the initial stage of learning of directing the learner's attention to a limited and specific set of stimuli. This is important for two reasons: First, novice learners typically cannot distinguish between relevant and irrelevant stimuli associated with a new task. Second, the typical motor learning environment—the gymnasium, playing field, and industrial plant—has an enormous number of distracting stimuli. With so many stimuli, it is not unusual for learners to have difficulty understanding directions and demonstrations from the instructor.

With regard to controlling stimuli, it is the instructor's responsibility to reduce the amount of irrelevant stimuli in a learning situation so the student will be free to concentrate attention on the relevant stimuli. If the learner's attention is not directed to appropriate stimuli, communication of any kind will be ineffective. One method of directing attention and limiting stimuli is for instructors to present the general movement demands, rather than the details of the movements, in their initial communications to the learner. As the learner practices and becomes more adroit, the details of the task and the tactics associated with its use can be added gradually.

One technique that the instructor might use when it is not possible to reduce the irrelevant stimuli is to call the learner's attention to what to look for—to point out which stimuli are relevant. Thus, one of the requirements of good motor skills instructors is that they know which information within the sensory display is worth attending to. For example, they might instruct learners to "keep your eyes on the ball" because they think that this is the most important source of information in the display.

As noted in earlier chapters, there is good evidence that learners have limited information-processing capabilities. Therefore, the amount of material and the speed with which it is presented to learners should be carefully controlled. Otherwise they will be unable to process the instructional information. Beginners who are given an elaborate explanation on how to execute a skill and who are asked to watch the details of a demonstration at the same time may not process all the information simply because they are not capable of doing so.

Once the preresponse period is complete and the learner begins the initial practice trials, the role of the instructor becomes one of movement diagnosis and movement prescription (this role is discussed in some detail in chapter 18). The instructor must be a careful observer of movement and provider of appropriate feedback. To suggest that feedback is essential in the cognitive phase of learning would be to state the obvious. The topic of feedback has appeared in several places throughout the book and was the subject of chapter 18, so a discussion of specific ways and means of employing feedback will not be presented here.

Associative or Intermediate Phase

The **associative,** or intermediate, **phase of motor learning** can be characterized as a period during which the movements begin to fuse into well-coordinated movement patterns. Spatial and temporal organization becomes fixed, and the motor program becomes more fully developed. Components of the movement pattern, independent at first, become fused and integrated as the interrelated aspects of the task are refined. Extraneous movements are eliminated and gross errors gradually attenuated.

It is in this phase that the effect of previously learned movement responses can affect the rate of learning of the new skill most markedly. If the new movement pattern requires a response opposite to a previously learned movement pattern when the stimulus situation is similar, the rate of learning may be slowed, a so-called negative transfer of skill. But if the new skill requires similar motor responses to similar stimulus situations, rate of learning will be enhanced, and positive transfer is said to occur. This topic is discussed in detail in chapter 19.

Proprioceptive feedback appears to become increasingly important after extended motor practice, and there is less reliance on visual cues as learning of a motor task progresses. The shifting nature of abilities that underlie performance is discussed in chapter 16, and the role of kinesthesis during motor skill acquisition is described in chapter 11.

For closed skills, wherein performance takes place in a stable, constant environment, the learner attempts gradually to reduce the variability in the movement pattern to achieve consistently the desired movements. On the other hand, for open skills, since various movements must be used to accomplish the desired goal, diverse movement patterns need to be practiced in an effort to learn to match the variable environmental contexts to appropriate movements.

While emphasis has been given to cognitive activity on the part of the learner during the initial phase of skill acquisition, it should not be inferred that cognitive factors are unimportant in the succeeding phases. Human learners are active problem solvers, decision makers, and processors of information, so cognitive factors do not diminish in their influence with practice (Adams 1981).

The length of time this phase lasts will vary considerably. In learning a skill such as serving a tennis ball, some novices may show rapid improvement, while others flounder along with little improvement for a long time before their performance improves appreciably. Such factors as prior experience with similar skills, complexity of the skill, practice schedules, teaching methods, feedback, and motivation of the learner will determine the length of this phase of skill learning.

Instructional Techniques

The instructor should know enough about the component parts of the skill being taught to be able to identify movement errors and prescribe corrections. When the instructor does not possess this error-detection proficiency, feedback information will be based on faulty diagnoses and have little chance for promoting learning. This role of **movement diagnostician** and **movement prescriptor** is at the heart of teaching motor activities, and the ability to identify correctly and precisely movement errors and communicate accurate instructions for corrective actions is the mark of a competent instructor.

The same communication media that were available and useful during the cognitive phase can be employed at this phase. Demonstrations are especially useful at this stage for showing tactics, if the skill is to be used in a game. In addition, learners can serve as their own demonstrators via the replay of their performance on film or videotape.

Figure 22.1   *The effects of instruction on learning a tracking task. The task required subjects to keep a dot in the center of an oscillograph display while at the same time trying to keep a pointer centered on an instrument dial.*

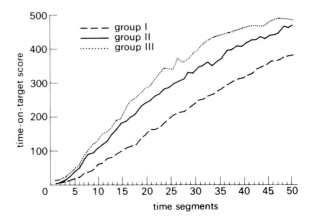

As learning progresses, verbal descriptions, analyses, and various verbal cues come to be more meaningful to learners because they have enough comprehension of the objectives of the task and its demands to utilize verbal information. Even the sounds associated with the execution of the skill—the "swish" of the tennis racket, the "click" of the golf club—begin to provide meaningful auditory information to the learner.

The advantage of modifying verbal guidance as learning progresses was nicely shown by Parker and Fleishman (1961). Three groups of subjects learned a complex tracking task under different guidance methods. Group One received no formal guidance at all; Group Two received "common-sense," or traditional, guidance, and Group Three received the same guidance as Group Two but also received special guidance at certain points in the learning process. For Group Three, the visual-spatial aspects of the task were emphasized in the early learning, kinesthetic-coordination aspects were emphasized later in the learning, and knowledge of various task components was emphasized near the end of learning. Group Three performed best throughout the study (figure 22.1). These results suggest that different verbal emphases may be more appropriate during different stages of learning.

Since skill acquisition problems are quite different for open and closed skills, instructional techniques—especially feedback—must be adapted to the types of skills being taught. In chapter 18 this issue is discussed in detail. Suffice to say here that both knowledge of results (KR) and knowledge of performance (KP) can be used with both types of skills, but the instructor needs to be particularly attuned to the use of KR with open skills and KP with closed skills. The instructor needs to have prepared well for the application of the appropriate feedback.

As noted in chapter 17, mental practice has been found to be an effective means of promoting motor learning in a wide variety of tasks. The introduction of covert rehearsal of the movement patterns seems to be appropriate in this phase since, presumably, the learner will have developed an understanding of the task and now needs the benefits that practice, both physical and mental, can bring.

Since the proficiency of a group of learners can become more heterogeneous as they practice, it behooves instructors increasingly to individualize their instruction. Close observation of individual learners will enable instructors to identify individual problems and prescribe corrections.

Autonomous Phase

The final, or **autonomous, phase of motor learning** occurs as the spatial and temporal aspects of the skill become highly organized and component processes become increasingly autonomous. There is a development of motor programs of increasing length and integration. As the movement pattern becomes automatic, conscious introspection about the component parts of the pattern during this phase of learning often results in the "paralysis from analysis" phenomenon.

Of course, occasionally learners may have to use a component analysis of their movement pattern if they wish to improve further their proficiency or correct an error that has crept into their execution. Temporal organization tends to be the last organizational characteristic of skilled behavior to be mastered by learners and it is the most fragile and most easily disrupted. Timing is usually the first aspect of a skill to be impaired under stressful conditions.

With practice, and as motor programs employed in performing a task become more consolidated, less attention needs to be given to movement execution. Stelmach (1980) notes: "As one progresses from an inexperienced to a skilled state, dramatic changes seem to occur in motor performance. Perhaps the most evident is the transition of motor control from a conscious mode to an automatic mode." One main advantage of this is that it allows the attentional mechanisms to be devoted to other stimuli in the environment.

Selective attention also becomes much more sophisticated at this stage. Highly skilled performers are able to reduce the amount of information to be processed and to focus attention on only the relevant aspects of the environment. According to Welford (1968), "Practice seems to enable the skilled performer to select from among the mass of data impinging on his sense organs so that he neglects much of what is, to an unskilled person, striking, and reacts strongly to data that a normal observer would fail to notice."

In the case of athletics, as beginners develop into skilled sports performers they also modify their selective attention in order to discriminate more precisely between accurate and false information. Indeed, perceiving the appropriate stimuli while the opposition is attempting to conceal and confuse is critical for skillful performance in most sports. Also, with increased experience sports performers must learn how to deceive their opposition with false (or irrelevant) information.

Much of the art of competitive play consists of misleading the opposition by confounding the display. As beginners develop into competent players, they learn both to deceive and to discriminate between accurate and false information. The "old pro" is not bothered by distractions (except in golf and tennis, where performers have come to expect no distractions) because during this phase the movement pattern is less directly subject to cognitive regulation, and less subject to interference from extraneous activities in the environment.

In the later stages of learning a closed motor skill, the emphasis is on refinement of technique. Practice involves repeated attempts to produce precisely the correct movement pattern. For open skills, the emphasis is on adaptation of movements to the various environmental conditions. One of the distinguishing characteristics of a skillful performer of an open skill is the ability to execute the skill in various ways depending on variations in the environment.

Old habits are remarkably resistant to new learning, and even in the autonomous stage of learning old movement patterns will occasionally reappear, usually during periods of stress. Swimmers who have recently changed their stroke and kick for greater efficiency frequently revert to their old movement pattern under the stress of competition. Basketball players who have recently changed their shooting movements for the jump shot may revert to their old shooting technique when confronted by a defensive player.

Instructional Techniques

Many of the instructional techniques employed during the previous phases can be used in this phase, with modifications to account for individual differences in learning style, task being learned, and particular problems of learners. The major responsibility of the instructor of highly skilled performers is to organize practice so proficiency continues to improve, provide appropriate feedback, and motivate for continued skill improvement. With both closed and open skills, ensuring that practice conditions simulate conditions under which actual performance will occur is important. In open skills, instructional emphasis should concentrate on developing the skill of learners to interpret environmental events so they can make quick and accurate decisions about which specific motor program, and its parameters, to employ. This can be done by providing the learner with opportunities to practice in a wide variety of situations that require many variations of the skill to meet the environmental demands.

Instructors continue to serve as movement diagnosticians and prescribers, frequently suggesting variations in a movement pattern for greater proficiency. They also must detect errors that may be reducing performance effectiveness. Finally, in sports, instructors serve as sources for strategy planning before competition and as tacticians during the contest.

A great deal of effective performance in sports depends upon the performers' ability to anticipate environmental stimuli, especially the relevant stimuli. Thus, anything that instructors can do to assist their performers to direct their attention to the relevant cues and anticipate them will be beneficial to their performance. Instructors can do this by providing performers with knowledge about typical tactics used by opponents and about certain movements that precede certain actions by the opponents. Arnold (1981) has described a method of structuring realistic practice of sports that she calls the "mini-game method." It involves a repeating cycle of game play, identification of an area of skill deficiency, mini-game practice drills, and application of the skill in game play (see Arnold for more details about the use of this method).

Summary

Although the main focus of this book has been on helping the reader understand the mechanisms, processes, and factors involved in motor control and learning, it seems appropriate to devote the last chapter to a discussion of instructional techniques, since many readers will be instructors of motor activities. The primary job of an instructor is to optimize learning, but there is no such thing as *the* way to teach. The four components to the teaching-learning process are the learner, teacher, task, and situation. The interaction of these components necessitates various instructional methodologies.

Learners typically go through several phases while learning a motor skill. In this chapter, the three phases identified by Fitts are used as a model. The three phases are: cognitive, associative, and autonomous. Each phase presents unique problems for both the learner and instructor.

The main task of the learner during the cognitive phase is to understand the goal of the task, movements to accomplish the goal, and the strategy that will produce the desired movements. In this phase the main task of the instructor is to help the learner understand the task through demonstrations, verbal descriptions, and manual guidance. Once the learner begins practicing, the instructor must provide appropriate feedback.

The associative phase is a period during which movements begin to fuse into well-coordinated movement patterns. The use of previously learned skills can often facilitate the learning of a new skill. Response-produced feedback is used by the learner to match the intended goal with the movements that are executed with each practice. Discrepancies necessitate modifications in motor programs to achieve the desired goal. Movement diagnosis and prescription are important functions of an instructor during this phase. Also, the use of mental practice can enhance learning rate.

During the autonomous phase, the learner has developed motor programs of increasing length and integration, and the spatial and temporal aspects of the skill are highly organized. Less attention needs to be given to movement execution, and selective attention becomes more sophisticated. The major role of the instructor of highly skilled performers is to organize practice so learning continues, provide appropriate feedback, and motivate the learner. In competitive motor activities the instructor also helps the learner with the tactics and strategies.

References

Abbs, J. H. "The Influence of the Gamma Motor System on Jaw Movements during Speech: A Theoretical Framework and Some Preliminary Observations." *Journal of Speech and Hearing Research* 16 (1973):175–200.

Abraham, L. D. "Neuronal Basis for Vestibulo-Proprioceptive Interactions in Motor Control." In D. M. Landers and R. W. Christina, eds. *Psychology of Motor Behavior and Sport, 1976.* Champaign, Ill.: Human Kinetics Publishers, 1977.

Adams. G. L. "Effect of Eye Dominance on Baseball Batting." *Research Quarterly* 36 (1965):3–9.

Adams, J. A. "Acquisition of Motor Responses." In M. H. Marx, ed. *Learning: Processes.* Toronto: Macmillan, 1969.

Adams, J. A. "A Closed-Loop Theory of Motor Learning." *Journal of Motor Behavior* 3 (1971):111–50.

Adams, J. A. "Issues for a Closed-Loop Theory of Motor Learning." In G. E. Stelmach, ed. *Motor Control: Issues and Trends.* New York: Academic Press, 1976a.

Adams, J. A. *Learning and Memory: An Introduction.* Homewood, Ill.: Dorsey Press, 1976b.

Adams, J. A. "Do Cognitive Factors in Motor Performance Become Nonfunctional with Practice?" *Journal of Motor Behavior* 13 (1981):262–73.

Adams, J. A., and Creamer, L. R. "Anticipatory Timing of Continuous and Discrete Responses." *Journal of Experimental Psychology* 63 (1962):84–90.

Adams, J. A., and Dijkstra, S. "Short-Term Memory for Motor Responses." *Journal of Experimental Psychology* 71 (1966):314–18.

Adams, J. A.; Gopher, D.; and Lintern, G. "Effects of Visual and Proprioceptive Feedback on Motor Learning." *Journal of Motor Behavior* 9 (1977):11–22.

Adams, J. A., and Hufford, L. E. "Contributions of a Part-Task Trainer to the Learning and Relearning of a Time-Shared Flight Maneuver." *Human Factors* 4 (1962):159–70.

Adams, J. A., and Reynolds, B. "Effect of Shift in Distribution of Practice Conditions Following Interpolated Rest." *Journal of Experimental Psychology* 47 (1954):32–36.

Alderson, G. J. K. "Variables Affecting the Perception of Velocity in Sports Situations." In H. T. A. Whiting, ed. *Readings in Sports Psychology* London: Henry Kimpton, 1972.

Allport, D. A.; Antonis, B.; and Reynolds, P. "On the Division of Attention: A Disproof of the Single Channel Hypothesis." *Quarterly Journal of Experimental Psychology* 24 (1972):225–35.

Ammons, R. B. "Effects of Knowledge of Performance: A Survey and Tentative Theroretical Formulation." *Journal of General Psychology* 54 (1956):279–99.

Ammons, R. B. "Le Mouvement." In G. H. Seward and J. P. Seward, eds. *Current Psychological Issues.* New York: Holt, Rinehart and Winston, 1958.

Andrew, B. L., and Dodt, E. "The Deployment of Sensory Nerve Endings at the Knee Joint of the Cat." *Acta Physiol. Scand.* 28 (1953):287–97.

Angel, R. W. "Efference Copy in the Control of Movement." *Neurology* 26 (1976):1164–68.

Arnold, R. K. S. *Developing Sport Skills.* Monograph 2, *Motor Skills: Theory Into Practice.* 1981.

Ascoli, K. M., and Schmidt, R. A. "Proactive Interference in Short-Term Motor Retention." *Journal of Motor Behavior* 1 (1969):29–35.

Ashby, A. A.; Shea, C. H.; and Tolson, H. "Memory Characteristics of Two-Dimensional Movement Information." *Research Quarterly for Exercise and Sport* 53 (1982):93–100.

Atkinson, R. C., and Shiffrin, R. M. "The Control of Short-Term Memory." *Scientific American* 225 (August 1971):82–90.

Bachman, J. C. "Specificity versus Generality in Learning and Performing Two Large Muscle Motor Tasks." *Research Quarterly* 32 (1961):3–11.

Bacon, S. J. "Arousal and the Range of Cue Utilization." *Journal of Experimental Psychology* 102 (1974):81–87.

Baddeley, A. D. "The Trouble with Levels: A Re-examination of Craik and Lockhart's Framework for Memory Research." *Psychological Review* 85 (1978):139–52.

Baker, K. E.; Wylie, R. C.; and Gagne, R. M. "Transfer of Training to a Motor Skill as a Function of Variation in Rate of Response." *Journal of Experimental Psychology* 40 (1950):721–32.

Bandura, A. "Self-Efficacy: Toward a Unifying Theory of Behavioral Change." *Psychological Review* 84 (1977):191–215.

Bandura, A. *Social Learning Theory.* Englewood Cliffs: Prentice-Hall, 1977.

Bannister, L. H. "Sensory Terminals of Peripheral Nerves." In D. W. Landon, ed. *The Peripheral Nerve.* London: Chapman and Hall, 1976.

Barclay, C. R., and Newell, K. M. "Children's Processing of Information in Motor Skill Acquisition." *Journal of Experimental Child Psychology* 30 (1980):98–108.

Barlow, H.; Blakemore, C. B.; and Pettigrew, J. D. "The Neural Mechanism of Binocular Depth Discrimination." *Journal of Physiology* 193 (1967):327–42.

Baron, R. S.; Moore, D.; and Sanders, G. S. "Distraction as a Source of Drive in Social Facilitation Research." *Journal of Personality and Social Psychology* 36 (1978):816–24.

Bartlett, F. C. *Remembering, A Study in Experimental and Social Psychology.* Cambridge: Cambridge University Press, 1932.

Bastian, H. C. "The 'Muscle Sense'; Its Nature and Cortical Localization." *Brain* 10 (1888):1–137.

Battig, W. F. "The Flexibility of Human Memory." In L. S. Cermak and F. I. M. Craik, eds. *Levels of Processing and Human Memory.* Hillsdale, N.J.: Erlbaum, 1979.

Beals R. P. et al. "The Relationship between Basketball Shooting Performance and Certain Visual Attributes." *American Journal of Optometry* 45 (1971):585–90.

Bell, V. L. "Augmented Knowledge of Results and Its Effect upon Acquisition and Retention of a Gross Motor Skill." *Research Quarterly* 39 (1968):25–30.

Beltel, P. A. "Multivariate Relationships among Visual-Perceptual Attributes and Gross-Motor Tasks with Different Environmental Demands." *Journal of Motor Behavior* 12 (1980):29–40.

Beverley, K. I., and Regan, D. "Evidence for the Existence of Neural Mechanisms Selectively Sensitive to the Direction of Movement in Space." *Journal of Physiology* 235 (1973):17–29.

Billing, J. "An Overview of Task Complexity." *Motor Skills: Theory Into Practice* 4 (1980):18–23.

Bills, A. G. "The Influence of Muscular Tension on the Efficiency of Mental Work." *American Journal of Psychology* 38 (1927):227–51.

Bilodeau, E. A. "Retention under Free and Stimulated Conditions." In E. A. Bilodeau and I. McD. Bilodeau, eds. *Principles of Skill Acquisition.* New York: Academic Press, 1969.

Bilodeau, E. A., and Bilodeau, I. McD. "Variable Frequency of Knowledge of Results and the Learning of a Simple Skill." *Journal of Experimental Psychology* 55 (1958a):379–83.

Bilodeau, E. A., and Bilodeau, I. McD. "Variation of Temporal Intervals among Critical Events in Five Studies of Knowledge of Results." *Journal of Experimental Psychology* 55 (1958b):603–12.

Bilodeau, E. A., and Bilodeau, I. McD. "Motor-Skills Learning." In P. Farnsworth, ed. *Annual Review of Psychology* 12 (1961):243–80.

Bilodeau, E. A.; Bilodeau, I. McD.; and Schumsky, D. A. "Some Effects of Introducing and Withdrawing Knowledge of Results Early and Late in Practice." *Journal of Experimental Psychology* 58 (1959):142–44.

Bilodeau, I. McD. "Accuracy of a Simple Positioning Response with Variation in the Number of Trials by Which Knowledge of Results Is Delayed." *American Journal of Psychology* 69 (1956):434–37.

Bizzi, E. "Central and Peripheral Mechanisms in Motor Control." In G. E. Stelmach and J. Requin, eds. *Tutorials in Motor Control.* Amsterdam: North Holland, 1980.

Boddy, J. *Brain Systems and Psychological Concepts.* New York: John Wiley, 1978.

Bossom, J. "Movement without Proprioception." *Brain Research* 71 (1974):285–96.

Botwinick, J., and Thompson, L. W. "Pre-motor and Motor Components of Reaction Time." *Journal of Experimental Psychology* 71 (1966):9–15.

Boucher, J. L. "Higher Processes in Motor Learning." *Journal of Motor Behavior* 6 (1974):131–37.

Boulter, L. R. "Evaluations of Mechanisms in Delay of Knowledge of Results." *Canadian Journal of Psychology* 18 (1964):281–91.

Bower, T. G. "The Visual World of Infants." *Scientific American* 215 (December 1966):80–92.

Bowerman, R. F., and Larimer, J. L. "Command Fibers in the Circumoesophageal Connectives of Crayfish. I. Tonic Fibers." *Journal of Experimental Biology* 60 (1974):95–117.

Boyd, I. A., and Roberts, T. D. M. "Proprioceptive Discharges from Stretch-Receptors in the Knee Joint of the Cat." *Journal of Physiology* 122 (1953):38–58.

Boyd, L. P. "A Comparative Study of the Effects of Ankle Weights on Vertical Jumping Ability." Master's thesis, Springfield College, 1969.

Brace, D. K. *Measuring Motor Ability.* New York: A. S. Barnes, 1927.

Brace, D. K. "Studies in the Rate of Learning Gross Bodily Motor Skills." *Research Quarterly* 12 (1941):181–85.

Broadbent, D. E. *Perception and Communication.* New York: Pergamon Press, 1958.

Broer, M. "Effectiveness of a General Basic Skills Curriculum for Junior High School Girls." *Research Quarterly* 29 (1958):379–88.

Brooks, V. B. "Motor Programs Revisited." In R. E. Talbott and D. R. Humphrey, eds. *Posture and Movement.* New York: Raven Press, 1979.

Brown, B. B. *Stress and the Art of Biofeedback.* New York: Bantam Books, 1978.

Brown, I. D. "Measuring the 'Spare Mental Capacity' of Car Drivers by a Subsidiary Auditory Task." *Ergonomics* 5 (1962):247–50.

Brown, T. G. "The Intrinsic Factors in the Act of Progression in the Mammal." *Proc. Roy. Soc. London Ser. B* 84 (1911):308–19.

Browne, K.; Lee, J.; and Ring, P. A. "The Sensation of Passive Movement at the Metatarso-Phalangeal Joint of the Great Toe in Man." *Journal of Physiology* 126 (1954):448–58.

Bryan, J. F., and Locke, E. A. "Goal Setting as a Means of Increasing Motivation." *Journal of Applied Psychology* 51 (1967):274–77.

Bryan, W. L., and Harter, N. "Studies in the Physiology and Psychology of Telegraphic Language." *Psychological Review* 4 (1897):27–53.

Bryan, W. L., and Harter, N. "Studies on the Telegraphic Language: The Acquisition of a Hierarchy of Habits." *Psychological Review* 6 (1899):345–75.

Burdenshaw, D.; Spragens, J. E.; and Weis, P. A. "Evaluation of General versus Specific Instruction of Badminton Skills to Women of Low Motor Ability." *Research Quarterly* 41 (1970):472–77.

Burg, A. "Visual Acuity as Measured by Dynamic and Static Tests: Comparative Evaluation." *Journal of Applied Psychology* 50 (1966):460–66.

Burgess, P. R., and Clark, J. F. "Characteristics of Knee Joint Receptors in the Cat." *Journal of Physiology* 203 (1969):317–35.

Burgess, P. R. et al. "Signaling of Kinesthetic Information by Peripheral Sensory Receptors" *Annual Review of Neuroscience* 5 (1982):171–87.

Burrows, D., and Murdock, B. B. "Effects of Extended Practice on High Speed Scanning." *Journal of Experimental Psychology* 82 (1969):231–37.

Buzas, H. P., and Ayllon, T. "Differential Reinforcement in Coaching Tennis Skills." *Behavior Modification* 5 (1981):372–85.

Campbell, D. J., and Ilgen, D. R. "Additive Effects of Task Difficulty and Goal Setting on Subsequent Task Performance." *Journal of Applied Psychology* 61 (1976):319–24.

Campbell, F. W., and Maffei, L. "Electrophysiological Evidence for the Existence of Orientation and Size Detectors in the Human Visual System." *Journal of Physiology* 207 (1970):635–52.

Campos, J. "The Fear of Falling." *Human Behavior* 8 (January 1979):49.

Cannon, W. B. *The Wisdom of the Body.* New York: Norton, 1932.

Carlton, L. G. "Processing Visual Feedback Information for Movement Control." *Journal of Experimental Psychology: Human Perception and Performance* 7 (1981):1019–30.

Carron, A. V. "Motor Performance under Stress." *Research Quarterly* 39 (1968):463–68.

Carron, A. V. "Performance and Learning in a Discrete Motor Task under Massed vs. Distributed Practice." *Research Quarterly* 40 (1969):481–89.

Carron, A. V. *Social Psychology of Sport.* Ithaca, N.Y.: Mouvement Publication, 1980.

Carson, L. M., and Wiegand, R. L. "Motor Schema Formation and Retention in Young Children: A Test of Schmidt's Schema Theory." *Journal of Motor Behavior* 11 (1979):247–51.

Catalano, J. F. "Arousal as a Factor in Reminiscence." *Perceptual and Motor Skills* 24 (1967):1171–80.

Catalano, J. F., and Whalen, P. M. "Factors in Recovery from Performance Decrements: Activation, Inhibition, Warm-up." *Perceptual and Motor Skills* 24 (1967):1223–31.

Cermak, L. S., and Craik, F. I. M. eds. *Levels of Processing in Human Memory.* Hillsdale, N.J.: Erlbaum, 1979.

Chambers, M. R. et al. "The Structure and Function of the Slowly Adapting Type II Mechanoreceptor in Hairy Skin." *Quarterly Journal of Experimental Physiology* 57 (1972):417–45.

Chase, R. A.; Harvey, S.; Standfast, S.; Rapin, I.; and Sutton, S. "Studies on Sensory Feedback: I. Effect of Delayed Auditory Feedback on Speech and Keytapping." *Quarterly Journal of Experimental Psychology* 13 (1961a):141–52.

Chase, R. A. et al. "Sensory Feedback Influences on Motor Performance." *J. Audit. Res.,* 1 (1961b):212–23.

Chase, R. A. et al. "Studies on sensory feedback: II. Sensory Feedback Influence on Keytapping Motor Tasks." *Quarterly Journal of Experimental Psychology* 13 (1961c):153–67.

Chernikoff, R., and Taylor, F. V. "Reaction Time to Kinesthetic Stimulation Resulting from Sudden Arm Displacement." *Journal of Experimental Psychology* 43 (1952):1–8.

Cherry, C. "Some Experiments on the Recognition of Speech with One and with Two Ears." *J. Acoust. Soc. Amer.,* 25 (1953):957–79.

Chi, M. "Short-Term Memory Limitations in Children: Capacity or Processing Deficits? *Memory and Cognition* 4 (1976):559–72.

Christina, R. W. "The Side Arm Positional Test of Kinesthetic Sense." *Research Quarterly* 38 (1967):177–83.

Christina, R. W., and Anson, J. G. "The Learning of Programmed- and Feedback-Based Processes Controlling the Production of a Positioning Response in Two Dimensions." *Journal of Motor Behavior* 13 (1981):48–64.

Christina, R. W.; Feltz, D. L.; Hatfield, B. D.; and Daniels, F. S. "Demographic and Physical Characteristics of Shooters." In G. C. Roberts and D. M. Landers, eds. *Psychology of Motor Behavior and Sport.* Champaign, Ill.: Human Kinetics Publishers, 1981.

Christina, R. W.; Fischman, M. G.; Vercruyssen, M. J. P.; and Anson, J. G. "Simple Reaction Time as a Function of Response Complexity: Memory Drum Theory Revisited.: *Journal of Motor Behavior* 14 (1982):301–21.

Christina, R. W.; Lambert, P. J.; and Fischman, M. G. "Hand Position as a Variable Determining the Accuracy of Aiming Movements." *Journal of Experimental Psychology: Human Perception and Performance* 8 (1982):341–48.

Clark, F. J., and Burgess, P. R. "Slowly Adapting Receptors in the Cat Knee Joint: Can They Signal Joint Angle?" *Journal of Neurophysiology* 38 (1975):1448–63.

Clark, F. J.; Landgren, S.; and Silfvenius, H. "Projections to the Cat's Cerebral Cortex from Low Threshold Joint Afferents." *Acta Physiol. Scand.* 89 (1973):504–21.

Clawson, A. L. "The Effect of Three Types of Competitive Motivating Conditions upon the Scores of Archery Students." Doctoral dissertation, University of Texas, 1965.

Cobb, R. A. "Effects of Selected Visual Conditions on Throwing Accuracy." Doctoral dissertation, Springfield College, 1969.

Cofer, C. N., and Appley, M. H. *Motivation: Theory and Research.* New York: John Wiley, 1964.

Coleman, D. M. "The Effect of a Unit of Movement Education Upon the Level of Achievement in the Specialized Skill of Bowling." Doctoral dissertation, Texas Women's University, 1967.

Cooper, L. K., and Rothstein, A. L. "Videotape Replay and the Learning of Skills in Open and Closed Environments." *Research Quarterly for Exercise and Sport* 52 (1981):191–99.

Corballis, M. "Laterality and Myth." *American Psychologist* 35 (1980):284–95.

Cotten, D. J. et al. "Temporary Fatigue Effects in a Gross Motor Skill." *Journal of Motor Behavior* 4 (1972):217–22.

Cottrell, N. B. "Performance in the Presence of Other Human Beings: Mere Presence, Audience, and Affiliation Effects." In E. C. Simmel, R. A. Hoppe, and G. A. Milton, eds. *Social Facilitation and Imitative Behavior.* Boston: Allyn and Bacon, 1968.

Coville, F. H. "The Learning of Motor Skills as Influenced by Knowledge of Mechanical Principles." *Journal of Educational Psychology* 48 (1957):321–27.

Cox, R. H. "Consolidation of Pursuit Rotor Learning under Conditions of Induced Arousal." Paper presented at the annual AAHPERD convention, Houston, Tex., 1982.

Cozens, F. W. *The Measurement of General Athletic Ability in College Men.* Eugene, Oreg.: University of Oregon Press, 1929.

Crago, P. E.; Houk, J. C.; and Rymer, W. Z. "Sampling of Total Muscle Force by Tendon Organs." *Journal of Neurophysiology* 47 (1982):1069–83.

Craik, F. I. M. "The Fate of Primary Items in Free Recall." *Journal of Verbal Learning and Verbal Behavior* 9 (1970):143–48.

Craik, F. I. M. "Depth of Processing in Recall and Recognition." In S. Dornic, ed. *Attention and Performance VI.* Hillsdale, N.J.: Erlbaum, 1977.

Craik, F. I. M., and Lockhart, R. "Levels of Processing: A Framework for Memory Research." *Journal of Verbal Learning and Verbal Behavior* 11 (1972):671–76.

Cratty, B. J. "Transfer of Small-Pattern Practice to Large-Pattern Learning." *Research Quarterly* 33 (1962):523–35.

Cratty, B. J. *Movement Behavior and Motor Learning.* Philadelphia: Lea & Febiger, 1973.

Cratty, B. J., and Hutton, R. S. "Figural After-Effects, Resulting from Gross Action Patterns." *Research Quarterly* 35 (1964):147–60.

Cronbach, L. J. *Essentials of Psychological Testing.* 2d ed. New York: Harper and Row, 1960.

Cross, M. J., and McCloskey, D. I. "Position Sense Following Surgical Removal of Joints in Man." *Brain Research* 55 (1973):443–45.

Crossman, E. R. F. "A Theory of the Acquisition of Speed-Skill." *Ergonomics* 2 (1959):153–66.

Crouch, J. E. *Functional Human Anatomy.* Philadelphia: Lea & Febiger, 1965.

Crowder, R. G. "Sensory Memory Systems." In E. C. Carterette and M. P. Friedman, eds. *Handbook of Perception.* New York: Academic Press, 1978.

Cynader, M., and Regan, D. "Neurons in Cat Parastriate Cortex Sensitive to the Direction of Motion in Three-Dimensional Space." *Journal of Physiology* 274 (1978):549–69.

Danskin, D. G., and Crow, M. A. *Biofeedback.* Palo Alto, Calif.: Mayfield Publishers, 1981.

Davis, R. C. "The Pattern of Muscular Action in Simple Voluntary Movement." *Journal of Experimental Psychology* 31 (1942):347–66.

DeCoursey, R. M. *The Human Organism.* 3d ed. New York: McGraw-Hill, 1968.

DeLong, M. R., and Strick, P. L. "Relation of Basal Ganglia, Cerebellum, and Motor Cortex Units to Ramp and Ballistic Limb Movements." *Brain Research* 71 (1974):327–35.

DelRey, P. "Effects of Video-Taped Feedback on Form, Accuracy, and Latency in an Open and Closed Environment." *Journal of Motor Behavior* 3 (1971):281–88.

DelRey, P.; Wughalter, E. H.; and Whitehurst, M. "The Effects of Contextual Interference on Females with Varied Experience in Open Sport Skills." *Research Quarterly for Exercise and Sport* 53 (1982):108–15.

Deutsch, D., and Deutsch, J. A. *Short-Term Memory.* New York: Academic Press, 1975.

Deutsch, J. A. "The Cholenergic Synapse and the Site of Memory." In J. A. Deutsch, ed. *The Physiological Basis of Memory.* New York: Academic Press, 1973.

Deutsch, J. A., and Deutsch, D. "Attention: Some Theoretical Considerations." *Psychological Review* 70 (1963):80–90.

DeValois, R. L. "Analysis and Coding of Color Vision in the Primate Visual System." *Sensory Receptors.* Cold Spring Harbor, N.Y.: Laboratory of Quantitative Biology, 1965.

deVries H. A. *Physiology of Exercise.* Dubuque, Ia.: Wm. C. Brown Publishers, 1980.

Dewhurst, D. J. "Neuromuscular Control System." *IEEE Transactions on Biomedical Engineering* 14 (1967):167–71.

Dickinson, J. "The Training of Mobile Balancing under a Minimal Visual Cue Situation." *Ergonomics* 11 (1968):69–75.

Dickinson, J. *A Behavioral Analysis of Sport.* Princeton, N.J.: Princeton Book Company, 1977.

Dickinson, J. "Retention of Intentional and Incidental Motor Learning." *Research Quarterly* 49 (1978):437–41.

Diewert, G. L. "Retention and Coding in Motor Short-Term Memory: A Comparison of Storage Codes for Distance and Location Information." *Journal of Motor Behavior* 7 (1975):183–90.

Diewert, G. L., and Stelmach, G. E. "Perceptual Organization in Motor Learning." In G. E. Stelmach, ed. *Information Processing in Motor Control and Learning.* New York: Academic Press, 1978.

Digman, J. M. "Growth of a Motor Skill as a Function of Distribution of Practice." *Journal of Experimental Psychology* 57 (1959):310–16.

Dimond, S. J. *Introducing Neuropsychology: The Study of Brain and Mind.* Springfield, Ill.: Charles C Thomas, 1978.

Donahue, J. A.; Gillis, J. H.; and King, K. "Behavior Modification in Sport and Physical Education: A Review." *Journal of Sport Psychology* 2 (1980):311–28.

Drowatzky, J. N., and Schwartz, R. M. "Effect of Physical Work on Static Depth Perception." *International Journal of Sport Psychology* 2 (1971):135.

Duffy, E. *Activation and Behavior.* New York: John Wiley, 1962.

Duffy, E. "Activation." In H. S. Greenfield and R. A. Sternbach, eds. *Handbook of Psychophysiology.* New York: Holt, Rinehart and Winston, 1972.

Dunham, P. "Learning and Performance." *Research Quarterly* 42 (1971):334–37.

Dunham, P. "Distribution of Practice as a Factor Affecting Learning and/or Performance." *Journal of Motor Behavior* 8 (1976):305–7.

Dunham, P. "Retention of Bilateral Performance as a Function of Practice Order." *Perceptual and Motor Skills* 46 (1978):43–46.

Dunn, A. J. "Neurochemistry of Learning and Memory: An Evaluation of Recent Data." *Annual Review of Psychology* 31 (1980):343–90.

Durentini, C. L. "The Relationship of a Purported Measure of Kinesthesis to the Learning of a Simple Motor Skill, the Basketball Free Throw, Projected with and without Vision." Master's thesis, University of Massachusetts, 1967.

Easton, T. A. "On the Normal Use of Reflexes." *American Scientist* 60 (1972):591–99.

Easton, T. A. "Coordinative Structures—the Basis for a Motor Program." In D. M. Landers and R. W. Christina, eds. *Psychology of Motor Behavior and Sport.* Champaign, Ill.: Human Kinetics Publishers, 1978.

Eccles, J. C. "The Synapse." *Scientific American* 212 (January 1965):56–66.

Eccles, J. C. *The Understanding of the Brain.* 2d ed. New York: McGraw-Hill, 1977.

Eccles, R. M., and Lundberg, A. "Supraspinal Control of Interneurons Mediating Spinal Reflexes." *Journal of Physiology* 147 (1959):565–84.

Eckert, H. M. "Linear Relationships of Isometric Strength to Propulsive Force, Angular Velocity, and Angular Acceleration in the Standing Broad Jump." *Research Quarterly* 35 (1964):298–306.

Edington, D. W., and Edgerton, V. R. *The Biology of Physical Activity.* Boston: Houghton Mifflin, 1976.

Elliott, R., and McMichael, R. E. "Effect of Specific Training on Frame Dependence." *Perceptual and Motor Skills* 17 (1963):363–67.

Elwell, J. L., and Grindley, G. C. "The Effect of Knowledge of Results on Learning and Performance. I. A Coordinated Movement of the Two Hands." *British Journal of Psychology* 29 (1938):39–53.

Ericsson, K. A.; Chase, W. G.; and Faloon, S. "Acqusition of a Memory Skill." *Science* 208 (1980):1181–82.

Esterbrook, J. A. "The Effect of Emotion on Cue Utilization and the Organization of Behavior." *Psychological Review* 66 (1959):183–201.

Evarts, E. V. "Motor Cortex Reflexes Associated with Learned Movements." *Science* 179 (1973):501–3.

Evarts, E. V. "Brain Mechanisms of Movement." *Scientific American* 241 (September 1979):164–79.

Evarts, E. V., and Fromm, C. "The Pyramidal Tract Neuron as Summing Point in a Closed-Loop Control System in the Monkey." In J. E. Desmedt, ed. *Cerebral Motor Control in Man: Long Loop Mechanisms.* Basel: Karger, 1978.

Evarts, E. V., and Tanji, J. "Gating of Motor Cortex Reflexes by Prior Instruction." *Brain Research* 71 (1974):479–94.

Evarts E. V., and Tanji, J. "Reflex and Intended Responses in Motor Cortex Pyramidal Tract Neurons of the Monkey." *Journal of Neurophysiology* 39 (1976):1069–80.

Eysenck, H. J. *The Biological Basis of Personality.* Springfield, Ill.: Charles C Thomas, 1967.

Eysenck, H. J., and Frith, C. D. *Reminiscence, Motivation, and Personality.* New York: Plenum Press, 1977.

Eysenck, M. W. "Levels of Processing: A Critique." *British Journal of Psychology* 69 (1978):157–69.

Fantz, R. L. "The Origin of Form Perception." *Scientific American.* 204 (May 1961):66–72.

Feltz, D. L. "The Effects of Age and Number of Demonstrations on Modeling of Form and Performance." *Research Quarterly for Exercise and Sport* 53 (1982):291–96.

Feltz, D. L., and Landers, D. M. "Informational-Motivational Components of a Model's Demonstration." *Research Quarterly* 48 (1977):525–33.

Feltz, D. L.; Landers, D. M.; and Raeder, U. "Enhancing Self-Efficacy in High-Avoidance Motor Tasks: A Comparison of Modeling Techniques." *Journal of Sport Psychology* 1 (1979):112–22.

Fentress, J. C. "Development of Grooming in Mice with Amputated Forelimbs." *Science* 179 (1973):704–5.

Filskov, S. B.; Grimm, B. H.; and Lewis, J. A. "Brain-Behavior Relationships." In S. B. Filskov and T. J. Boll, *Handbook of Clinical Neuropsychology.* New York: John Wiley, 1981.

Fishman, S. "A Procedure for Recording Augmented Feedback in Physical Education Classes." Doctoral dissertation, Teachers College, Columbia University, 1974.

Fitts, P. M. "Perceptual-Motor Skill Learning." In A. W. Melton, ed. *Categories of Human Learning.* New York: Academic Press, 1964.

Fitts, P. M. "Factors in Complex Skill Training." In R. Glasser, ed. *Training Research and Education.* New York: John Wiley, 1965.

Fitts, P. M., and Posner, M. I. *Human Performance.* Belmont, Calif.: Brooks/Cole, 1967.

Fleishman, E. A. "Performance Assessment of an Empirically Derived Task Taxonomy." *Human Factors* 9 (1967):349–66.

Fleishman, E. A. "On the Relation Between Abilities, Learning, and Human Performance." *American Psychologist* 27 (1972):1017–32.

Fleishman, E. A. "Relating Individual Differences to the Dimensions of Human Tasks." *Ergonomics* 21 (1978):1007–19.

Fleishman, E. A., and Hempel, W. E., Jr. "Changes in Factor Structure of a Complex Psychomotor Test as a Function of Practice." *Psychometrika* 19 (1954):239–52.

Fleishman, E. A., and Hempel, W. E., Jr. "The Relation between Abilities and Improvement with Practice in a Visual Discrimination Reaction Task." *Journal of Experimental Psychology* 49 (1955):301–12.

Fleishman, E. A., and Parker, J. F., Jr. "Factors in the Retention and Relearning of Perceptual-Motor Skill." *Journal of Experimental Psychology* 64 (1962):215–26.

Fleishman, E. A., and Rich, S. "Role of Kinesthetic and Spatial-Visual Abilities in Perceptual-Motor Learning." *Journal of Experimental Psychology* 66 (1963):6–11.

Fox, M. G. "Lateral Dominance in the Teaching of Bowling." *Research Quarterly* 28 (1957):327–31.

Fox, M. G., and Lamb, E. "Improvement during a Non-practice Period in a Selected Physical Education Activity." *Research Quarterly* 33 (1962):381–85.

Fox, M. G., and Young, V. P. "Effect of Reminiscence on Learning Selected Badminton Skills." *Research Quarterly* 33 (1962):386–94.

Frackenpohl, H., and McCarthy, J. F. *Reading 300 instructor's manual.* New York: McGraw-Hill. Educational Developmental Laboratories, 1969.

Freeman, G. L. "Mental Activity and the Muscular Process." *Psychological Review* 38 (1931):428–49.

Freeman, G. L. "The Facilitative and Inhibitory Effects of Muscular Tension." *American Journal of Psychology* 45 (1933):17–52.

Freeman, G. L. "The Optimal Muscular Tensions for Various Performances." *American Journal of Psychology* 51 (1938):146–50.

Fukuda, T. "Studies on Human Dynamic Postures from the Viewpoint of Postural Reflexes." *Acta Oto-Laryngologica* 161 (1961):1–52.

Fundamentals of Progress. Scientific Research on Transcendental Meditation. Maharishi International University, 1974.

Fuster, J. M. "Effects of Stimulation of Brain Stem on Tachistoscopic Perception." *Science* 127 (1958):150.

Gallagher, J. D., and Thomas, J. R. "Effects of Varying Post-KR Intervals upon Children's Motor Performance." *Journal of Motor Behavior* 12 (1980):41–46.

Gallahue, D. L.; Werner, P. H.; and Luedke, G. C. *A Conceptual Approach to Moving and Learning.* New York: John Wiley, 1975.

Gallistel, C. R. *The Organization of Action: A New Synthesis.* Hillsdale, N.J.: Erlbaum, 1980.

Gallwey, W. T. *The Inner Game of Tennis.* New York: Random House, 1974.

Gandevia, S. C., and McCloskey, D. I. "Joint Sense, Muscle Sense, and Their Combination as Position Sense, Measured at the Distal Interphalangeal Joint of the Middle Finger." *Journal of Physiology* 260 (1976):387–407.

Gandevia, S. C., and McCloskey, D. I. "Sensations of Heaviness." *Brain* 100 (1977):345–54.

Gardner, E. *Fundamentals of Neurology.* 5th ed. Philadelphia: W. B. Saunders, 1969.

Gardner, E. B. "Proprioceptive Reflexes and Their Participation in Motor Skills." *Quest* 12 (1969):1–25.

Garner, A. I. "An Overlooked Problem: Athletes' Visual Needs." *The Physician and Sportsmedicine* 5 (4)(1977):74–83.

Gazzaniga, M. S. *The Bisected Brain.* New York: Appleton-Century-Crofts, 1970.

Gelfan, S., and Carter, S. "Muscle Sense in Man." *Experimental Neurology* 18 (1967):469–73.

Gentile, A. M. "A Working Model of Skill Acquisition with Application to Teaching." *Quest* 17 (1972):3–23.

Gentile, A. M. et al. "The Structure of Motor Tasks." *Mouvement.* Actes du 7e symposium en apprentissage psycho-moteur et psychologie due sport, Quebec City, 1975.

Gentile, A. M., and Nacson, J. "Organizational Processes in Motor Control." In J. Keogh and R. S. Hutton, eds. *Exercise and Sport Sciences Reviews.* vol. 4. Santa Barbara, Calif.: Journal Publishing Affiliates, 1976.

George, C. "Effects of the Asymmetrical Tonic Neck Posture upon Grip Strength of Normal Children." *Research Quarterly* 41 (1970):361–64.

George, C. "Facilitative and Inhibitory Effects of the Tonic Neck Reflex upon Grip Strength of Right- and Left-Handed Children." *Research Quarterly* 43 (1972):157–66.

George, F. H. "Errors of Visual Recognition." *Journal of Experimental Psychology* 43 (1952):202–6.

Gibbs, C. B., and Brown, I. D. "Increased Production from the Information Incentive in a Repetitive Task." *Medical Research Council, Appl. Psychological Res. Unit* Great Britain, 230, March, 1955.

Gibson, E. J., and Bergman, R. B. "The Effect of Training on Absolute Estimation of Distances over the Ground." *Journal of Experimental Psychology* 48 (1954):137–49.

Gibson, E. J., and Walk, R. D. "The Visual Cliff." *Scientific American* 202 (April 1960):64–71.

Gibson, J. J. "Adaptation, After-effect and Contrast in the Perception of Curved Lines." *Journal of Experimental Psychology* 16 (1933):1–33.

Gibson, J. J. *The Senses Considered as Perceptual Systems.* New York: Houghton Mifflin, 1966.

Gill, D. L. "Knowledge of Results Precision and Motor Skill Acquisition." *Journal of Motor Behavior* 7 (1975):191–98.

Gire, E., and Espenschade, A. "Relation between Measures of Motor Educability and Learning of Specific Motor Skills." *Research Quarterly* 13 (1942):43–56.

Glanzer, M., and Koppenaal, L. "The Effect of Encoding Tasks on Free Recall: Stages and Levels." *Journal of Verbal Learning and Verbal Behavior* 16 (1977):21–28.

Glencross, D. J. "Control of Skilled Movements." *Psychological Bulletin.* 84 (1977):14–29.

Glencross, D. J., and Oldfield, S. R. "The Use of Ischemic Nerve Block Procedures in the Investigation of the Sensory Control of Movements." *Biological Psychology* 2 (1975):227–36.

Godwin, M. A., and Schmidt, R. A. "Muscular Fatigue and Learning a Discrete Motor Skill." *Research Quarterly* 42 (1971):374–82.

Goldsheider, A. "Untersuchungen über den muskelsinn." *Arch. Anat. Physiol., Leipzig.* 3 (1889):369–502. (Ministry Supply, U.K., Transl. No. 20825T).

Goodwin, G. M. "The Sense of Limb Position and Movement." In J. Keogh and R. S. Hutton, eds. *Exercise and Sport Sciences Reviews.* vol. 4. Santa Barbara, Calif.: Journal Publishing Affiliates, 1976.

Goodwin, G. M.; McCloskey, D. I.; and Matthews, P. B. C. "The Contribution of Muscle Afferents to Kinesthesia Shown by Vibration Induced Illusions of Movement and by the Effects of Paralysing Joint Afferents." *Brain* 95 (1972):705–48.

Goslin, D. A. *The Search for Ability* New York: Russell Sage Foundation, 1963.

Gould, D. R., and Roberts, G. C. "Modeling and Motor Skill Acquisition." *Quest* 33 (1981):214–30.

Graboi, D. "Searching for Targets: The Effects of Specific Practice." *Perception and Psychophysics* 10 (1971):300–4.

Granit, R. "Constant Errors in the Execution and Appreciation of Movement." *Brain* 95 (1972):451–60.

Granit, R. *The Purposive Brain.* Cambridge: MIT Press, 1977.

Granit, R.; Holmgren, B.; and Merton, P. A. "The Two Routes for Excitation of Muscle and Their Subservience to the Cerebellum." *Journal of Physiology* 130 (1955):213–24.

Graw, H. M. A. "The Most Efficient Usage of a Fixed Work plus Rest Practice Period in Motor Learning." Doctoral dissertation, University of California, Berkeley, 1968.

Graybiel, A.; Jokl, E.; and Trapp, C. "Russian Studies of Vision in Relation to Physical Activity and Sports." *Research Quarterly* 26 (1955):480–85.

Greenough, W. T.; Juraska, J. M.; and Volkmar, F. R. "Maze Training Effects on Dendritic Branching in Occipital Cortex of Adult Rats." *Behavioral and Neural Biology* 26 (1979):287–97.

Greenwald, A. G. "Sensory Feedback Mechanisms in Performance Control: With Special Reference to the Ideo-motor Mechanisms." *Psychological Review* 77 (1970):73–99.

Gregorc, A. F. "Learning/Teaching Styles." In *Student Learning Styles: Diagnosing and Prescribing Programs.* Reston, Va.: National Association of Secondary School Principals, 1979.

Gregory, R. L., and Wallace, J. G. "Recovery from Early Blindness: A Case Study." *Experimental Psychology and Sociology Monographs,* no. 2. Cambridge: 1963.

Grigg, P. "Mechanical Factors Influencing Response of Joint Afferent Neurons from Cat Knee." *Journal of Neurophysiology.* 38 (1975):1473–84.

Grigg, P.; Finerman, G. A.; and Riley, L. H. "Joint Position Sense After Total Hip Replacement." *Journal of Bone and Joint Surgery* 55A (1973):1016–25.

Grigg, P., and Greenspan, B. J. "Response of Primate Joint Afferent Neurons to Mechanical Stimulation of Knee Joint." *Journal of Neurophysiology* 40 (1977):1–8.

Grillner, S., and Zangger, P. "Locomotor Movements Generated by the Deafferented Spinal Cord." *Acta Physiol. Scand.* 91 (1974):38A–39A.

Gruen, A. "The Relation of Dancing Experience and Personality to Perception." *Psychological Monographs* 69 (no. 14, Whole no. 399) 1955.

Gutin, B. "Effect of Systemic Exertion on Rotary Pursuit and Maze Performance and Learning." In G. S. Kenyon, ed. *Contemporary Psychology of Sport.* Chicago: The Athletic Institute, 1970.

Gutin, B., and DiGennaro, J. "Effect of One-Minute and Five-Minute Step-ups on Performance of Simple Addition." *Research Quarterly* 39 (1968):81–85.

Gutin, B. et al. "Steadiness as a Function of Prior Exercise." *Journal of Motor Behavior* 6 (1974):69–76.

Guyton, A. C. *Basic Human Physiology: Normal Function and Mechanisms of Disease.* 2d ed. Philadelphia: W. B. Saunders, 1977.

Guyton, A. C. *Textbook of Medical Physiology.* 6th ed. Philadelphia: W. B. Saunders, 1981.

Gyllenhammar, P. G. *People at Work.* Reading, Mass.: Addison-Wesley, 1977.

Halstead, W., and Rucker, W. "Memory: A Molecular Maze." *Psychology Today* 2 (June 1968):38–41.

Hamilton, E. L. "The Effect of Delayed Incentives on the Hunger Drive of the White Rat." *Genetic Psychology Monographs* 5 (1929):131–207.

Harari, H. "Level of Aspiration and Athletic Performance." *Perceptual and Motor Skills* 28 (1969):519–24.

Hart, B. L. *Experimental Neuropsychology.* San Francisco: W. H. Freeman and Company, 1969.

Hatze, H. "Biomechanical Aspects of a Successful Motion Optimization." In P. V. Komi, ed. *Biomechanics V-B.* Baltimore: University Park Press, 1976.

Haywood, K. M. "Eye Movements during Coincidence-Anticipation Performance." *Journal of Motor Behavior* 9 (1977):313–18.

Haywood, K. M., and Glad, H. L. "Relative Effects of Three Knowledge of Results Treatments on the Ability to Perform a Coincidence-Anticipation Task." Paper presented at the AAHPER Convention, Anaheim, California, 1974.

Heath, C. J.; Hore, J.; and Phillips, C. G. "Inputs from Low Threshold Muscle and Cutaneous Afferents of Hand and Forearm to Area 3a and 3b of Baboon's Cerebral Cortex." *Journal of Physiology* 257 (1976):199–227.

Hebb, D. O. *Textbook of Psychology.* 3d ed. Philadelphia: W. B. Saunders, 1972.

Hecaen, H., and Albert, M. L. *Human Neuropsychology.* New York: John Wiley, 1978.

Held, R., and Bauer, J. "Visually Guided Reaching in Infant Monkeys after Restricted Rearing." *Science* 155 (1967):718–20.

Hellebrandt, F., and Waterland, J. "Expansion of Motor Patterning under Exercise Stress." *American Journal of Physical Medicine* 41 (1962):56–66.

Hellebrandt, F. M.; Schade, M.; and Carns, M. "Methods of Evoking the Tonic Neck Reflexes in Normal Human Subjects." *American Journal of Physical Medicine* 41 (1962):90–139.

Hendrickson, G., and Schroeder, W. H. "Transfer of Training in Learning to Hit a Submerged Target." *Journal of Educational Psychology* 32 (1941):205–13.

Henry, F. M. "Variable and Constant Performance Errors within a Group of Individuals." *Journal of Motor Behavior.* 6 (1974):149–54.

Henry, F. M. "Absolute Error vs. 'E' in Target Accuracy." *Journal of Motor Behavior* 7 (1975):227–28.

Henry, F. M., and Rogers, D. E. "Increased Response Latency for Complicated Movements and a Memory Drum Theory of Neuromotor Reaction." *Research Quarterly* 31 (1960):448–58.

Hernandez-Peon, R. "Physiological Mechanisms in Attention." In R. W. Russell, ed. *Frontiers in Physiological Psychology.* New York: Academic Press, 1967.

Higgins, J. R., and Angel, R. W. "Correction of Tracking Errors without Sensory Feedback." *Journal of Experimental Psychology.* 84 (1970):412–16.

Higgins, J. R., and Spaeth, R. K. "Relationship between Consistency of Movement and Environmental Condition." *Quest* 17 (1972):61–69.

Hilgard, E. R. *Introduction to Psychology.* New York: Harcourt, Brace, 1957.

Ho, L., and Shea, J. B. "Levels of Processing and the Coding of Position Cues in Motor Short-Term Memory." *Journal of Motor Behavior* 10 (1978):113–21.

Holding, D. H. "Transfer between Difficult and Easy Tasks." *British Journal of Psychology* 53 (1962):397–407.

Holding, D. H. *Principles of Training.* New York: Pergamon Press, 1965.

Hole, J. W. *Human Anatomy and Physiology.* 2nd ed. Dubuque, Ia.: Wm. C. Brown Publishers, 1981.

Holson, R., and Henderson, M. T. "A Preliminary Study of Visual Fields in Athletes." *Iowa Academy of Science* 48 (1941):331–37.

Holzman, P. S., and Klein, G. S. "Cognitive System-Principles of Leveling and Sharpening; Individual Differences in Assimilation Effects in Visual Time-Error." *Journal of Psychology* 37 (1954):105–122.

Hore, J. et al. "Response of Cortical Neurons (areas 3a and 4) to Ramp Stretch of Hindlimb Muscles of the Baboon." *Journal of Neurophysiology* 39 (1976):484–500.

Hornak, J. E. "The Effects of Three Methods of Teaching on the Learning of a Motor Skill." Doctoral dissertation, University of Northern Colorado, 1971.

Houk, J., and Henneman, E. "Responses of Golgi Tendon Organs to Active Contractions of the Soleus Muscle of the Cat." *Journal of Neurophysiology* 30 (1967):466–81.

Howard, I. P., and Templeton, W. B. *Human Spatial Orientation.* New York: John Wiley, 1966.

Howell, M. T. "Use of Force-Time Graphs for Performance Analysis in Facilitating Motor Learning." *Research Quarterly* 27 (1956):12–22.

Hsu, S. H., and Payne, R. B. "Effector Localization and Transfer of Reactive Inhibition." *Journal of Motor Behavior* 11 (1979):153–58.

Hubbard, A. W., and Seng, C. N. "Visual Movements of Batters." *Research Quarterly* 25 (1954):42–57.

Hubel, D. H., and Wiesel, T. N. "Receptive Fields, Binocular Interaction, and Functional Architecture in the Cat's Visual Cortex." *Journal of Physiology* 160 (1962):106.

Hubel, D. H., and Wiesel, T. N. "Receptive Fields and Functional Architecture in Monkey Striate Cortex." *Journal of Physiology* 195 (1968):215–43.

Hubel, D. H., and Wiesel, T. N. "Brain Mechanisms of Vision." *Scientific American* 241 (September 1979):150–62.

Hull, C. *Principles of Behavior.* New York: Appleton-Century-Crofts, 1943.

Hunt, D. E. "Learning Styles and Student Needs: An Introduction to Conceptual Level." In *Student Learning Styles: Diagnosing and Prescribing Programs.* Reston, Va.: National Association of Secondary School Principals, 1979.

Hutton, R. S.; Stevens, J. L.; and Stevens, F. "The Effect of Strenuous and Exhaustive Exercise on Learning: A Theoretical Note and Preliminary Findings." *Journal of Motor Behavior* 4 (1972):207–16.

Isaacs, L. D. "Effects of Ball Size, Ball Color, and Preferred Color on Catching by Young Children." *Perceptual and Motor Skills* 51 (1980):583–86.

Ismail, A. H., and Gruber, J. J. *Motor Aptitude and Intellectual Performance.* Columbus, Ohio: Charles E. Merrill, 1967.

Ismail, A. H.; Kane, J.; and Kirkendall, D. R. "Relationships among Intellectual and Non-intellectual Variables." *Research Quarterly* 40 (1969):83–92.

Jacobson, E. "Electrical Measurements of Neuromuscular States during Mental Activities. II. Imagination and Recollection of Various Muscular Acts." *American Journal of Physiology* 94 (1930):27–34.

Jacobson, E. "Electrophysiology of Mental Activities." *American Journal of Psychology* 44 (1932):677–94.

Jacobson, E. *Progressive Relaxation.* Chicago: University of Chicago Press, 1938.

Jacobson, E. "Electrophysiology of Mental Activities and Introduction to the Psychological Process of Thinking." In F. J. McGuigan and R. A. Schoonover, eds. *The Psychophysiology of Thinking.* New York: Academic Press, 1973.

Jahnke, J. C., and Duncan, C. P. "Reminiscence and Forgetting in Motor Learning after Extended Rest Intervals." *Journal of Experimental Psychology* 52 (1956):273–82.

James, W. *The Principles of Psychology.* New York: Henry Holt, 1890.

James, W. *Talks to Teachers on Psychology.* New York: Henry Holt, 1899.

Jensen, B. E. "Pretask Speed Training and Movement Complexity as Factors in Rotary Pursuit Skill Acquisition." *Research Quarterly* 46 (1975):1–11.

Jensen, B. E. "Pretask Speed Training and Movement Complexity." *Research Quarterly* 47 (1976):657–65.

John, E. R. "Switchboard versus Statistical Theories of Learning and Memory." *Science* 177 (1972):850–64.

John, E. R. "How the Brain Works—a New Theory." *Psychology Today.* 9 (May 1976):48–52.

John, E. R. et al. "Neural Readout from Memory." *Journal of Neurophysiology* 36 (1973):893–924.

Johnson, G. B. "Physical Skill Tests for Sectioning Classes into Homogeneous Units." *Research Quarterly* 3 (March 1932):128–36.

Johnson, R. W.; Wicks, G.; and Ben-Sira, D. "Practice in the Absence of Knowledge of Results: Skill Acquisition and Retention." In G. C. Roberts and D. M. Landers, eds. *Psychology of Motor Behavior and Sport.* Champaign, Ill.: Human Kinetics Publishers, 1981.

Johnson, W. G. "Peripheral perception of athletes and non-athletes and the effect of practice." Master's thesis, University of Illinois, 1952.

Jones, B. "The Role of Central Monitoring of Efference in Short-Term Memory for Movements." *Journal of Experimental Psychology* 102 (1974):37–43.

Jordan, T. C. "Characteristics of Visual and Proprioceptive Response Times in the Learning of a Motor Skill." *Quarterly Journal of Experimental Psychology* 24 (1972):536–43.

Jorgensen, J. M. "The Relationship between Perceptual Style and the Rate of Learning a Novel Movement Task." Master's thesis, University of Wisconsin, 1972.

Judd, C. H. "The Relation of Special Training to General Intelligence." *Educational Review* 36 (1908):28–42.

Kahneman, D. *Attention and Effort.* Englewood Cliffs: Prentice-Hall, 1973.

Kalat, J. W. *Biological Psychology.* Belmont, Calif.: Wadsworth Publishing Company, 1981.

Kay, H. "Information Theory in the Understanding of Skills." *Occupational Psychology* 31 (1957):218–24.

Keele, S. W. *Attention and Human Performance.* Pacific Palisades, Calif.: Goodyear, 1973.

Keele, S. W. "Learning and Control of Coordinated Motor Patterns: The Programming Perspective." In J. A. S. Kelso, ed. *Human Motor Behavior: An Introduction.* Hillsdale, N.J.: Erlbaum, 1982.

Keele, S. W., and Hawkins, H. L. "Explorations of Individual Differences Relevant to High Level Skill." *Journal of Motor Behavior* 14 (1982):3–23.

Keele, S. W., and Posner, M. I. "Processing of Visual Feedback in Rapid Movements." *Journal of Experimental Psychology* 77 (1968):155–58.

Keller, F. S. "The Phantom Plateau." *Journal of Experimental Anal. Behavior* 1 (1958):1–13.

Kelso, J. A. S. "Planning and Efferent Components in the Coding of Movement." *Journal of Motor Behavior* 9 (1977a):33–47.

Kelso, J. A. S. "Motor Control Mechanisms Underlying Human Movement Reproduction." *Journal of Experimental Psychology: Human Perception and Performance* 3 (1977b):529–43.

Kelso, J. A. S.; Holt, K. G.; and Flatt, A. E. "The Role of Proprioception in the Perception and Control of Human Movement: Toward a Theoretical Reassessment." *Perception and Psychophysics.* 28 (1980):45–52.

Kelso, J. A. S.; Southard, D. L.; and Goodman, D. "On the Nature of Human Interlimb Coordination." *Science* 203 (1979):1029–31.

Kelso, J. A. S., and Stelmach, G. E. "Behavioral and Neurological Parameters of the Nerve Compression Block." *Journal of Motor Behavior* 6 (1974):179–90.

Kelso, J. A. S., and Wallace, S. "Conscious Mechanisms in Movement." In G. E. Stelmach, ed. *Information Processing in Motor Control and Learning.* New York: Academic Press, 1978.

Kerr, B. "Processing Demands during Movement." *Journal of Motor Behavior* 7 (1975):15–27.

King, B.; Streufert, S.; and Fiedler, F. E., eds. *Managerial Control and Organizational Democracy.* New York: Halsted Press, 1978.

Kinsbourne, M. "Single-Channel Theory." In D. H. Holding, ed. *Human Skills.* New York: John Wiley, 1981.

Klapp, S. T. "Short-Term Memory as a Response-Preparation State." *Memory and Cognition* 4 (1976):721–29.

Klapp, S. T. "Reaction Time Analysis of Programmed Control." In R. S. Hutton, ed. *Exercise and Sport/ Sciences Reviews.* vol. 5. Santa Barbara, Calif.: Journal Publishing Affiliates, 1977.

Klatzky, R. L. *Human Memory: Structures and Processes.* San Francisco: Freeman Publications, 1975.

Klavora, P. "Customary Arousal for Peak Athletic Performance." In P. Klavora and J. V. Daniel, eds. *Coach, Athlete, and the Sport Psychologist.* Champaign, Ill.: Human Kinetics Publishers, 1979.

Klein, R. M. "Attention and Movement." In G. Stelmach, ed. *Motor Control: Issues and Trends.* New York: Academic Press, 1976.

Klein, R. M. "Attention and Visual Dominance: A Chronometric Analysis." *Journal of Experimental Psychology: Human Perception and Performance* 3 (1977):365–78.

Klein, R. M., and Posner, M. I. "Attention to Visual and Kinesthetic Components of Skills." *Brain Research* 71 (1974):401–11.

Knapp, B.N. "A Note on Skill." *Occupational Psychology* 35 (1961):76–78.

Knibestol, M. "Stimulus-Response Functions of Slowly Adapting Mechanoreceptors in the Human Glabrous Skin Area." *Journal of Physiology* 245 (1975):63–80.

Knibestol, M., and Vallbo, A. B. "Single Unit Analysis of Mechanoreceptor Activity from Human Glabrous Skin." *Acta Physiol. Scand.* 80 (1970):178–95.

Kohl, R. M., and Roenker, D. L. "Bilateral Transfer as a Function of Mental Imagery." *Journal of Motor Behavior* 12 (1980):197–206.

Komaki, J., and Barnett, F. T. A. "A Behavioral Approach to Coaching Football: Improving the Play Execution on the Offensive Backfield on a Youth Football Team." *Journal of Applied Behavior Analysis* 10 (1977):657–64.

Korman, A. K. *The Psychology of Motivation.* Englewood Cliffs: Prentice-Hall, 1974.

Kornhuber, H. H. "Cerebral Cortex, Cerebellum and Basal Ganglia: An Introduction to Their Motor Functions." In F. O. Schmitt, ed. *The Neurosciences III.* Cambridge: MIT Press, 1974.

Kreiger, J. C. "The Influence of Figure-Ground Perception on Spatial Adjustment in Tennis." Master's thesis, University of California, Los Angeles, 1962.

Kupfermann, I., and Weiss, K. R. "The Command Neuron Concept." *The Behavioral and Brain Sciences* 1 (1978):3–39.

Kushnir, T., and Duncan, K. D. "An Analysis of Social Facilitation Effects in Terms of Signal Detection Theory." *The Psychological Record* 28 (1978):535–41.

Laabs, G. J. "Retention Characteristics of Different Reproduction Cues in Motor Short-Term Memory." *Journal of Experimental Psychology* 100 (1973):168–77.

Laabs, G. J., and Simmons, R. W. "Motor Memory." In D. H. Holding, ed. *Human Skills.* New York: John Wiley, 1981.

Lakatos, J. S. "Eye Dominance in Batting Performance." *Athletic Journal* 49 (November 1968):76.

Landers, D. M. "Observational Learning of a Motor Skill: Temporal Spacing of Demonstrations and Audience Presence." *Journal of Motor Behavior* 7 (1975): 281–87.

Landers, D. M. "The Arousal-Performance Relationship Revisited." *Research Quarterly for Exercise and Sport* 51 (1980):77–90.

Landers, D. M. "Arousal, Attention, and Skilled Performance: Further Considerations." *Quest* 33 (1982):271–83.

Landers, D. M., and Landers, D. M. "Teacher versus Peer Models: Effects of Model's Presence and Performance Level on Motor Behavior." *Journal of Motor Behavior* 5 (1973):129–39.

Landers, D. M., and McCullagh, P. D. "Social Facilitation of Motor Performance." In J. Keogh and R. S. Hutton, eds. *Exercise and Sport Sciences Reviews*. vol. 4. Santa Barbara, Calif. Journal Publishing Affiliates, 1976.

Langley, L. L.; Telford, I. R.; and Christensen, J. B. *Dynamic Anatomy and Physiology*. 3d ed. New York: McGraw-Hill, 1969.

Lashley, K. S. "The Accuracy of Movement in the Absence of Excitation from the Moving Organ." *American Journal of Physiology* 43 (1917):169–94.

Lashley, K. S. "In Search of the Engram." *Symp. Soc. Exp. Biology*. 4 (1950):454–83.

Laszlo, J. I. "The Performance of a Simple Motor Task with Kinesthetic Sense Loss." *Quarterly Journal of Experimental Psychology* 18 (1966):1–8.

Laszlo, J. I. "Training of Fast Tapping with Reduction of Kinesthetic, Tactile, Visual, and Auditory Sensations." *Quarterly Journal of Experimental Psychology* 19 (1967):344–49.

Laszlo, J. I., and Bairstow, P. J. "Accuracy of Movement, Peripheral Feedback and Efference Copy." *Journal of Motor Behavior* 3 (1971):241–52.

Laszlo, J. I.; Shamoon, J. S.; and Sanson-Fisher, R. "Reacquisition and Transfer of Motor Skills with Sensory Feedback Reduction." *Journal of Motor Behavior* 1 (1969):195–209.

Lavery, J. J. "The Effect of One-Trial Delay in Knowledge of Results on the Acquisition and Retention of a Tossing Skill." *American Journal of Psychology* 77 (1964):437–43.

Lavery, J. J., and Suddon, F. H. "Retention of Simple Motor Skills as a Function of the Number of Trials by Which KR Is Delayed." *Perceptual and Motor Skills* 15 (1962):231–37.

Lee, D. N. "The Functions of Vision." In H. L. Pick and E. Saltzman, eds. *Modes of Perceiving and Processing Information*. New York: John Wiley, 1978.

Lemon, R. N., and Porter, R. "Short-Latency Peripheral Afferent Inputs to Pyramidal and Other Neurons in the Precentral Cortex of Conscious Monkeys." In G. Gordon, ed. *Active Touch*. Oxford: Pergamon Press, 1978.

Lersten, K. C. "Transfer of Movement Components in a Motor Learning Task." *Research Quarterly* 39 (1968):575–81.

Lersten, K. C. "Retention of Skill on the Rho Apparatus After One Year." *Research Quarterly* 40 (1969):418–19.

Levitt, S. "The Effects of Exercise-Induced Activation upon Simple, Two-Choice, and Five-Choice Reaction Time and Movement Time." Doctoral dissertation, Teachers College, Columbia University, 1972.

Levitt, S., and Gutin, B. "Multiple Choice Reaction Time and Movement Time during Physical Exertion." *Research Quarterly*. 42 (1971):405–10.

Lewellen, J. O. "A Comparative Study of Two Methods of Teaching Beginning Swimming." Doctoral dissertation, Stanford University, 1951.

Lewis, M. "Culture and Gender Roles: There's No Unisex in the Nursery." *Psychology Today* 5 (May 1972):54–57.

Liebowitz, H. W., and Appelle, S. "The Effect of a Central Task on Luminance Thresholds for Peripherally Presented Stimuli." *Human Factors* 11 (1969):387–92.

Lindeberg, F. A. "A Study of the Degree of Transfer between Quickening Exercises and Other Coordinated Movements." *Research Quarterly* 20 (1949):180–95.

Lindeburg, F. A., and Hewitt, J. E. "Effect of Oversized Basketball on Shooting Ability and Ball Handling." *Research Quarterly* 36 (1965):164–67.

Llewellyn, J. H. "Effects of Hand and Eye Dominance Combinations on Hitting Performance." *VAHPER Research Journal* 1 (1, 1972):8–11.

Llinas, R. "The Cortex of the Cerebellum." *Scientific American* 232 (January 1975):56–71.

Llinas, R., and Wolfe, J. W. "Functional Linkage between the Electrical Activity in the Vermal Cerebellar Cortex and Saccadic Eye Movements." *Experimental Brain Research* 29 (1977):1–14.

Lloyd, A. J., and Caldwell, L. S. "Accuracy of Active and Passive Positioning of the Leg on the Basis of Kinesthetic Cues." *Journal of Comparative and Physiological Psychology* 60 (1965):102–6.

Lloyd, A. J., and Voor, J. H. "The Effect of Training on Performance Efficiency during a Competitive Isometric Exercise." *Journal of Motor Behavior* 5 (1973):17–24.

Locke, E. A. "Motivational Effects of Knowledge of Results: Knowledge or Goal Setting." *Journal of Applied Psychology* 51 (1967):324–29.

Locke, E. A. "Toward a Theory of Task Motivation and Incentives." *Organizational Behavior and Human Performance* 3 (1968):157–89.

Locke, E. A., and Bryan, J. F. "Cognitive Aspects of Psychomotor Performance: The Effects of Performance Goals on Level of Performance." *Journal of Applied Psychology* 50 (1966a):286–91.

Locke, E. A., and Bryan, J. F. "The Effects of Goal-Setting, Rule Learning and Knowledge of Score on Performance." *American Journal of Psychology* 79 (1966b):451–57.

Locke, E. A.; Cartledge, N.; and Koeppel, J. "Motivational Effects of Knowledge of Results: A Goal Setting Phenomenon?" *Psychological Bulletin* 70 (1968):474–85.

Loftus, E. F., and Loftus, G. R. "On the Permanence of Stored Information in the Human Brain." *American Psychologist* 35 (1980):409–20.

London, M., and Oldham, G. R. "Effects of Varying Goal Types and Incentive Systems on Performance and Satisfaction." *Academy of Management Journal* 19 (1976):537–46.

Lorge, I. *Influence of Regularly Interpolated Time Intervals upon Subsequent Learning.* Teachers College Contributions to Education, no. 438, 1930.

Lorge, I., and Thorndike, E. L. "The Influence of Delay in the After-Effect of a Connection." *Journal of Experimental Psychology* 18 (1935):186–94.

Low, F. N. "Some Characteristics of Peripheral Visual Performance." *American Journal of Physiology* 146 (1946):573–84.

Ludvigh, E., and Miller, J. W. "Study of Visual Acuity during the Ocular Pursuit of Moving Test Objects: I. Introduction." *Journal Opt. Soc. Amer.* 48 (1958):799–802.

Lund, F. H. "The Dependence of Eye-Hand Coordination upon Eye Dominance." *American Journal of Psychology* 44 (1932):756–62.

Lundberg, A. "Integration in the Reflex Pathway." In R. Granit, ed. *Muscular Afferents and Motor Control.* New York: John Wiley, 1966.

Lundberg, A.; Malmgren, K.; and Schomburg, E. D. "Convergence from Ib, Cutaneous, and Joint Afferents in Reflex Pathways to Motoneurons." *Brain Research* 87 (1975):81–84.

Luria, A. R. *Human Brain and Psychological Processes* New York: Harper and Row, 1966.

Luria, A. R. "Functional Organization of the Brain." *Scientific American* 222 (March 1970):66–78.

Luria, A. R. *The Working Brain.* New York: Basic Books, 1973.

McBride, E. R., and Rothstein, A. L. "Mental and Physical Practice and the Learning and Retention of Open and Closed Skills." *Perceptual and Motor Skills* 49 (1979):359–65.

McCaughan, L. R., and Gimbert, B. "Social Reinforcement as a Determinant of Performance, Performance Expectancy and Attributions." *Journal of Motor Behavior* 13 (1981):91–101.

McCloskey, D. I. "Kinesthetic Sensibility." *Physiological Reviews* 58 (1978):763–820.

McCloskey, D. I.; Ebeling, P.; and Goodwin, G. M. "Estimation of Weights and Tensions and Apparent Involvement of a 'Sense of Effort.'" *Experimental Neurology* 42 (1974):220–32.

McCloskey, D. I., and Torda, T. A. G. "Corollary Motor Discharges and Kinesthesia." *Brain Research* 100 (1975):467–70.

McCloy, C. H. "An Analytical Study of the Stunt Type Tests as a Measure of Motor Educability." *Research Quarterly* 8 (October 1937):46–55.

McCracken, H. D., and Stelmach, G. E. "A Test of Schema Theory of Discrete Motor Learning." *Journal of Motor Behavior* 9 (1977):193–201.

McGaugh, J. L., and Herz, M. J. *Memory Consolidation.* San Francisco: Albion, 1972.

McGeer, P. L., and McGeer, E. G. "The Control of Movement by the Brain." *Trends in Neural Sciences* (November 1980):111–14.

MacGillivary, W. W. "Perceptual Style and Ball Skill Acquisition." *Research Quarterly* 50 (1979):222–29.

McGown, C. M., and Schmidt, R. A. "Coordination in Two-Handed Movements." Paper presented at the annual meeting of the North American Society for the Psychology of Sport and Physical Activity, Asilomar, California, 1981.

McIntyre, J. S. et al. "Transfer of Work Decrement in Motor Learning." *Journal of Motor Behavior* 4 (1972):223–29.

McKenzie, T. L., and Rushall, B. S. "Effects of Self-recording on Attendance and Performance in a Competitive Swimming Training Environment." *Journal of Applied Behavior Analysis* 7 (1974):199–206.

Mackworth, J. F. *Vigilance and Habituation.* Baltimore: Penguin Books, 1969.

McNaught, A. B., and Callander, R. *Illustrated Physiology.* Baltimore: Williams and Wilkins, 1963.

MacNichol, E. F. "Retinal Mechanisms of Color Vision." *Vision Research* 4 (1964):119–33.

Magill, R. A. "The Post-KR Interval: Time and Activity Effects and the Relationship of Motor Short-Term Memory Theory." *Journal of Motor Behavior* 5 (1973):49–56.

Magill, R. A. "The Processing of Knowledge of Results for a Serial Motor Task." *Journal of Motor Behavior* 9 (1977):113–18.

Magill, R. A., and Dowell, M. N. "Serial Position Effects in Motor Short-Term Memory." *Journal of Motor Behavior* 9 (1977):319–23.

Maharishi Mahesh Yogi. *Maharishi Mahesh Yogi on the Bhagavad-Gita: A New Translation and Commentary.* Baltimore: Penguin Books, 1969.

Mail, P. D. "The Influence of Binocular Depth Perception in the Learning of a Motor Skill." Master's thesis, Smith College, 1965.

Malina, R. M. "Effects of Varied Information Feedback Practice Conditions on Throwing Speed and Accuracy." *Research Quarterly* 40 (1969):134–45.

Marks, L. E. "Synesthesia: The Lucky People with Mixed-up Senses." *Psychology Today* 9 (June 1975):48–52.

Marsden, C. D.; Merton, P. A.; and Morton, H. B. "Servo Action in Human Voluntary Movement." *Nature* 238 (1972):140–43.

Marteniuk, R. G. "Individual Differences in Motor Performance and Learning." In Jack H. Wilmore, ed. *Exercise and Sport Sciences Reviews.* vol. 2. New York: Academic Press, 1974.

Marteniuk, R. G. *Information Processing in Motor Skills.* New York: Holt, Rinehart and Winston, 1976.

Marteniuk, R. G., and MacKenzie, C. L. "Information Processing in Movement Organization and Execution." In R. S. Nickerson, ed. *Attention and Performance VIII.* New York: Academic Press, 1980.

Marteniuk, R. G., and Roy, E. A. "The Codability of Kinesthetic Location and Distance Information." *Acta Psychologica* 36 (1972):471–79.

Marteniuk, R. G., and Wenger, H. A. "Facilitation of Pursuit Rotor Learning by Induced Stress." *Perceptual and Motor Skills* 31 (1970):471–77.

Martens, R. "Arousal and Motor Performance." In J. H. Wilmore, ed. *Exercise and Sport Sciences Reviews.* vol. 2. New York: Academic Press, 1974.

Martens, R. *Sport-Competitive Anxiety Test.* Champaign, Ill.: Human Kinetics Publishers, 1977.

Martens, R.; Burwitz, L.; and Newell, K. M. "Money and Praise: Do They Improve Motor Learning and Performance?" *Research Quarterly* 43 (1972):429–42.

Martens, R.; Burwitz, L.; and Zuckerman, J. "Modeling Effects of Motor Performance." *Research Quarterly* 47 (1976):277–91.

Matthews, P. B. C. "Muscle Spindles and Their Motor Control." *Physiological Reviews* 44 (1964):219–88.

Matthews, P. B. C. *Mammalian Muscle Receptors and Their Central Actions.* London: Arnolds, 1972.

Matthews, P. B. C. "Muscle Afferents and Kinesthesia." *British Medical Bulletin* 33 (1977):137–42.

Matthews, P. B. C. "Where Does Sherrington's 'Muscle Sense' Originate? Muscles, Joints, Corollary Discharges?" *Annual Review of Neuroscience* 5 (1982):189–218.

Meday, H. W. "The Influence of Practice on Kinesthetic Discrimination." Master's thesis, University of California, 1952.

Meek, F., and Skubic, V. "Spatial Perception of Highly Skilled and Poorly Skilled Females." *Perceptual and Motor Skills* 33 (1971):1309–10.

Megaw, E. D. "Directional Errors and Their Correction in a Discrete Tracking Task." *Ergonomics* 15 (1972):633–43.

Melnick, M. J. "Effects of Overlearning on the Retention of a Gross Motor Skill." *Research Quarterly* 42 (1971):60–69.

Mengelkoch, R. F.; Adams, J. A.; and Gainer, C. A. "The Forgetting of Instrument Flying Skills." *Human Factors* 13 (1971):397–405.

Merton, P. A. "How We Control the Contraction of Our Muscles." *Scientific American* 226 (May 1972):30–37.

Meyers, J. L. "Retention of Balance Coordination Learning as Influenced by Extended Layoffs." *Research Quarterly* 38 (1967):72–78.

Millar, J. "Flexion-Extension Sensitivity of Elbow Joint Afferents in Cat." *Experimental Brain Research* 24 (1975):209–14.

Miller, D. M. "The Relationship between Some Visual-Perceptual Factors and the Degree of Success Realized by Sports Performers." Doctoral dissertation, University of Southern California, 1960.

Miller, G. A. "The Magical Number Seven, Plus or Minus Two: Some Limits on Our Capacity for Processing Information." *Psychological Review* 63 (1956):81–97.

Miller, G. A.; Galanter, R.; and Pribram, K. H. *Plans and the Structure of Behavior.* New York: Holt, Rinehart and Winston, 1960.

Miller, J. W., and Ludvigh, E. J. "The Effect of Relative Motion on Visual Acuity." *Surv. Ophth.* 7 (1962):83–116.

Milner, B. "Hemispheric Specialization: Scope and Limits." In F. O. Smith and F. C. Worden, eds. *The Neurosciences: Third Study Program.* Cambridge: MIT Press, 1974.

Minas, S. C. "Mental Practice of a Complex Perceptual-Motor Skill." *Journal of Human Movement Studies* 4 (1978):102–7.

Minas, S. C. "Acquisition of a Motor Skill following Guided Mental and Physical Practice." *Journal of Human Movement Studies* 6 (1980):127–41.

Mitchell, T. R. "Organizational Behavior." In M. R. Rosenzweig and L. W. Porter, eds. *Annual Review of Psychology* Palo Alto: Annual Reviews, 1979.

Mitchell, W. M. *The Use of Hypnosis in Athletics.* printed by Valley Oaks Printers, Stockton, Calif., 1972.

Mohr, D. "The Contributions of Physical Activity to Skill Learning." *Research Quarterly* 31 (1960):321–50.

Mohr, D. R., and Barrett, M. E. "Effect of Knowledge of Mechanical Principles in Learning to Perform Intermediate Swimming Skills." *Research Quarterly* 33 (1962):574–80.

Montebello, R. A. "The Role of Stereoscopic Vision in Some Aspects of Baseball Playing Ability." Master's thesis, Ohio State University, 1953.

Moray, N. *Listening and Attention.* Harmondsworth: Penguin Books, 1969.

Moritani, T., and deVries, H. A. "Neural Factors vs. Hypertrophy in the Time Course of Muscle Strength Gain." *American Journal of Physical Medicine* 58 (1979):115–30.

Morris, G. S. D. "Effects Ball and Background Color Have upon the Catching Performance of Elementary School Children." *Research Quarterly* 47 (1976):409–16.

Morris, G. S. D., and Kreighbaum, E. "Dynamic Visual Acuity of Varsity Women Volleyball and Basketball Players." *Research Quarterly* 48 (1977):480–83.

Moruzzi, G., and Magoun, H. W. "Brain Stem Reticular Formation and Activation of the EEG." *Electroencephalography and Clinical Neurophysiology* 1 (1949):455–73.

Mott, F. W., and Sherrington, C. S. "Experiments on the Influence of Sensory Nerves upon Movement and Nutrition of Limbs: Preliminary Communication." *Proceedings of the Royal Society of London* 57 (1895):481–88.

Mountcastle, V. B., and Darian-Smith, I. "Neural Mechanisms in Somesthesia." In V. B. Mountcastle, ed. *Medical Physiology.* 12th ed., vol. 2. St. Louis: C. V. Mosby, 1968.

Müller, G. E., and Pilzecker, A. "Experimentelle beiträge zur lehre vom gedächtniss." *Zeitshrift für Psychologie and Physiologie der Sinnesorgone.* Ergan zungsband, 1 (1900):1–288.

Murray, M. J. "Matching Preferred Cognitive Mode with Teaching Methodology in Learning a Novel Motor Skill." *Research Quarterly* 50 (1979):80–87.

Nashner, L. M., and Woolacott, M. "The Organization of Rapid Postural Adjustments of Standing Humans: An Experimental-Conceptual Model." In R. E. Talbott and D. R. Humphrey, eds. *Posture and Movement.* New York: Raven Press, 1979.

Nathan, P. W., and Sears, T. A. "Effects of Posterior Root Section on the Activity of Some Muscles in Man." *Journal of Neurol. Neurosurg. Psychiat.* 23 (1960):10–22.

Naylor, J. C., and Briggs, G. E. "Long-Term Retention of Learned Skills, and Review of the Literature." *Lab. of Aviation Psychology.* Ohio State University Research Foundation, 1961.

Neisser, U. *Cognitive Psychology.* New York: Appleton-Century-Crofts, 1967.

Neisser, U. Cognition and Reality: Principles and Implications of Cognitive Psychology. San Francisco: Freeman, 1976.

Nelson, D. O. "Effects of Swimming on the Learning of Selected Gross Motor Skills." *Research Quarterly* 28 (1957):374–78.

Nelson, R. C., and Fahrney, R. A. "Relationships between Strength and Speed of Elbow Flexion." *Research Quarterly* 36 (1965):455–63.

Nelson, R. C., and Nofsinger, M. R. "Effect of Overload on Speed of Elbow Flexion and the Associated Side-Effects." *Research Quarterly* 36 (1965):174–82.

Nelson, T. O. "Repetition and Depth of Processing." *Journal of Verbal Learning and Verbal Behavior* 16 (1977):151–71.

Nessler, J. "Length of Time Necessary to View a Ball while Catching It." *Journal of Motor Behavior* 5 (1973):179–85.

Newell, K. M. "Knowledge of Results and Motor Learning." *Journal of Motor Behavior* 6 (1974):235–44.

Newell, K. M. "More on Absolute Error, Etc." *Journal of Motor Behavior* 8 (1976):139–42.

Newell, K. M. "Skill Learning." In D. H. Holding. ed. *Human Skills.* New York: John Wiley, 1981.

Newell, K. M., and Chew, R. A. "Visual Feedback and Positioning Movements." *Journal of Motor Behavior* 7 (1975):153–58.

Newell, K. M., and Kennedy, J. A. "Knowledge of Results and Children's Motor Learning." *Developmental Psychology* 14 (1978):531–36.

Newmeister, G. H. "Effects of a Visually Directed Sensory-Motor Training Program of Depth Perception of Children." *Research Quarterly* 48 (1977):129–33.

Nicklaus, J., and Bowden, K. *Golf My Way.* New York: Simon and Schuster, 1974.

Nideffer, R. M. *The Inner Athlete.* New York: Thomas Y. Crowell, 1976.

Niemeyer, R. K. "Part versus Whole Methods and Massed versus Distributed Practice in the Learning of Selected Large Muscle Activities." *62d Proceedings of the NCPEAM,* 1959, pp. 122–25.

Nixon, J. E., and Locke, L. F. "Research on Teaching Physical Education." In R. M. W. Travers ed. *Second Handbook of Research on Teaching.* Chicago: Rand McNally, 1973.

Norback, C. R., and Demarest, R. J. *The Human Nervous System.* 2d ed. New York: McGraw-Hill, 1975.

Norman, D. A. "Towards a Theory of Memory and Attention." *Psychological Review* 75 (1968):522–36.

Norman, D. A. *Memory and Attention: An Introduction to Human Information Processing.* New York: John Wiley, 1976.

Nottebohm, F. "The Ontogeny of Bird Song." *Science* 167 (1970):950–56.

Olds, J. *Drives and Reinforcements: Behavioral Studies of Hypothalamic Functions.* New York: Raven Press, 1977.

Olds, J. et al. "Learning Centers of Rat Brain Mapped by Measuring Latencies of Conditioned Unit Responses." *Journal of Neurophysiology* 35 (1972):202–19.

Olsen, E. A. "Relationship between Psychological Capacities and Success in College Athletics." *Research Quarterly* 27 (1956):79–89.

Ornstein, P. A., and Naus, M. J. "Rehearsal Processes in Children's Memory." In P. A. Ornstein, ed. *Memory Development in Children.* Hillsdale, N.J.: Erlbaum, 1978.

Oscarsson, O., and Rosen, I. "Projection to Cerebral Cortex of Large Muscle-Spindle Afferents in Forelimb Nerves of the Cat." *Journal of Physiology* 169 (1963):924–45.

Pack, M.; Cotten, D. J.; and Biasiotto, J. "Effect of Four Fatigue Levels on Performance and Learning of a Novel Dynamic Balance Skill." *Journal of Motor Behavior* 6 (1974):179–90.

Papcsy, F. E. "The Effect of Understanding a Specific Mechanical Principle upon Learning a Physical Education Skill." Doctoral dissertation, New York University, 1968.

Pargman, D.; Bender, P.; and Deshaies, P. "Correlation between Visual Disembedding and Basketball Shooting by Male and Female Varsity College Athletes." *Perceptual and Motor Skills* 41 (1975):956.

Pargman, D.; Schreiber, L. E.; and Stein, F. "Field Dependence of Selected Athletic Subgroups." *Medicine and Science in Sport* 6 (1974):283–86.

Parke, R. D. "Some Effects of Punishment of Children's Behavior." *Young Children* 24 (1969):225–40.

Parker, J. F., and Fleishman, E. A. "Use of Analytical Information Concerning Task Requirements to Increase the Effectiveness of Skill Training." *Journal of Applied Psychology* 45 (1961):295–302.

Patrick, J. "The Effect of Interpolated Motor Activities in Short-Term Motor Memory." *Journal of Motor Behavior* 3 (1971):39–48.

Pearson, K. G. "The Control of Walking." *Scientific American* 235 (December 1976):72–87.

Pemberton, C., and Cox, R. H. "Consolidation Theory and the Effects of Stress and Anxiety on Motor Behavior." *International Journal of Sport Psychology* 12 (1981):131–39.

Percival, L. "Question Clinic and Commentary on Part 3." in J. W. Taylor, ed. *Proceedings of the First International Symposium on the Art and Science of Coaching.* Willowdale, Ontario, Canada: F. I. Productions, 1971.

Petrie, A. *Individuality in Pain and Suffering.* Chicago: University of Chicago Press, 1967.

Pew, R. W. "Acquisition of Hierarchical Control over the Temporal Organization of a Skill." *Journal of Experimental Psychology* 71 (1966):764–71.

Pew, R. W. "Human Perceptual-Motor Performance." In B. H. Kantowitz, ed. *Human Information Processing: Tutorials in Performance and Cognition.* Hillsdale, N.J.: Erlbaum, 1974.

Phillips, C. G.; Powell, T. P. S.; and Wiesendanger, M. "Projection from Low-Threshold Muscle Afferents of Hand and Forearm to Area 3a of Baboon's Cortex." *Journal of Physiology* 217 (1971):419–46.

Phillips, M., and Summers, D. "Relation of Kinesthetic Perception to Motor Learning." *Research Quarterly* 25 (1954):456–69.

Phillips, W. H. "Influence of Fatiguing Warm-up Exercises on Speed of Movement and Reaction Latency." *Research Quarterly* 34 (1963):370–78.

Picton, T. W. et al. "Human Auditory Attention: A Central or Peripheral Process?" *Science* 173 (1971):351–53.

Picton, T. W., and Hillyard, S. A. "Human Auditory Evoked Potentials. II. Effects of Attention." *Electroenceph. Clin. Neurophysiol.* 36 (1974):191–99.

Pineda, A., and Adkisson, M. "Electroencephalographic Studies in Physical Fatigue." *Texas Reports in Biology and Medicine* 19 (1961):332–42.

Polit, A., and Bizzi, E. "Processes Controlling Arm Movements in Monkeys." *Science* 201 (1978):1235–37.

Polit, A., and Bizzi, E. "Characteristics of Motor Programs Underlying Arm Movements in Monkeys." *Journal of Neurophysiology* 42 (1979):183–94.

Poppelreuter, A. "Analysis der erziehung zur exaktheitsarbeit nach experimental-psychologischer methods." *Zeitschrift fur Angewandte Psychologie* vol. 29, 1928.

Posner, M. I. "Characteristics of Visual and Kinesthetic Memory Codes." *Journal of Experimental Psychology* 75 (1967): 103–7.

Posner, M. I., and Konick, A. F. "Short-Term Retention of Visual and Kinesthetic Information." *Organizational Behavior and Human Performance* 1 (1966):71–86.

Posner, M. I.; Nissen, M. J.; and Klein, R. M. "Visual Dominance: An Information-Processing Account of Its Origins and Significance." *Psychological Review* 83 (1976):157–71.

Poulton, E. C. "On Prediction in Skilled Movements." *Psychological Bulletin* 54 (1957):467–78.

Poulton, E. C. "Skill in Fast Ball Games." *Biology and Human Affairs* 3 (1965):1–5.

Proske, U. "The Golgi Tendon Organ." *Trends in Neurosciences* January 1979, pp. 7–8.

Provins, K. "The Effect of Peripheral Nerve Block on the Appreciation and Execution of Finger Movements." *Journal of Physiology* 143 (1958):55–67.

Puff, C. R., ed. *Memory Organization and Structure*. New York: Academic Press, 1979.

Purdy, B. J., and Lockhart, A. "Retention and Relearning of Gross Motor Skills after Long Periods of No Practice." *Research Quarterly* 33 (1962):265–72.

Quartermain, D. "The Influence of Drugs on Learning and Memory." In M. R. Rosenzweig and E. L. Bennett, eds. *Neural Mechanisms of Learning and Memory*. Cambridge: MIT Press, 1976.

Ragsdale, C. E. *The Psychology of Motor Learning*. Ann Arbor, Mich.: Edward Brothers Press, 1930.

Rainbow, T. C. "Role of RNA and Protein Synthesis in Memory Formation." *Neurochemical Research* 4 (1979):297–312.

Ranson, S. W., and Clark, S. L. *The Anatomy of the Nervous System*. 10th ed. Philadelphia: W. B. Saunders, 1959.

Rarick, G. L. "Cognitive-Motor Relationships in the Growing Years." *Research Quarterly for Exercise and Sport* 51 (1980):174–92.

Reed, E. S. "An Outline of a Theory of Action Systems." *Journal of Motor Behavior* 14 (1982):98–134.

Regan, D. *Evoked Potentials in Psychology, Sensory Physiology, and Clinical Medicine*. London: Chapman and Hall, 1972.

Regan, D., and Beverley, K. I. "Illusory Motion in Depth: Aftereffect of Adaptation to Changing Size." *Vision Research* 18 (1978):209–12.

Reynolds, H. L. "The Effects of Augmented Levels of Stress on Reaction Time in the Peripheral Visual Field." *Research Quarterly* 47 (1976):768–75.

Ridini, L. M. "Relationship between Psychological Functions Tests and Selected Sports Skills of Boys in Junior High School. *Research Quarterly* 39 (1968):674–83.

Rikli, R., and Smith, G. "Videotape Feedback Effects on Tennis Serving Form." *Perceptual and Motor Skills* 50 (1980):895–901.

Robb, M. D. "Feedback and Skill Learning." *Research Quarterly* 39 (1968):175–84.

Roberts, W. H. "The Effect of Delayed Feeding on White Rats in a Problem Cage." *Journal of Genetic Psychology* 37 (1930):35–38.

Robinson, E. S. "The 'Similarity' Factor in Retroaction." *American Journal of Psychology* 39 (1927):297–312.

Roediger, H. L.; Knight, J. L.; and Kantowitz, B. "Inferring Decay in Short-Term Memory: The Issue of Capacity." *Memory and Cognition* 5 (1977):167–76.

Rogers, C. A., Jr. "Feedback Precision and Postfeedback Interval Duration." *Journal of Experimental Psychology* 102 (1974):604–8.

Roland, P. E. "Do Muscular Receptors in Man Evoke Sensations of Tension and Kinesthesia?" *Brain Research* 99 (1975):162–65.

Roland, P. E., and Ladegaard-Peterson, H. "A Quantitative Analysis of Sensations of Tension and of Kinesthesia in Man: Evidence for a Peripherally Originating Muscular Sense and Sense of Effort." *Brain* 100 (1977):671–92.

Roland, P. E. et al. "The Role of Different Cortical Areas in the Organization of Voluntary Movements in Man." In D. H. Ingvar and N. A. Lassen, eds. *Cerebral Function: Metabolism and Circulation*. Copenhagen: Munksgaard, 1977.

Rose, J. E., and Mountcastle, V. B. "Touch and Kinesthesis." In J. Field, ed. *Handbook of Physiology: Neurophysiology* Section I (Vol. I). Washington, D.C.: American Physiological Society, 1959.

Rose, M. C., and Glad, H. L. "Relationship of Some Traditional Methods and a Unique Procedure for Measuring Kinesthesis." Paper presented at AAHPER Convention, Anaheim, California, 1974.

Rose, S. P. R., and Longstaff, A. "Neurochemical Aspects of Learning and Memory." In J. L. McGaugh and R. Thompson, eds. *Neurobiology of Learning and Memory*. New York: Plenum Press, 1979.

Rosenberg, M. *Conceiving the Self*. New York: Basic Books, 1979.

Rosenzweig, M. R.; Bennett, E. L.; and Diamond, M. C. "Brain Changes in Response to Experience." *Scientific American* 226 (February 1972):22–29.

Rothstein, A. L., and Arnold, R. K. "Bridging the Gap: Application of Research on Videotape Feedback and Bowling." *Motor Skills: Theory into Practice*. 1 (1976):35–62.

Roy, E. A. "Role of Preselection in Memory for Movement Extent." *Journal of Experimental Psychology: Human Learning and Memory*. 4 (1978):397–405.

Ruch, T. C., and Fulton, J. F., eds. *Medical Physiology and Biophysics*. 18th ed. Philadelphia: W. B. Saunders, 1960.

Rushall, B. S., and Siedentop, D. *The Development and Control of Behavior in Sport and Physical Education*. Philadelphia: Lea & Febiger, 1972.

Russell, W. R. *Brain: Memory and Learning.* London: Oxford University Press, 1959.

Ryan, E. D. "Retention of Stabilometer and Pursuit Rotor Skills." *Research Quarterly* 33 (1962):593–98.

Ryan, E. D. "Retention of Stabilometer Performance over Extended Periods of Time." *Research Quarterly* 36 (1965):46–51.

Ryan, E. D. "Perceptual Characteristics of Vigorous People." In B. J. Cratty and R. C. Brown, eds. *New Perspectives of Man in Action.* Englewood Cliffs: Prentice Hall, 1969.

Ryan, E. D., and Simons, J. "Cognitive Demand, Imagery, and Frequency of Mental Rehearsal as Factors Influencing Acquisition of Motor Skills." *Journal of Sport Psychology.* 3 (1981):35–45.

Safrit, M. J.; Spray, J. A.; and Diewert, G. L. "Methodological Issues in Short-Term Motor Memory Research." *Journal of Motor Behavior* 12 (1980):13–28.

Sage, G. H., and Bennett, B. "The Effects of Induced Arousal on Learning and Performance of a Pursuit Motor Skill." *Research Quarterly* 44 (1973):140–49.

Sage, G. H., and Hornak, J. E. "Progressive Speed Practice in Learning a Continuous Motor Skill." *Research Quarterly* 49 (1978):190–96.

Sanderson, F. H., and Whiting, H. T. A. "Dynamic Visual Acuity and Performance in a Catching Task." *Journal of Motor Behavior* 6 (1974):87–94.

Sanderson, F. H., and Whiting, H. T. A. "Dynamic Visual Acuity: A Possible Factor in Catching Performance." *Journal of Motor Behavior* 10 (1978):7–14.

Scanlan, T. K. "Social Evaluation: A Key Developmental Element in the Competition Process." In R. A. Magill; J. J. Ash; and F. L. Smoll, eds. *Children in Sport: A Contemporary Anthology.* Champaign, Ill.: Human Kinetics Publishers, 1978.

Scannell, R. J. "Transfer of Accuracy Training When Difficulty Is Controlled by Varying Target Size." *Research Quarterly* 39 (1968):341–50.

Schmidt, R. A. "Performance and Learning of a Gross Motor Skill under Conditions of Artificially Induced Fatigue." *Research Quarterly* 40 (1969):185–90.

Schmidt, R. A. "The Case against Learning and Forgetting Scores." *Journal of Motor Behavior* 4 (1972):79–88.

Schmidt, R. A. "A Schema Theory of Discrete Motor Skill Learning." *Psychological Review* 82 (1975):225–60.

Schmidt, R. A. "Control Processes in Motor Skills." In J. Keogh and R. S. Hutton, eds. *Exercise and Sport Sciences Reviews.* vol. 4. Santa Barbara, Calif.: Journal Publishing Affiliates, 1976a.

Schmidt, R. A. "The Schema as a Solution to Some Persistent Problems in Motor Learning Theory." In G. E. Stelmach, ed. *Motor Control: Issues and Trends.* New York: Academic Press, 1976b.

Schmidt, R. A. "Past and Future Issues in Motor Programming." *Research Quarterly for Exercise and Sport* 51 (1980):122–40.

Schmidt, R. A. *Motor Control and Learning.* Champaign, Ill.: Human Kinetics Publishers, 1981.

Schmidt, R. A. "More on Motor Programs." In J. A. S. Kelso, ed. *Human Motor Behavior: An Introduction.* Hillsdale, N.J.: Erlbaum, 1982.

Schmidt, R. A.; Christenson, R.; and Rogers, P. "Some Evidence for the Independence of Recall and Recognition in Motor Behavior." In D. M. Landers; D. V. Harris; and R. W. Christina, eds. *Psychology of Motor Behavior and Sport.* Penn State Series. State College, Pennsylvania: 1975.

Schmidt, R. A., and McCabe, J. F. "Motor Program Utilization over Extended Practice." *Journal of Human Movement Studies* 2 (1976):239–47.

Schmidt, R. A. and McGown, C. M. "Terminal Accuracy of Unexpected Loaded Rapid Movements: Evidence for a Mass-Spring Mechanism in Programming." *Journal of Motor Behavior* 12 (1980):149–61.

Schmidt, R. A., and Shea, J. B. "A Note on Delay of Knowledge of Results in Positioning Responses." *Journal of Motor Behavior* 8 (1976):129–31.

Schneider W., and Shiffrin, R. M. "Controlled and Automatic Human Information Processing: I. Detection, Search, and Attention." *Psychological Review* 84 (1977):1–66.

Schultz, D. D. *Sensory Restriction: Effects on Behavior.* New York: Academic Press, 1965.

Schultz, J. A. *Das autogenne training. Konzentrative selbstentspannung* [The Self-Training. The Concentrative Self-Relaxation]. Stuttgart, Germany, 1956.

Schutz, R. W. "Absolute, Constant, and Variable Error: Problems and Solutions." In D. Mood, ed. *Proceedings of the Colorado Measurement Symposium.* Boulder, Colo.: University of Colorado, 1977.

Schutz, R. W., and Roy, E. A. "Absolute Error: The Devil in Disguise." *Journal of Motor Behavior* 5 (1973):141–53.

Schwartz, S. "A Learning-Based System to Categorize Teacher Behavior." *Quest* 17 (1972):52–55.

Scott, M. G. "Measurement of Kinesthesis." *Research Quarterly* 26 (1955):324–41.

Sekuler, R., and Levinson, E. "The Perception of Moving Targets." *Scientific American* 236 (January 1977):60–73.

Shapiro, D. C. "Bilateral Transfer of a Motor Program." Paper presented at the annual meeting of the AAHPER, Seattle, Washington, 1977.

Shapiro, D. C., and Schmidt, R. A. "The Schema Theory: Recent Evidence and Developmental Implications." In J. A. S. Kelso and J. E. Clark, eds. *The Development of Movement Control and Co-ordination*. New York: John Wiley, 1982.

Shea, J. B. "Interresponse Interval Length and the Development of an Error Detection Mechanism: A Test of Adams' Closed-Loop Theory of Motor Learning." Paper presented at the AAHPER convention, 1975.

Shea, J. B. "Effects of Labeling on Motor Short-Term Memory." *Journal of Experimental Psychology: Human Learning and Memory.* 3 (1977):92–99.

Shea, J. B., and Morgan, R. L. "Contextual Interference Effects on the Acquisition, Retention, and Transfer of a Motor Skill." *Journal of Experimental Psychology: Human Learning and Memory* 5 (1979):179–87.

Shea, J. B., and Upton, G. "The Effects of Skill Acquisition of an Interpolated Motor Short-Term Memory Task during the KR-Delay Interval." *Journal of Motor Behavior* 8 (1976):277–81.

Shelton, T. O., and Mahoney, M. J. "The Content and Effect of 'Psyching-up' Strategies in Weight Lifters." *Cognitive Therapy and Research* 2 (1978):275–84.

Sherrington, C. *The Integrative Action of the Nervous System*. New Haven: Yale University Press, 1906.

Sherrington, C. "Flexion-Reflex of the Limb, Crossed Extension Reflex, and Reflex Stepping and Standing." *Journal of Physiology* 40 (1910):28–121.

Shick, J. "Effects of Mental Practice on Selected Volleyball Skills for College Women." *Research Quarterly* 41 (1970):88–94.

Shick, J. "Relationship between Depth Perception and Hand-Eye Dominance and Free-throw Shooting in College Women." *Perceptual and Motor Skills* 33 (1971):539–42.

Shik, M. L., and Orlovskii, G. N. "Neurophysiology of a Locomotor Automatism." *Physiological Reviews* 56 (1976):465–501.

Shugart, B. S.; Souder, M. A.; and Bunker, L. K. "Relationship between Vertical Space, Perception and a Dynamic Non-locomotor Balance Task." *Perceptual and Motor Skills* 34 (1972):43–46.

Siedentop, D. *Developing Teaching Skills in Physical Education*. Boston: Houghton Mifflin, 1976.

Siegel, D., and Davis, C. "Transfer Effects of Learning at Specific Speeds on Performance over a Range of Speeds." *Perceptual and Motor Skills* 50 (1980):83–89.

Sills, F. D., and Troutman, D. C. "Peripheral Vision and Accuracy in Shooting a Basketball." *69th Proceedings of the NCPEAM*, 1966, pp. 112–14.

Simmons, R. W., and Snyder, R. J. "The Effects of Varying Knowledge of Results Delay upon the Acquisition of a Discrete Skill." In G. C. Roberts and D. M. Landers, eds. *Psychology of Motor Behavior and Sport*. Champaign, Ill.: Human Kinetics Publishers, 1980.

Sinclair, C. B., and Smith, I. M. "Laterality in Swimming and Its Relationship to Dominance of Hand, Eye, and Foot." *Research Quarterly* 28 (1957):395–401.

Singer, R. N. "Transfer Effects and Ultimate Success in Archery Due to Degree of Difficulty of the Initial Learning." *Research Quarterly* 37 (1966):532–39.

Sjoberg, H. "Relations between Different Arousal Levels Induced by Graded Physical Work and Psychological Efficiency." Report from the Psychological Laboratories, No. 251, University of Stockholm, Sweden, 1968.

Skinner, B. F. *The Technology of Teaching*. New York: Appleton-Century-Crofts, 1968.

Skinner, B. F. *Contingencies of Reinforcement*. New York: Appleton-Century-Crofts, 1969.

Skinner, J. E. *Neuroscience: A Laboratory Manual*. Philadelphia: W. B. Saunders Company, 1971.

Skoglund, S. "Anatomical and Physiological Studies of Knee Joint Innervation in the Cat." *Acta Physiol. Scandinav.* 36 (1956):(suppl. 124): 1–101.

Slater-Hammel, A. T. "Reaction Time to Light Stimulus in the Peripheral Visual Field." *Research Quarterly* 26 (1955):82–87.

Smith, A. "Sport Is a Western Yoga." *Psychology Today* 9 (October 1975):48.

Smith, J. L. "Kinesthesis: A Model for Movement Feedback." In R. C. Brown and B. J. Cratty, eds. *New Perspectives of Man in Action*. Englewood Cliffs: Prentice-Hall, 1969.

Smith, J. L. "Sensorimotor Integration during Motor Programming." In G. E. Stelmach, ed. *Information Processing in Motor Control and Learning*. New York: Academic Press, 1978.

Smith, J. L.; Roberts, E. M.; and Atkins, E. "Fusimotor Neuron Block and Voluntary Arm Movement in Man." *American Journal of Physical Medicine.* 51 (1972):225–39.

Smith, K. U. *Delayed Sensory Feedback and Behavior*. Philadelphia: W. B. Saunders, 1962.

Smith, K. U., and Smith, W. M. *Perception and Motion.* Philadelphia: W. B. Saunders, 1962.

Smith, W. M., and Bowen, K. F. "The Effects of Delayed and Displaced Visual Feedback on Motor Control." *Journal of Motor Behavior* 12 (1980):91–101.

Smode, A. "Learning and Performance in a Tracking Task under Two Levels of Achievement Information Feedback." *Journal of Experimental Psychology* 56 (1958):297–304.

Smoll, F. L. "Effects of Precision of Information Feedback upon Acquisition of a Motor Skill." *Research Quarterly* 43 (1972):489–93.

Smyth, M. M. "Attention to Visual Feedback in Motor Learning." *Journal of Motor Behavior* 10 (1978):185–90.

Smyth, M. M., and Marriott, A. M. "Vision and Proprioception in Simple Catching." *Journal of Motor Behavior* 14 (1982):143–52.

Solomon, P. et al., eds. *Sensory Deprivation.* Cambridge: Harvard University Press, 1961.

Sperling, G. "The Information Available in Brief Visual Presentations." *Psychological Monographs* 74 (11, Whole no. 498), 1960.

Sperry, R. W. "Lateral Specialization in the Surgically Separated Hemispheres." In F. O. Schmitt and F. G. Worden, eds. *The Neurosciences: Third Study Program.* Cambridge: MIT Press, 1974.

Spielberger, C. D. "Theory and Research on Anxiety." In C. D. Spielberger, ed. *Anxiety and Behavior.* New York: Academic Press, 1966.

Speilberger, C. D.; Gorsuch, R. L.; and Lushene, R. E. *State-Trait Anxiety Inventory.* Palo Alto, Calif.: Consulting Psychologists Press, 1970.

Stabler, J. R., and Dyal, J. A. "Discriminative Reaction-Time as a Joint Function of Manifest Anxiety and Intelligence." *American Journal of Psychology* 76 (1963):484–87.

Stallings, L. M. "The Role of Visual-Spatial Abilities in the Performance of Certain Motor Skills." *Research Quarterly* 39 (1968):708–13.

Stein, P. S. G. "Motor Systems, with Specific Reference to the Control of Locomotion." *Annual Review of Neuroscience* 1 (1978):61–81.

Stelmach, G. E. "Prior Positioning Responses as a Factor in Short-Term Retention of a Simple Motor Task." *Journal of Experimental Psychology* 81 (1969a):523–26.

Stelmach, G. E. "Efficiency of Motor Learning as a Function of Intertrial Rest." *Research Quarterly* 40 (1969b):198–202.

Stelmach, G. E. "Learning and Response Consistency with Augmented Feedback." *Ergonomics* 13 (1970):421–25.

Stelmach, G. E. "Retention of Motor Skills." In J. H. Wilmore, ed. *Exercise and Sport Sciences Reviews.* vol. 2. New York: Academic Press, 1974.

Stelmach, G. E. "A New Perspective on Motor Skill Automation." *Research Quarterly for Exercise and Sport* 51 (1980):141–57.

Stennett, R. G. "The Relationship of Performance Level to Level of Arousal." *Journal of Experimental Psychology* 54 (1957):54–61.

Stevens, C. F. *Neurophysiology: A Primer.* New York: John Wiley, 1966.

Stockfelt, T. "Mental Performance during Varied Physiological Exertion." In G. S. Kenyon, ed. *Contemporary Psychology of Sport.* Chicago: The Athletic Institute, 1970.

Stockholm, A. J., and Nelson, R. "The Immediate After-effects of Increased Resistance upon Physical Performance." *Research Quarterly* 36 (1965):337–41.

Straub, W. F. "Effect of Overload Training Procedures upon Velocity and Accuracy of the Overarm Throw." *Research Quarterly* 39 (1968):370–79.

Suinn, R. M. "Psychology for Olympic Champs." *Psychology Today* 10 (July 1976):38–43.

Suinn, R. M. *Psychology in Sports: Methods and Applications.* Minneapolis: Burgess Publishing, 1980.

Summers, J. J. "Motor Programs." In D. H. Holding, ed. *Human Skills.* New York: John Wiley, 1981.

Swift, E. J. "Studies in the Psychology and Physiology of Learning." *American Journal of Psychology.* 14 (1903):201–51.

Szekely, A.; Czech, G.; and Voros, G. "The Activity Pattern of Limb Muscles in Freely Moving Normal and Deafferented Newts." *Experimental Brain Research* 9 (1969):53–72.

Taub, E., and Berman, A. J. "Movement and Learning in the Absence of Sensory Feedback." In S. J. Freedman, ed. *The Neuropsychology of Spatially Oriented Behavior.* Homewood, Ill.: Dorsey Press, 1968.

Taub, E.; Heitmann, E.; and Barro, G. "Alertness, Level of Activity, and Purposive Movement following Somatosensory Deafferentation in Monkeys." *Annals of the New York Academy* 290 (1977):348–65.

Taub, E.; Perrella, P.; and Barro, G. "Behavioral Development after Forelimb Deafferentation on Day of Birth in Monkeys with and without Blinding." *Science.* 181 (1973):959–60.

Taylor, A., and Cody, F. W. J. "Jaw Muscle Spindle Activity in the Cat during Normal Movements of Eating and Drinking." *Brain Research* 71 (1974):523–30.

Tecce, J. J. "Contingent Negative Variation (CNV) and Psychological Processes in Man." *Psychological Bulletin* 77 (1972):73–108.

Temple, I. G., and Williams, H. G. "Rate and Level of Learning as Functions of Information-Processing Characteristics of the Learner and the Task." *Journal of Motor Behavior* 9 (1977):179–92.

Thach, W. T. "Discharge of Cerebellar Neurons Related to Two Maintained Postures and Two Prompt Movements. II. Purkinje Cell Output and Input." *Journal of Neurophysiology* 33 (1970):537–47.

Thayer, R. E. "Measurement of Activation through Self-report." Monograph Suppl. 1–V20. *Psychology Reports.* 20 (1967):663–78.

Thayer, R. E. "Activation States as Assessed by Verbal Report and Four Psychophysiological Variables." *Psychophysiology* 7 (1970):86–94.

Thomas, J. R.; Mitchell, B.; and Solomon, M. A. "Precision Knowledge of Results and Motor Performance: Relationship to Age." *Research Quarterly* 50 (1979):687–98.

Thomas, J. R.; Pierce, C.; and Ridsdale, S. "Age Differences in Children's Ability to Model Motor Behavior." *Research Quarterly* 48 (1977):592–97.

Thompson, R. "Localization of the 'Maze Memory System' in the White Rat." *Physiological Psychology* 2 (1974):1–17.

Thorndike, E. L. *Educational Psychology.* New York: Lemcke and Buechner, 1903.

Thorndike, E. L. *Animal Intelligence.* New York: Macmillan, 1911.

Toole, T., and Arink, E. A. "Movement Education: Its Effect on Motor Skill Performance." *Research Quarterly for Exercise and Sport* 53 (1982):156–62.

Toole, T.; Christina, R. W.; and Anson, J. G. "Preselected Movement Accuracy as a Function of Movement Time, Distance, and Velocity." *Journal of Human Movement Studies* 8 (1982):93–102.

Tracey, D. J. "Joint Receptors and the Control of Movement." *Trends in Neurosciences* (November 1980):253–55.

Trowbridge, M. H., and Cason, H. "An Experimental Study of Thorndike's Theory of Learning." *Journal of General Psychology* 7 (1932):245–58.

Trumbo, D.; Ulrich, L.; and Noble, M. "Verbal Coding and Display Coding in the Acquisition and Retention of Tracking Skill." *Journal of Applied Psychology* 49 (1965):368–75.

Tulving, E. "Subjective Organization and Effects of Repetition in Multi-trial Free-Recall Learning. *Journal of Verbal Learning and Verbal Behavior* 5 (1966):193–97.

Tulving, E. "Cue-Dependent Forgetting." *American Scientist* 62 (1974):74–82.

Turvey, M. T. "Preliminaries to a Theory of Action with Reference to Vision." In R. Shaw and J. Bransford, eds. *Perceiving, Acting, and Knowing: Towards an Ecological Psychology.* Hillsdale, N.J.: Erlbaum, 1977.

Tyldesley, D. T. "Timing in motor skills." Doctoral dissertation, University of Leeds, 1978.

Vance, M. A. "Corrective Movements in a Pursuit Task." *Quarterly Journal of Experimental Psychology* 1 (1948):85–103.

Vandell, R. A.; Davis, R. A.; and Clugston, H. A. "The Function of Mental Practice in the Acquisition of Motor Skills." *Journal of General Psychology* 29 (1943):243–50.

Vander, A. J.; Sherman, J. H.; and Luciano, D. S. *Human Physiology: The Mechanisms of Body Function.* New York: McGraw-Hill, 1970.

Vincent, W. J. "Transfer Effects between Motor Skills Judged Similar in Perceptual Components." *Research Quarterly* 39 (1968):380–88.

Walker, E. L., and Tarte, R. D. "Memory Storage as a Function of Arousal and Time with Homogeneous and Heterogeneous Lists." *Journal of Verbal Learning and Verbal Behavior* 2 (1963):113–19.

Wallace, R. K., and Benson, H. "The Physiology of Meditation." *Scientific American* 226 (February 1972):85–90.

Wallace, S. A., and Hagler, R. W. "Knowledge of Performance and the Learning of a Closed Motor Skill." *Research Quarterly* 50 (1979):265–71.

Wallace, S. A., and McGhee, R. C. "The Independence of Recall and Recognition in Motor Learning." *Journal of Motor Behavior* 11 (1979):141–51.

Walsh, W. D. et al. "Memory for Constrained and Preselected Movement Location and Distance: Effects of Starting Position and Length." *Journal of Motor Behavior* 11 (1979):201–14.

Walters, G. C. and Grusec, J. E. *Punishment.* San Francisco: W. H. Freeman and Company, 1977.

Weinberg, D. R.; Guy, D. E.; and Tupper, R. W. "Variation of Postfeedback Interval in Simple Motor Learning." *Journal of Experimental Psychology* 67 (1964):98–99.

Weinberg, R. S. "The Effects of Success and Failure on the Patterning of Neuromuscular Energy." *Journal of Motor Behavior* 10 (1978):53–61.

Weinberg, R. S. "The Relationship between Mental Preparation Strategies and Motor Performance: A Review and Critique." *Quest* 33 (1981):195–213.

Weinberg, R. S.; Gould, D.; and Jackson, A. "Expectations and Performance: An Empirical Test of Bandura's Self-efficacy Theory." *Journal of Sport Psychology* 1 (1979):320–31.

Weinberg, R. S.; Gould, D.; and Jackson, A. "Cognition and Motor Performance: Effect of Psyching-up Strategies on Three Motor Tasks." *Cognitive Therapy and Research* 4 (1980):239–45.

Weinberg, R. S., and Hunt, V. V. "The Interrelationships between Anxiety, Motor Performance and Electromyography." *Journal of Motor Behavior* 8 (1976):219–24.

Weinberg, R. S., and Ragan, J. "Motor Performance under Three Levels of Trait Anxiety and Stress." *Journal of Motor Behavior* 10 (1978):169–76.

Weinberg, R. S.; Yukelson, D.; and Jackson, A. "Effect of Public and Private Efficacy Expectations on Competitive Performance." *Journal of Sport Psychology* 2 (1980):340–49.

Weiner, B. "Motivation and Memory." *Psychological Monographs.* 80 (18, Whole no. 626), 1966.

Weiner, B. "Motivation Factors in Short-Term Retention: II. Rehearsal or Arousal?" *Psychology Report* 20 (1967):1203–8.

Weiner, B., and Walker, E. L. "Motivational Factors in Short-Term Retention." *Journal of Experimental Psychology* 71 (1966):190–93.

Weingarten, G. "Mental Performance during Physical Exertion: The Benefit of Being Physically Fit." *International Journal of Sport Psychology.* 4 (1973):16–26.

Weingarten, G., and Alexander, J. P. "Effects of Physical Exertion on Mental Performance of College Males of Different Physical Fitness Level." *Perceptual and Motor Skills* 31 (1970):371–78.

Weissman, S., and Freeburne, C. M. "Relationship between Static and Dynamic Visual Acuity. *Journal of Experimental Psychology.* 70 (1965):141–46.

Welford, A. T. *Fundamentals of Skill.* London: Methuen, 1968.

Welford, A. T. *Skilled Performance: Perceptual and Motor Skills.* Glenview, Ill.: Scott, Foresman, 1976.

Weltman, G., and Egstrom, G. H. "Perceptual Narrowing in Novice Divers." *Human Factors* 8 (1966):499–506.

Werner, P. "Integration of Physical Education Skills with the Concept of Levers at Intermediate Grade Levels." *Research Quarterly* 43 (1972):423–28.

White, K. D.; Ashton, R.; and Lewis, S. "Learning a Complex Skill: Effects of Mental Practice, Physical Practice, and Imagery Ability." *International Journal of Sport Psychology* 10 (1979):71–78.

Whiting, H. T. A. "Training in a Continuous Ball Throwing and Catching Task." *Ergonomics* 11 (1968):375–82.

Whiting, H. T. A. "Overview of the Skill Learning Process." *Research Quarterly* 43 (1972):266–94.

Whiting, H. T. A.; Alderson, G. J. K.; and Sanderson, F. H. "Critical Time for Viewing and Individual Differences in Performance of a Ball-Catching Task." *International Journal of Sport Psychology* 4 (1973):155–64.

Whiting, H. T. A.; Gill, B.; and Stephenson, J. "Critical Time Intervals for Taking in Flight Information in a Ball-Catching Task." *Ergonomics* 13 (1970):265–72.

Whiting, H. T. A., and Sanderson, F. H. "The Effect of Exercise on the Visual and Auditory Acuity of Table-tennis Players." *Journal of Motor Behavior* 4 (1972):163–70.

Whitley, J. D. "Effects of Practice Distribution on Learning a Fine Motor Task." *Research Quarterly* 41 (1970):576–83.

Whorf, B. L. "Science and Linguistics." In S. Saporta, ed. *Psycholinguistics.* New York: Holt, Rinehart and Winston, 1961.

Wiesendanger, M. "The Pyramidal Tract. Recent Investigations on Its Morphology and Function." *Ergebnisse der Physiologie, Biologischen Chemie und Experimentellen Pharmakologie* 61 (1969):72–136.

Wiesendanger, M. "Input from Muscle and Cutaneous Nerves of the Hand and Forearm to Neurons of the Precentral Gyrus of Baboons and Monkeys." *Journal of Physiology* 228 (1973):203–19.

Wilberg, R. B., and Girard, N. C. "A Further Investigation into the Serial Position Curve for Short-Term Motor Memory." *Proceedings of the IX Canadian Psychomotor Learning and Sport Psychology Symposium.* Banff, Alberta, Canada, 1977.

Williams, H. G., and Helfrich, J. "Saccadic Eye Movement Speed and Motor Response Execution." *Research Quarterly* 48 (1977):598–605.

Williams, J., and Singer, R. N. "Muscular Fatigue and the Learning and Performance of a Motor Control Task." *Journal of Motor Behavior.* 7 (1975):265–69.

Williams, J. M. "Perceptual Style and Fencing Skill." *Perceptual and Motor Skills* 40 (1975):282.

Williams, J. M., and Thirer, J. "Vertical and Horizontal Peripheral Vision in Male and Female Athletes and Non-athletes." *Research Quarterly* 46 (1975):200–205.

Wilson, D. M. "The Central Nervous Control of Flight in a Locust." *Journal of Experimental Biology* 38 (1961):471–90.

Winningham, S. N. "Effect of Training with Ankle Weights on Running Skill." Doctoral dissertation, University of Southern California, 1966.

Witkin, H. A. et al. *Personality through Perception.* New York: Harper and Row, 1954.

Wood, G. A. "An Electrophysiological Model of Human Visual Reaction Time." *Journal of Motor Behavior* 9 (1977):267–74.

Woods, J. B. "The Effect of Varied Instructional Emphasis upon the Development of a Motor Skill." *Research Quarterly* 38 (1967):132–42.

Woodworth, R. S. "The Accuracy of Voluntary Movement." *Psychological Review* 3 (2, Whole no. 13), 1899.

Woodworth, R. S. *Le Mouvement.* Paris: Dain, 1903.

Yerkes, R. M., and Dodson, J. D. "The Relation of Strength of Stimulus to Rapidity of Habit Formation." *Journal of Comparative Neur. Psychology* 18 (1908):459–82.

Young, J. Z. *Programs of the Brain.* New York: Oxford Press, 1978.

Yost, M.; Strauss, R.; and Davis, R. "The Effectiveness of the 'Golfer's Groove' in Improving Golfers' Scores." *Research Quarterly* 47 (1976):569–73.

Yukl, G. A., and Latham, G. P. "Interrelationships among Employee Participation, Individual Differences, Goal Difficulty, Goal Acceptance, Instrumentality, and Performance." *Personnel Psychology* 31 (1978):305–23.

Zaichkowsky, L. D., and Sime, W. E., eds. *Stress Management for Sport.* Reston, Va.: AAHPERD, 1982.

Zajonc, R. B. "Social Facilitation." *Science* 149 (1965): 269–74.

Zajonc, R. B. *Social Psychology: An Experimental Approach.* Belmont, Calif.: Brooks/Cole, 1966.

Zander, A. F. *Motives and Goals in Groups.* New York: Academic Press, 1971.

Zeki, S. "Cells Responding to Changing Image Size and Disparity in the Cortex of the Rhesus Monkey." *Journal of Physiology* 242 (1974):827–41.

Zelaznik, H. N., Hawkins, B., and Kisselburgh, L. "Rapid Visual Feedback Processing in Single-Aiming Movements." *Journal of Motor Behavior* 15 (1983):217–36.

Zelaznik, H. N.; Shapiro, D. C.; and Newell, K. M. "On the Structure of Motor Recognition Memory." *Journal of Motor Behavior* 10 (1978):313–23.

Zelazo, P. R. "From Reflexive to Instrumental Behavior." In L. Lipsitt, ed. *Developmental Psychobiology: The Significance of Infancy.* Hillsdale, N.J.: Erlbaum, 1976.

Credits

Table 2.2 Gentile, A. M. et al. "Structure of motor tasks." *Mouvement, Actes du 7ᵉ symposium en apprentissage psychomoteur et psychologie du sport.* October, 1975, pp. 11–28.

Figure 2.1 From *Experimental Psychology: a Laboratory Manual* edited by Benjamin L. Hart. W. H. Freeman and Company. Copyright © 1976.

Figure 2.2 From J. E. Skinner. *Neuroscience: a Laboratory Manual,* Philadelphia: W. B. Saunders, 1971. Reproduced with permission of publisher.

Figure 2.4 From G. A. Wood. "An Electrophysical Model of Human Visual Reaction Time." *Journal of Motor Behavior.* 9:267–274, 1977. Reproduced by permission of publisher.

Figure 2.6 Adapted from Figure 1, page 336, *Research Quarterly* 1963, *34,* from "Reaction Time and Speed of Movement in Males and Females of Various Ages," by Jean Hodgkins. Used by permission.

Figure 2.12 Based on Noble, C. E., "Selective Learning." In E. A. Bilodeau (ed.) *Acquisition of Skill.* New York: Academic Press, pp. 47–97. Reprinted by permission.

Figure 4.1 From Langley, L. L., I. R. Telford & J. B. Christensen 1969. *Dynamic Anatomy and Physiology,* 3rd ed. Copyright 1969 by McGraw-Hill Book Company. Reprinted by permission.

Figure 4.3 From Crouch, J. D. (1965). *Functional Human Anatomy.* Philadelphia: Lea & Febiger. Reprinted by permission.

Figure 4.4 From Langley, L. L., I. R. Telford & J. B. Christensen 1969. *Dynamic Anatomy and Physiology,* 3rd ed. Copyright 1969 by McGraw-Hill Book Company. Reprinted by permission.

Figure 4.5 From C. R. Noback, *The Human Nervous System.* © 1967 McGraw-Hill Book Company, New York, New York. Reprinted by permission.

Figure 4.6 From Langley, L. L., I. R. Telford & J. B. Christensen. *Dynamic Anatomy and Physiology,* 3rd ed. Copyright 1969 by McGraw-Hill Book Company. Reprinted by permission.

Figure 4.7 From Hole, John W., Jr., *Human Anatomy and Physiology* 2nd ed. © 1978, 1981 Wm. C. Brown Publishers, Dubuque, Iowa. All Rights Reserved. Reprinted by permission.

Figure 4.8 From Langley, L. L., I. R. Telford & J. B. Christensen. *Dynamic Anatomy and Physiology,* 3rd ed. Copyright 1969 by McGraw-Hill Book Company. Reprinted by permission.

Figure 4.9 Based on McNaught, A. B. & Callander, R. *Illustrated Physiology.* Baltimore: Williams & Wilkins, 1963.

Figure 4.10 From Langley, L. L., I. R. Telford & J. B. Christensen. *Dynamic Anatomy and Physiology,* 3rd ed. Copyright 1969 by McGraw-Hill Book Company. Reprinted by permission.

Figure 4.12 From Langley, L. L., I. R. Telford & J. B. Christensen. *Dynamic Anatomy and Physiology,* 3rd ed. Copyright 1969 by McGraw-Hill Book Company. Reprinted by permission.

Figure 4.13 From Langley, L. L., I. R. Telford & J. B. Christensen. *Dynamic Anatomy and Physiology,* 3rd ed. Copyright 1969 by McGraw-Hill Book Company. Reprinted by permission.

Figure 4.14 From C. R. Noback, *The Human Nervous System.* © 1967, McGraw-Hill Book Company, New York, New York. Reprinted by permission.

Figure 4.15 From Langley, L. L., I. R. Telford & J. B. Christensen. *Dynamic Anatomy and Physiology,* 3rd ed. Copyright 1969 by McGraw-Hill Book Company. Reprinted by permission.

Figure 4.16 From Langley, L. L., I. R. Telford & J. B. Christensen. *Dynamic Anatomy and Physiology,* 3rd ed. Copyright 1969 by McGraw-Hill Book Company. Reprinted by permission.

Figure 4.17 From Langley, L. L., I. R. Telford & J. B. Christensen. *Dynamic Anatomy and Physiology,* 3rd ed. Copyright 1969 by McGraw-Hill Book Company. Reprinted by permission.

Figure 10.9 From: Matthews, *Mammalian Muscle Receptors and Their Central Actions,* 1972. Used with permission of Edward Arnold (Publishers) Ltd.

Figure 10.10 McNaught, A. B. & Callander, R. (1983). *Illustrated Physiology* 4th edn. Edinburgh: Churchill Livingstone.

Figure 10.11 Based on Guyton, A. C. 1966. *Textbook of Medical Physiology* (3rd ed.) Philadelphia: W. B. Saunders. Reprinted by permission.

Figure 10.13 Based on Woodburne, L. S., 1967. *The Neural Basis of Behavior.* Columbus, Ohio: Charles E. Merrill Publishing Co. Reprinted by permission.

Figure 10.14 McNaught, A. B. & Callander, R. (1983). *Illustrated Physiology* 4th edn. Edinburgh: Churchill Livingstone.

Figure 10.15 McNaught, A. B. & Callander, R. (1983). *Illustrated Physiology* 4th edn. Edinburgh: Churchill Livingstone.

Figure 10.16 McNaught, A. B. & Callander, R. (1983). *Illustrated Physiology* 4th edn. Edinburgh: Churchill Livingstone.

Figure 11.1 Based on Fleishman, E. A. "A relationship between incentive motivation and ability level in psycho-motor performance." *Journal of Experimental Psychology, 56:*78–81, 1958. Copyright 1958 by the American Psychological Association. Adapted by permission of the author.

Table 11.1 Adapted from Temple, I. G. & Williams, H. G. "Rate and level of learning as functions of information-processing characteristics of the learner and the task." *Journal of Motor Behavior.* 9:179–192, 1977, a publication of the Helen Dwight Reid Educational Foundation.

Figure 11.2 From Bossom, Joseph, "Movement Without Proprioception." *Brain Research,* Vol 71, pp. 285–296, 1974. Used with permission of Elsevier Biomedical Press B.V. Amsterdam.

Figure 11.3 From Fleishman, E. A. & Rich, S. 1963. "Role of kinesthetic & spatial-visual abilities in perceptual-motor learning." *Journal of Experimental Psychology.* 66:6–11.

Figure 11.4 From Temple, I. G. and Williams, H. G., "Rate and level of learning as functions of information-processing characteristics of the learner and the task." *Journal of Motor Behavior,* Vol. 9, 1977. Used with permission of Journal Publishing Affiliates, Santa Barbara, California.

Figure 12.1 From Langley, L. L., I. R. Telford & J. B. Christensen. *Dynamic Anatomy and Physiology,* 3rd ed. Copyright 1969 by McGraw-Hill Book Company. Reprinted by permission.

Figure 12.2 McNaught, A. B., & R. Callander (1983). *Illustrated Physiology* 4th edn. Edinburgh: Churchill Livingstone.

Figure 12.3 From Hole, John W., Jr., *Human Anatomy and Physiology* 2nd ed. © 1978, 1981 Wm. C. Brown Publishers, Dubuque, Iowa. All Rights Reserved. Reprinted by permission.

Figure 12.4 From D. P. Kimble, *Physiological Psychology: A Unit for Introductory Psychology,* © 1963, Addison-Wesley, Reading, Massachusetts. Pgs. 161, 229, 240, 262, 285 & 325. Reprinted with permission.

Figure 12.5 From *Physiology of the Human Body* 5th Ed. by Arthur C. Guyton, M.D. Copyright © 1979 by W. B. Saunders Company. Reprinted by permission of Holt, Rinehart and Winston, CBS College Publishing.

Figure 12.6 From Langley, L. L., I. R. Telford & J. B. Christensen. *Dynamic Anatomy and Physiology,* 3rd ed. Copyright 1969 by McGraw-Hill Book Company. Reprinted by permission.

Figure 12.7 McNaught, A. B., & R. Callander (1983). *Illustrated Physiology* 4th edn. Edinburgh: Churchill Livingstone.

Figure 12.8 From Langley, L. L., I. R. Telford & J. B. Christensen. *Dynamic Anatomy and Physiology,* 3rd ed. Copyright 1969 by McGraw-Hill Book Company. Reprinted by permission.

Figure 13.1 From *Biological Psychology* by James W. Kalat. © 1981 by Wadsworth, Inc. Reprinted by permission of Wadsworth Publishing Company, Belmont, California 94002.

Figure 13.2 McNaught, A. B., & Callander, R. (1983). *Illustrated Physiology* 4th edn. Edinburgh: Churchill Livingstone.

Figure 13.3 From Hole, John W., Jr., *Human Anatomy and Physiology* 2nd ed. © 1978, 1981 Wm. C. Brown Publishers, Dubuque, Iowa. All Rights Reserved. Reprinted by permission.

Figure 13.4 From: Gardner, E. *Fundamentals of Neurology,* W. B. Saunders Publishers, (5th ed.) 1969. Reprinted by permission.

Figure 14.3 From Keogh, J. and Hutton, R. S. *Exercise and Sport Sciences Reviews,* Vol. 4, 1976. Used with permission of Journal Publishing Affiliates, Santa Barbara, California.

Figure 14.4 From Schmidt, R. A. "A Schema Theory of Discrete Motor Skill Learning," *Psychological Review,* 82:225–260. Copyright 1975 by the American Psychological Association. Reprinted by permission of the author.

Figure 15.3 From Adams, J. A. & S. Dijkstra, 1966. "Short-term memory for motor responses." *Journal of Experimental Psychology,* 71:314–318. Copyright 1966 by the American Psychological Association. Adapted by permission of the author.

Figure 15.4 From Stelmach, G. E. "Prior positioning responses as a factor in short-term retention of a simple motor task." *Journal of Experimental Psychology.* 81:523–526, 1969. Copyright © 1969 by the American Psychological Association. Reprinted by permission of the author.

Figure 15.6 From Craik, R. I. M. "The Fate of Primary Memory Items in Free Recall." *Journal of Verbal Learning and Verbal Behavior, 9,* p. 145, 1970. Used with permission of Academic Press and the author.

Figure 15.7 From Magill, A. A. and Dowell, M. N. *Journal of Motor Behavior,* Vol. 9,#4, 1977. Used with permission of Journal Publishing Affiliates, Santa Barbara, California.

Figure 15.8 Based on Crossman, E. R. F. 1959. "A theory of the acquisition of speed-skill." *Ergonomics 2:*153–166.

Figure 16.2 Reprinted from E. A. Fleishman & W. E. Hempel, Jr., "Changes in factor structure of a complex psychomotor test as a function of practice," *Psychometrika, 18,* 1954, pp. 239–252. Reprinted by permission.

Figure 16.4 Based on Parker, J. F. & Fleishman, E. A. "Use of analytical information concerning task requirements to increase the effectiveness of skill training." *Journal of Applied Psychology.* 45:295–302, 1961. Copyright © 1961 by the American Psychological Association. Reprinted by permission of the author.

Figure 17.1 From Landers, D. M. *Journal of Motor Behavior,* Vol. 7,#4, 1975. Used with permission of Journal Publishing Affiliates, Santa Barbara, California.

Figure 17.3 Based on Lorge, I. *Influence of Regularly Interpolated Time Intervals Upon Subsequent Learning.* Teachers College Contributions to Education, #438, 1930.

Figure 17.4 From Digman, J. M. "Growth of a motor skill as a function of distribution of practice." *Journal of Experimental Psychology.* 57:310–316, 1959. Copyright 1959 by the American Psychological Association. Adapted by permission of the author.

Figure 17.5 Adaptations of Figures 1 & 2, pages 200 & 201, *Research Quarterly* 1969, *40,* from "Efficiency of Motor Learning as a Function of Intertrial Rest," by George E. Stelmach. Used with permission.

Figure 17.6 From Durham, *Journal of Motor Behavior,* Vol. 8, #4, 1976. Used with permission of Journal Publishing Affiliates, Santa Barbara, California.

Figure 17.7 From "Muscular Fatigue and Learning a Discrete Motor Skill", by M. A. Godwin and R. A. Schmidt, *Research Quarterly,* 1971, *42:* 374–382. Published by AAHPERD. Reprinted with the permission of AAHPERD.

Figure 17.8 From Jacobson, E. "Electrophysiology of mental activities & introduction to the psychological process of thinking." *The Psychophysiology of Thinking,* 1973. New York: Academic Press. Reprinted by permission.

Figure 17.9 From McCracken, H. D. & Stelmach, G. E. "A test of schema theory of discrete motor learning." *Journal of Motor Behavior 9:*193–201, 1977. Reprinted by permission of Journal Publishing Affiliates.

Figure 18.2 From Stelmach, G. E., *Ergonomics,* Vol. 13, #4, pp. 421–425, 1970. Used with permission of Taylor & Francis Ltd. and the author.

Figure 18.4 Elwell, J. L. & G. C. Grindley 1938. "The effect of knowledge of results on learning and performance I. A coordinated movement of the two hands." *British Journal of Psychology 29:* 39–53. Reprinted by permission.

Figure 18.5 From Newell, K. M. *Journal of Motor Behavior,* Vol. 6, #4, pp. 235–244, 1974. Used with permission of Journal Publishing Affiliates, Santa Barbara, California.

Figure 18.7 From Shea, J. B. & Upton, G., *Journal of Motor Behavior, 8, #4,* pp. 277–281, 1976. Used with permission of Journal Publishing Affiliates, Santa Barbara, California.

Table 18.1 Sylvia E. Fishman, Ed.D.

Figure 18.8 Hatze, H., "Biomechanical Aspects of a Successful Motion Optimization." In P. V. Komi, ed. *Biomechanics V-B.* Baltimore: University Park Press, 1976. Reprinted by permission.

Figure 19.1 Based on Robinson, E. S. 1927. "The 'similarity' factor in retroaction." *American Journal of Psychology. 39:* 297–312.

Figure 19.2 From Sage, G. H. and Hornak, J. E. "Progressive speed practice in learning a continuous motor skill." *Research Quarterly. 49:*190–196, 1978.

Figure 19.3 Reprinted with permission of authors and publisher from: Siegel, D., & Davis, C. "Transfer effects of learning at specific speeds on performance over a range of speeds." *Perceptual and Motor Skills,* 1980, 50, 83–89, figure 1.

Figure 20.1 From D. P. Kimble, *Physiological Psychology: A Unit for Introductory Psychology,* © 1963, Addison-Wesley, Reading, Massachusetts. Pgs. 161, 229, 240, 262, 285 & 325. Reprinted with permission.

Figure 20.3 Based on Weinberg, R. S. & Ragan, J. "Motor Performance under Three Levels of Trait Anxiety & Stress." *Journal of Motor Behavior 10* (1978): 169–76, a publication of the Helen Dwight Reid Educational Foundation.

Figure 20.4 From Klavora, P. & Daniel, J. V. (eds.) *Coach, Athlete, and the Sport Psychologist.* Champaign, Il.: Human Kinetics Publishers, 1979. Used with the permission of Peter Klavora, University of Toronto.

Table 20.1 Based on Billing, J. "An Overview of Task Complexity." *Motor Skills: Theory into Practice* 4(1980):18–23. Reprinted by permission.

Figure 20.6 An adaptation of Figure 1, page 408, *Research Quarterly* 1971, *42,* from "Multiple Choice Reaction Time and Movement Time During Physical Exertion," by Stuart Levitt & Bernard Gutin, the adaptation representing only five-choice reaction time (RT). Used with permission.

Table 20.2 Based on Oxendine, J. B. *Quest, 13:* 23–32. Copyright 1970 by Human Kinetics Publishers. Reprinted by permission.

Figure 20.8 An adaptation of Figure 1, page 145, *Research Quarterly* 1973, *44,* from "The Effects of Induced Arousal on Learning & Performance of a Pursuit Motor Skill," by George H. Sage and Bonnie Bennett. Used with permission.

Figure 20.9 Based on Percival, L. 1971b. Question clinic and commentary on Part 2. In J. W. Taylor (ed.), "Proceedings of the 1st international symposium on the art & science of coaching." Willowdale, Ontario: F. I. Productions.

Figure 21.1 From Locke, E. A. & Bryan, J. R. *Journal of Applied Psychology.* "Cognitive aspects of psychomotor performance: The effects of performance goals on levels of performance." 50:286–291. Copyright © 1966 by the American Psychological Association. Reprinted by permission of the authors.

Figure 22.1 Based on Parker, J. F. & Fleishman, E. A. "Use of analytical information concerning task requirements to increase the effectiveness of skill training." *Journal of Applied Psychology.* 45:295–302, 1961. Copyright 1961 by the American Psychological Association. Reprinted by permission of the author.

Name Index

Subject Index